Jan, 2008 Joe Martin

ADVANCES IN NEUROLOGY

Volume 82

Advances in Neurology
Volume 82

Corticobasal Degeneration and Related Disorders

Editors

Irene Litvan, M.D.
Cognitive Neuropharmacology Unit
Defense and Veteran Head Injury Program
Henry M. Jackson Foundation
Bethesda, Maryland

Christopher G. Goetz, M.D.
Professor of Neurology
Department of Neurology
Rush Medical College
Chicago, Illinois

Anthony E. Lang, M.D.
Professor of Neurology
Toronto Western Hospital
Toronto, Ontario
Canada

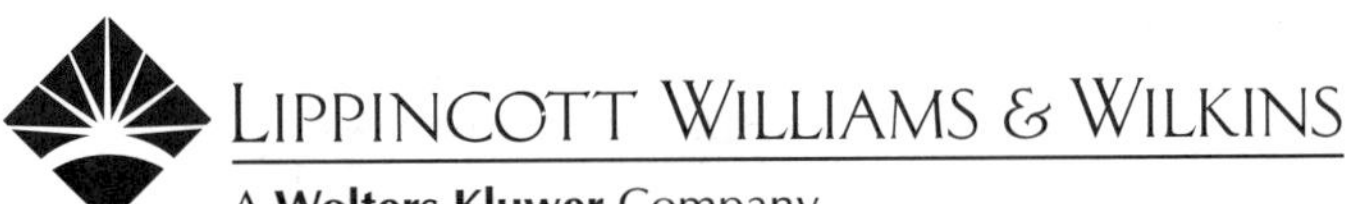
LIPPINCOTT WILLIAMS & WILKINS
A **Wolters Kluwer** Company
Philadelphia • Baltimore • New York • London
Buenos Aires • Hong Kong • Sydney • Tokyo

Acquisitions Editor: Anne M. Sydor
Developmental Editor: Mildred G. Ramos
Production Editor: Rakesh Rampertab
Manufacturing Manager: Tim Reynolds
Compositor: Circle Graphics
Printer: Maple Press

227 East Washington Square
Philadelphia, PA 19106-3780 USA
www.LWW.com

Printed in the USA

Library of Congress Cataloging-in Publication Data

ISBN 0-7817-2124-5
ISSN 0091-3592

---

10 9 8 7 6 5 4 3 2 1

Advances in Neurology Series

Vol. 81: Plasticity and Epilepsy: H. Stefan, P. Chauvel, F. Anderman, S.D. Sharvon, *editors*. 396 pp., 1999.
Vol. 80: Parkinson's Disease: *Gerald M. Stern, editor*. 704 pp., 1999
Vol. 79: Jasper's Basic Mechanisms of the Epilepsies. Third Edition: *A. Delgado-Escueta, W. Wilson, R. Olsen, R. Porter, editors*. 1,136 pp., 1999
Vol. 78: Dystonia 3: *S. Fahn, C. D. Marsden, M. R. DeLong, editors*. 374 pp., 1998.
Vol. 77: Consciousness: At the Frontiers of Neuroscience: *H. H. Jasper, L. Descarries, V. F. Castellucci, S. Rossignol, editors*. 300 pp., 1998.
Vol. 76: Antiepileptic Drug Development: *J. A. French, I. E. Leppik, M. A. Dichter, editors*. 276 pp., 1998.
Vol. 75: Reflex Epilepsies and Reflex Seizures: *B. G. Zifkin, F. Andermann, A. Beaumanoir, A. J. Rowan, editors*. 310 pp., 1998.
Vol. 74: Basal Ganglia and New Surgical Approaches for Parkinson's Disease: *J. A. Obeso, M. R. DeLong, C. Ohye, and C. D. Marsden, editors*. 286 pp., 1997.
Vol. 73: Brain Plasticity: *H. J. Freund, B. A. Sabel, and O. W. Witte, editors*. 448 pp., 1997.
Vol. 72: Neuronal Regeneration, Reorganization and Repair: *F. J. Seil, editor*. 416 pp., 1997.
Vol. 71: Cellular and Molecular Mechanisms of Ischemic Brain Damage: *B. K. Siesjö and T. Wieloch, editors*. 560 pp., 1996.
Vol. 70: Supplementary Sensorimotor Area: *H. O. Lüders, editor*. 544 pp., 1996.
Vol. 69: Parkinson's Disease: *L. Battistin, G. Scarlato, T. Caraceni, and S. Ruggieri, editors*. 752 pp., 1996.
Vol. 68: Pathogenesis and Therapy of Amyotrophic Lateral Sclerosis: *G. Serratrice and T. L. Munsat, editors*. 352 pp., 1995.
Vol. 67: Negative Motor Phenomena: *S. Fahn, M. Hallett, H. O. Lüders, and C. D. Marsden, editors*. 416 pp., 1995.
Vol. 66: Epilepsy and the Functional Anatomy of the Frontal Lobe: *H. H. Jasper, S. Riggio, and P. S. Goldman-Rakic, editors*. 400 pp., 1995.
Vol. 65: Behavioral Neurology of Movement Disorders: *W. J. Weiner and A. E. Lang, editors*. 368 pp., 1995.
Vol. 64: Neurological Complications of Pregnancy: *O. Devinsky, E. Feldmann, and B. Hainline, editors*. 288 pp., 1994.
Vol. 63: Electrical and Magnetic Stimulation of the Brain and Spinal Cord: *O. Devinsky, A. Beric, and M. Dogali, editors*. 352 pp., 1993.
Vol. 62: Cerebral Small Artery Disease: *P.M. Pullicino, L. R. Caplan, and M. Hommel, editors*. 256 pp., 1993.
Vol. 61: Inherited Ataxias: *A. E. Harding and T. Deufel, editors*. 240 pp., 1993.
Vol. 60: Parkinson's Disease: From Basic Research to Treatment: *H. Narabayashi, T. Nagatsu, N. Yanagisawa, and Y. Mizuno, Editors*. 800 pp., 1993.
Vol. 59: Neural Injury and Regeneration: *F. J. Seil, editor*. 384 pp., 1993.
Vol. 58: Tourette Syndrome: Genetics, Neurobiology, and Treatment: *T. N. Chase, A. J. Friedhoff, and D. J. Cohen, editors*. 400 pp., 1992.
Vol. 57: Frontal Lobe Seizures and Epilepsies: *P. Chauvel, A. V. Delgado-Escueta, E. Halgren, and J. Bancaud, editors*. 752 pp., 1992.
Vol. 56: Amyotrophic Lateral Sclerosis and Other Motor Neuron Diseases: *L. P. Rowland, editor*. 592 pp., 1991.
Vol. 55: Neurobehavioral Problems in Epilepsy: *D. B. Smith, D. Treiman, and M. Trimble, editors*. 512 pp., 1990.
Vol. 54: Magnetoencephalography: *S. Sato, editor*. 284 pp., 1990.
Vol. 52: Brain Edema: Pathogenesis, Imaging, and Therapy: *D. Long, editor*. 640 pp., 1990.
Vol. 51: Alzheimer's Disease: *R. J. Wurtman, S. Corkin, J. H. Growdon, and E. Ritter-Walker, editors*. 308 pp., 1990.

Vol. 48: Molecular Genetics of Neurological and Neuromuscular Disease: *S. DiDonato, S. DiMauro, A. Mamoli, and L. P. Rowland, editors.* 288 pp., 1987.
Vol. 47: Functional Recovery in Neurological Disease: *S. G. Waxman, editor.* 640 pp., 1987.
Vol. 46: Intensive Neurodiagnostic Monitoring: *R. J. Gumnit, editor.* 336 pp., 1987.
Vol. 45: Parkinson's Disease: *M. D. Yahr and K. J. Bergmann, editors.* 640 pp., 1986.
Vol. 44: Basic Mechanisms of the Epilepsies: Molecular and Cellular Approaches: *A. V. Delgado-Escueta, A. A. Ward, Jr., D. M. Woodbury, and R. J. Porter, editors.* 1,120 pp., 1986.
Vol. 43: Myoclonus: *S. Fahn, C. D. Marsden, and M. H. VanWoert, editors.* 752 pp., 1986.
Vol. 42: Progress in Aphasiology: *F. C. Rose, editor.* 384 pp., 1984.
Vol. 41: The Olivopontocerebellar Atrophies: *R. C. Duvoisin and A. Plaitakis, editors.* 304 pp., 1984.
Vol. 40: Parkinson-Specific Motor and Mental Disorders, Role of Pallidum: Pathophysiological, Biochemical, and Therapeutic Aspects: *R. G. Hassler and J. F. Christ, editors.* 601 pp., 1984.
Vol. 38: The Dementias: *R. Mayeux and W. G. Rosen, editors.* 288 pp., 1983.
Vol. 37: Experimental Therapeutics of Movement Disorders: *S. Fahn, D. B. Calne, and I. Shoulson, editors.* 339 pp., 1983.
Vol. 36: Human Motor Neuron Diseases: *L. P. Rowland, editor.* 592 pp., 1982.
Vol. 35: Gilles de la Tourette Syndrome: *A. J. Friedhoff and T. N. Chase, editors.* 476 pp., 1982.
Vol. 34: Status Epilepticus: Mechanism of Brain Damage and Treatment: *A. V. Delgado-Escueta, C. G. Wasterlain, D. M. Treiman, and R. J. Porter, editors.* 579 pp., 1983.
Vol. 31: Demyelinating Diseases: Basic and Clinical Electrophysiology: *S. Waxman and J. Murdoch Ritchie, editors.* 544 pp., 1981.
Vol. 30: Diagnosis and Treatment of Brain Ischemia: *A. L. Carney and E. M. Anderson, editors.* 424 pp., 1981.
Vol. 22: Complications of Nervous System Trauma: *R. A. Thompson and J. R. Green, editors.* 454 pp., 1979.

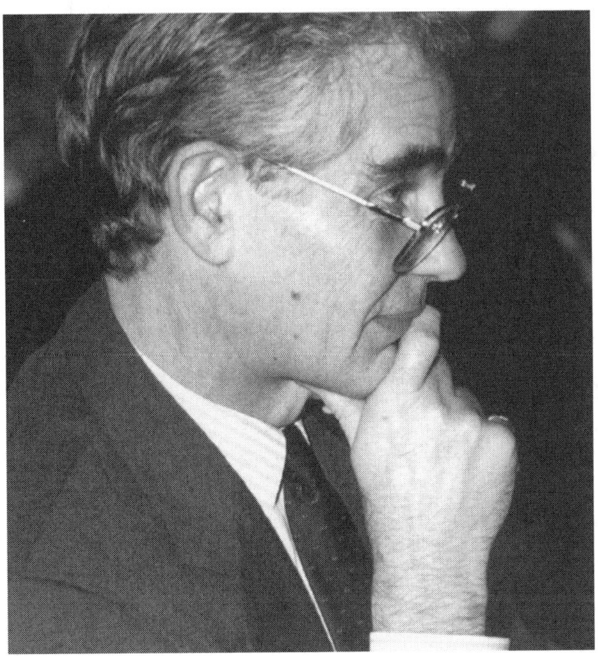

In tribute to C. David Marsden for his brilliant and timely contributions to our understanding of the functions and pathology of the basal ganglia. David had planned to write the forward for this book prior to his sudden and premature death. Not being able to read and debate his musings on Corticobasal Degeneration (CBD) in this volume is sad for all of us. Beyond his remarkable contributions to the basic and clinical aspects of CBD, his important legacy lives in the large number of investigators whom he inspired to continue the search for leads to better understand and treat this devastating disease.

An important component of David's legacy are the many research fellows who trained at the Institute of Psychiatry and King's College Hospital and then at the National Hospital at Queen's Square. It was there that one of the editors, Dr. Anthony E. Lang, had the good fortune of beginning his career in the field of movement disorders. Shortly after Dr. Lang arrived in London to start his fellowship, a very unusual patient was seen in the Friday clinic at the Maudsely, first in consultation by Dr. Lang, after which the patient was presented to the "prof." This patient was a sixty-seven year-old retired diesel engineer who had a two-year history of progressive neurological disability dominated by a fixed dystonia of the right hand with superimposed stimulus-sensitive myoclonic jerks of the hand and forearm. For want of a better term, the phenomenology was presented to David as "myoclonic dystonia." Although the term didn't stick (because David and colleagues were planning to use it to describe a distinctly different entity [1]), David admitted that this patient was unique in his experience, and that he had no idea of the nature of the underlying disorder. The patient was investigated extensively and the results of his electrophysiological studies (case 6) were published in a seminal paper by Obeso, Rothwell, and Marsden on the spectrum of cortical myoclonus (2). The patient was followed until he died and post mortem showed the characteristic pathological features of CBD. He was reported as Case 1 in the Gibb, Luthert, and Marsden paper first coining the term "corticobasal degeneration." Thus, the legacy in the field of CBD that David leaves began on a Friday morning in 1980 when he and his new Canadian research fellow unknowingly saw their first case together.

IL, CGG, AEL

1. Obeso JA, Rothwell JC, Lang AE et al. Myoclonic dystonia. *Neurology* 1983;33:825–830.
2. Obeso JA, Rothwell JC, Marsden CD. The spectrum of cortical myoclonus. From focal reflex jerks to spontaneous motor epilepsy. *Brain* 1985;108:193–224.
3. Gibb WRG, Luthert PJ, Marsden CD. Cortical basal degeneration. *Brain* 1989;112:1171–1192.

In memory of my Dad, Marcos,
whose intellectual serenades encouraged me to engage the challenges of life
and to better prepare for the mysteries of death.
To my Mom, Raquel,
who continues to inspire me with her warmth, curiosity, and independence.

IL

To the patients and caregivers who have suffered with the devastating disease that has come to be known as corticobasal degeneration (CBD), and have generously given of their time and energy so that we may learn how to improve the clinical management of CBD while we marvel at the brain's functional intricacy. We hope that this volume will assist in advancing the science further and will contribute to the eventual eradication of the disease.

IL, CGG, AEL

Contents

Contributing Authors

Yves Agid, M.D., Ph.D.
Fédération de Neurologie and INSERM U 289
Hôpital de la Salpêtrière
47 Boulevard de l'Hôpital
75013 Paris
France

Jorge Balej, Ph.D.
Department of Movement Disorders
Raúl Carrea Institute of Neurological Research, FLENI
Montañeses 2325
Buenos Aires
Argentina

Kailash P. Bhatia, M.D., Ph.D.
Senior Lecturer
University Department of Clinical Neurology
Institute of Neurology
Queen Square
London WC1N 3BG
United Kingdom

Sandra E. Black, M.D.
Head
Division of Neurology
Sunnybrook and Women's College Health Sciences Centre
2075 Bayview Avenue, A421
Toronto, Ontario M4N 3M5
Canada

David J. Brooks, M.D., DSc.
Harnett Professor of Neurology
MRC Cyclotron Unit
Imperial College School of Medicine
Du Cane Road
London W12 0NN
United Kingdom

Richard J. Caselli, M.D.
Assistant Professor
Department of Neurology
Mayo Clinic, Scottsdale
13400 East Shea Boulevard
Scottsdale, Arizona 85259

Jeffrey L. Cummings, M.D.
Augustus S. Rose Professor of Neurology
Department of Neurology
UCLA School of Medicine
710 Westwood Plaza
Los Angeles, California 90095-1769

Leo Davies, M.D.
Head
Department of Clinical Neurophysiology
Royal Prince Alfred Hospital
Missenden Road
Camperdown 2050
New South Wales
Australia

Dennis W. Dickson, M.D.
Professor
Pathology Department
Mayo Clinic Jacksonville
4500 San Pablo Road
Jacksonville, Florida 32224

Rachelle S. Doody, M.D., Ph.D.
Associate Professor
Department of Neurology
Baylor College of Medicine
6550 Fannin, Suite 1801
Houston, Texas 77030

Bruno Dubois, M.D.
Professor
Department of Neurology
Hôpital de la Salpêtrière
47 Boulevard de l'Hôpital
75013 Paris
France

Charles Duyckaerts, M.D.
Laboratoire de Neuropathologie
Raymond Escourolle
Hôpital de la Pitié-Salpêtrière
47 Boulevard de l'Hôpital
75651 Paris, Cedex 13
France

Carol M. Frattali, Ph.D.
Research Coordinator
Speech-Language Pathology Section
Rehabilitation Medicine Department
National Institutes of Health
10 Center Drive, Room 6S 235
Bethesda, Maryland 20892

Floriano Girotti, M.D.
Head
Department of Neuroradiology
Instituto Nazionale Neurologico "C. Besta"
Via Celoria, 11
20133 Milano
Italy

Christopher G. Goetz, M.D.
Professor
Department of Neurological Sciences
Rush-Presbyterian-St. Luke's Medical Center
1725 West Harrison Street, Suite 1106
Chicago, Illinois 60612

David A. Grimes, M.D., FRCPC
Assistant Professor
Department of Medicine
The Ottawa Hospital
D 715-1053 Carling Avenue
Ottawa, Ontario K1Y 4E9
Canada

Marina Grisoli, M.D.
Department of Neuroradiology
Instituto Nazionale Neurologico "C. Besta"
Via Celoria, 11
20133 Milano
Italy

Philip A. Hanna, M.D.
Assistant Professor
New Jersey Neuroscience Institute
JFK Medical Center
65 James Street
Edison, New Jersey 08818

Jean-Jacques Hauw, M.D.
Chief
Laboratoire de Neuropathologie
Raymond Escourolle
Hôpital de la Petié-Salpêtrière
47 Boulevard de l'Hôpital
75013 Paris, Cedex 13
France

Joseph Jankovic, M.D.
Professor of Neurology
Department of Neurology
Baylor College of Medicine
6550 Fannin, Suite 1801
Houston, Texas 77030

Andrew Kertesz, M.D., FRCPC
Director
Cognitive Neurology and Alzheimer Research Centre
St. Joseph's Health Centre
268 Grosvenor Street
London, Ontario N6A 4V2
Canada

Katie Kompoliti, M.D.
Assistant Professor
Department of Neurological Sciences
Rush University
1725 West Harrison Street, Suite #1106
Chicago, Illinois 60612

Hanna Ksiezak-Reding, Ph.D.
Department of Pathology
Albert Einstein College of Medicine
1300 Morris Park Avenue
Bronx, New York 10461

Anthony E. Lang, M.D.
Director
Division of Neurology
Toronto Western Hospital
399 Bathurst Street MP11
Toronto, Ontario M5T 2S8
Canada

Myung S. Lee, M.D.
University Department of Clinical Neurology
Institute of Neurology
Queen Square
London WC1N 3BG
United Kingdom

Ramón Leiguarda, M.D.
Chairman
Department of Neurology
Raúl Carrea Institute of Neurological Research, FLENI
Montañeses 2325
Buenos Aires
Argentina

Irene Litvan, M.D.
Chief
Cognitive Neuropharmacology Unit
Defense and Veteran Head Injury Program
Henry M. Jackson Foundation
The Champlain Building
6410 Rockledge Drive
Bethesda, Maryland 20817-1844

Wan-Kyng Liu, M.D.
Department of Pharmacology
Mayo Clinic Jacksonville
4500 San Pablo Road
Jacksonville, Florida 32224

C. David Marsden, M.D.
Deceased

Marcelo Merello, M.D.
Head
Movement Disorders Section
Raúl Carrea Institute of Neurological Research, FLENI
Montañeses 2325
Buenos Aires
Argentina

David G. Munoz, M.D., FRCPC
Director of Neuropathology
Department of Pathology
London Health Sciences Centre
339 Windermer Road
London, Ontario N6A 5A5
Canada

Bernard Pillon, Ph.D.
Director of Research
INSERM U 289
Hôpital de la Salpêtrière
47 Boulevard de l'Hôpital
75013 Paris
France

Tamas Revesz, M.D.
Department of Neuropathology
Institute of Neurology
Queen Square
London WC1N 3BG
United Kingdom

David E. Riley, M.D.
Department of Neurology
University Hospitals of Cleveland
Department of Neurology
11100 Euclid Avenue
Cleveland, Ohio 44106

Juha O. Rinne, M.D.
University Department of Clinical Neurology
Institute of Neurology
Queen Square
London WC1N 3BG
United Kingdom

Sophie Rivaud-Péchoux, Ph.D.
INSERM U 289
Hôpital de la Salpêtrière
47 Boulevard de l'Hôpital
75651 Paris, Cedex 13
France

Mario Savoiardo, M.D.
Chief
Department of Neuroradiology
Instituto Nazionale Neurologico "C. Besta"
Via Celoria, 11
20133 Milano
Italy

Francesco Scaravilli, M.D., Ph.D., DSc., MRCPath
Professor of Neuropathology
Department of Neuropathology
Institute of Neurology
Queen Square
London WC1N 3BG
United Kingdom

Hiroshi Shibasaki, M.D., Ph.D.
Professor
Department of Brain Pathophysiology
Kyoto University Graduate School of Medicine
Shogoin, Sakyo-Ku
Kyoto 606-8507
Japan

Barbara C. Sonies, Ph.D.
Chief
Speech-Language Pathology Section
Rehabilitation Medicine Department
National Institutes of Health
Clinical Center, Room 6S 235
Bethesda, Maryland 20892

Caroline M. Tanner, M.D., Ph.D.
Director
Department of Clinical Research
The Parkinson's Institute
1170 Morse Avenue
Sunnyvale, California 94089-1605

Philip D. Thompson, M.B., Ph.D., FRACP
Professor of Neurology
University Department of Medicine
University of Adelaide
North Terrace, Adelaide
South Australia 5000
Australia

Daniel M. Togasaki, M.D., Ph.D.
Movement Disorders Specialist
The Parkinson's Institute
1170 Morse Avenue
Sunnyvale, California 94089-1605

Zeba Fatima Vanek, M.D.
Assistant Professor
Department of Neurology
University of California, Los Angeles
710 Westwood Plaza
Los Angeles, California 90095-1769

Marie Vidailhet, M.D.
Professor
Department of Neurology
Hôpital Saint Antoine
184 rue du Faubourg Saint Antoine
75012 Paris, Cedex 13
France

Shu-Hui Yen, Ph.D.
Professor
Department of Pharmacology
Mayo Clinic Jacksonville
4500 San Pablo Road
Jacksonville, Florida 32224

Foreword

As the population ages, the spectrum of disease changes. Both parkinsonism and dementia are becoming much more common. There is a long list of diagnostic possibilities for both syndromes separately and together. Precision of diagnosis is becoming more important as relevant therapies emerge and will be critical when it is possible to implement measures to prevent onset or progression of disease. In regard to differential diagnosis it is appropriate now to focus on corticobasal degeneration as an entity. What is it? How can it be recognized? The pathophysiology and treatment are obvious targets for the future.

Corticobasal degeneration has been confusing. Even the name has been in evolution. Although there may have been some cases in earlier literature, the first clear definition was from Rebeiz, Kolodny, and Richardson in 1968 with a syndrome they named corticodentatonigral degeneration with neuronal achromasia (1). They reported three patients with asymmetric akinetic-rigid syndrome characterized by a dystonic, apraxic arm. The arm was also tremulous and myoclonic. Aphasia and dementia were features. Pathologically, there was frontal and parietal atrophy with cell loss and gliosis. Many residual neurons were swollen and chromatolyzed with eccentric nuclei, and this was termed achromasia. They recognized from the outset the similarities to Pick's Disease and progressive supranuclear palsy. Gibb, Luthert and Marsden (2) first used the term corticobasal degeneration which has been most commonly used since. While they acknowledged that they were describing cases similar to Rebeiz et al., they thought that their shorter name was better. They also described three patients who presented with a progressive disease with clinical resemblance to progressive supranuclear palsy, but pathological features of Pick's disease. These patients suffered from focal dystonia and myoclonus of an arm, the "alien hand" sign, or an akinetic-rigid syndrome and developed a supranuclear gaze palsy, parkinsonian features and mild cerebellar signs. Pathologically, they had frontoparietal atrophy with cortical cell loss, gliosis, and Pick cells. There was nerve cell loss and gliosis in the thalamus, lentiform nucleus, subthalamic nucleus, red nucleus, midbrain tegmentum, substantia nigra, and locus coeruleus. They also reported neuronal inclusions in the substantia nigra, termed corticobasal inclusions, reminiscent of the globose neurofibrillary tangle of progressive supranuclear palsy, and other pale inclusions resembling the pale body of Parkinson's disease. Some nigral inclusions were similar to those in Pick's disease. Gibb et al., like Rebeiz et al., saw similarities to other disorders, most importantly Pick's disease and progressive supranuclear palsy, but thought that the disorder was distinct. Other terms for the same disorder have been "cortical-basal ganglionic degeneration" (3), "corticobasal ganglionic degeneration" (4), and "corticonigral degeneration with neuronal achromasia" (5).

While the "classic" descriptions have been both clinical and pathological and suggested that there was a concordance between the two, it is clear that there are problems. A number of patients seen subsequently with non-classical clinical syndromes such as predominant dementia and have turned out to have the classical pathologic picture. Other patients have presented with the classical clinical syndrome and have something else pathologically including progressive supranuclear palsy, Pick's disease, Alzheimer's disease, Parkinson's disease, multiple system atrophy, Lewy body dementia or hemiatrophy-hemiparkinsonism. These problems of concordance between clinical features and pathology come up repeatedly in the book. The clinician is faced with unestablished sensitivity and specificity for getting the pathology right and various sets of clinical rules. This poses difficulties for epidemiology as Togasaki and Tanner recognize in their chapter. Like them, Riley and Lang in their chapter note the need for a biological marker of the disease.

There is considerable progress in the pathology and the pathological investigations in this disease, described well in the book, but there are still controversies including the formal relationship to Pick's disease as displayed by the "Diagnostic Controversies" chapters.

Neurologists and neuropathologists both need help, and it is good that this book has come along. The book has its genesis partially from a small meeting in 1995 that was sponsored by the Movement Disorder Society and organized by Dr. Lang. The editors have built substantially from that base and performed a valuable service in bringing all this data together. They advocate the reasonable point of view that the designation *corticobasal degeneration* should now be used for those cases meeting clinicopathologic criteria. As it emerges in the book, particularly in the chapter by Litvan, Grimes, and Lang, there are two clinical phenotypes that should be considered. The first is the "classic" one emphasizing a motor presentation that is asymmetric, and the second is a presentation emphasizing frontal dementia with symmetric motor signs.

Mark Hallett, M.D.
Clinical Director
NINDS/NIH
Bethesda, Maryland

REFERENCES

1. Rebeiz JJ, Kolodny EH, Richardson EP, Jr. Corticodentatonigral degeneration with neuronal achromasia. *Arch Neurol* 1968;18:20–33.
2. Gibb WR, Luthert PJ, Marsden CD. Corticobasal degeneration. *Brain* 1989;112:1171–1192.
3. Riley DE, Lang AE, Lewis A, et al. Cortical-basal ganglionic degeneration. *Neurology* 1990;40:1203–1212.
4. Gimenez-Roldan S, Mateo D, Benito C, Grandas F, Perez-Gilabert Y. Progressive supranuclear palsy and corticobasal ganglionic degeneration: differentiation by clinical features and neuroimaging techniques. *J Neural Transm Suppl* 1994;42:79–90.
5. Paulus W, Selim M. Corticonigral degeneration with neuronal achromasia and basal neurofibrillary tangles. *Acta Neuropathol* 1990;81:89–94.

Preface

This is the first volume solely dedicated to corticobasal degeneration (CBD), until recently thought to be a relatively rare degenerative disorder of the central nervous system. This disorder can affect several cortical, basal ganglia and brainstem areas, clinically manifested by a variety of features including unilateral ideomotor apraxia, parkinsonism, dystonia, myoclonus, ocular apraxia, alien limb syndrome, aphasia, dementia, pseudobulbar palsy and/or gait disturbances.

What is in a name? The nomenclature for this disorder has varied over time reflecting investigators' interpretation of the different areas affected, leading to names and phrases that are difficult to pronounce, such as corticodentatonigral degeneration with neuronal achromasia, corticonigral degeneration with neuronal achromasia, cortical-basal ganglionic degeneration, and corticobasal degeneration. The latter name was chosen by the editors because it accurately reflects the cortical and subcortical pathologic involvement and is the easiest to articulate (not an irrelevant issue for patients suffering this disease).

The purpose of this book is to aid clinicians in achieving an earlier diagnosis of patients with CBD as well as to help them differentiate CBD patients from those suffering from other movement disorders such as Parkinson's disease and progressive supranuclear palsy, or from other dementia disorders including Alzheimer's disease and Pick's disease. We also hope that the appearance of a single resource volume on CBD will accelerate research in this area, emphasizing what is known and agreed upon by raising controversial issues and highlighting areas that are sorely needing scientific attention.

Each chapter herein summarizes state of the art knowledge and research, and formulates questions to help stimulate research, both useful tools for practitioners and investigators. We hope that with this volume, CBD, until recently considered an obscure neurological disorder, will be better recognized and that clinical- and research-based neuroscientists will join us in the search for the causes of, and effective treatment for this fascinating and devastating disease.

Irene Litvan
Christopher G. Goetz
Anthony E. Lang

ADVANCES IN NEUROLOGY

Volume 82

Corticobasal Degeneration.
Advances in Neurology, Vol. 82,
edited by I. Litvan, C. G. Goetz, and A. E. Lang.
Lippincott Williams & Wilkins, Philadelphia © 2000.

1

Nineteenth Century Studies of Atypical Parkinsonism: Charcot and His Salpêtrière School

Christopher G. Goetz

Department of Neurological Sciences, Rush-Presbyterian-St. Luke's Medical Center, Chicago, Illinois, 60612

INTRODUCTION

Whereas James Parkinson (1) described Parkinson's disease in 1817, the full clinical description of archetypical cases was made later in the nineteenth century by the celebrated French neurologist, Jean-Martin Charcot (2). In his lectures at the Salpêtrière Hospital in Paris and in publications coauthored with A. Vulpian, Charcot outlined the cardinal features of tremor, bradykinesia, rigidity, and postural reflex compromise of Parkinson's disease, as well as arthritic and trophic change (3,4). Today, these documents serve as landmark medical descriptions of the variety of clinical signs seen in typical Parkinson's disease and their natural evolution without medical intervention.

In addition to the cases of typical Parkinson's disease, Charcot and his students, collectively known as the Salpêtrière School (5), also described a number of Parkinsonian variants. Today, unusual cases of Parkinsonism are generally grouped under the rubric of atypical Parkinsonian syndromes, including such entities as this volume's focus, corticobasal degeneration (CBD), as well as progressive supranuclear palsy (PSP), and multiple system atrophy. These diagnoses, all of recent date, have distinctive histopathological findings unappreciated with the early microscopic techniques of the nineteenth century. Even today, differentiation of disorders within the general class of atypical Parkinsonian syndromes is difficult on clinical grounds alone (6). Because of these limitations, the modern exercise of reading case material from the nineteenth century and imputing specific diagnoses among the broad class of atypical Parkinsonism is largely conjectural and without a means of pathological validation. In specific regard to corticobasal degeneration, the first definitive description by Rebeiz (7) dates to 1967, and allusions to extrapyramidal features among some of the cases described as Pick's disease in the 1930s suggest, but do not confirm, instances of corticobasal degeneration in the earlier German literature (8,9). Therefore, this chapter focuses on early distinctions drawn by Charcot and French neurologists to separate atypical Parkinsonism from classic Parkinson's disease, with the goal of introducing the subject of corticobasal degeneration in its historical context. Whereas Charcot did not coalesce the clinical hallmarks of corticobasal degeneration into a single syndrome, his nosographic division of "atypical Parkinson's disease" included several of the individual signs that distinguish corticobasal degeneration from Parkinson's disease.

Charcot and "Atypical Parkinson's Disease"

Throughout Charcot's career, Parkinson's disease was considered a *névrose,* a neurological disorder without a known pathological lesion (2).

Although Charcot relied heavily on autopsy study and anatomoclinical correlations, he did not discover the characteristic degeneration of the substantia nigra seen in Parkinson's disease (10). As such, Charcot always considered atypical Parkinsonism as being Parkinson's disease, but suitably different from the archetype to deserve separate mention and analysis. He distinguished a number of categories that are pertinent to a discussion of corticobasal degeneration: cases without typical tremor, cases with atypical postures (extension rather than flexion), and cases with marked asymmetry with seeming hemiplegia. In all these categories, modern neurologists can see characteristics that typify corticobasal degeneration. Because other important hallmarks such as apraxia, myoclonus, and cortical sensory loss were not regular parts of the neurological examination performed by Charcot (11), these features cannot be well evaluated in an historical study.

Parkinsonism without Prominent Rest Tremor

Charcot recognized resting tremor as the most distinctive feature of typical Parkinson's disease, and placed patients who had unusual, intermittent, or no tremor into a single clinical category termed "Parkinson's disease without tremor" (2,3). Many of these cases actually had some tremor or other involuntary jerking, but the movements were atypical of classic Parkinson's disease because they were either mild in severity or often induced or exacerbated by emotion, surprise, or action (2). In current studies of the clinical spectrum of CBD, a variety of tremors are described, and mixed resting/postural/action tremors that can be seen in CBD would have been placed in this category by Charcot and his school (6).

It is also possible that myoclonus, a feature frequently seen in CBD, would have been categorized within this nosography as a form of unusual, intermittent tremors. As a neurological term, "myoclonus" was appreciated in the era of Charcot, but the early studies were largely German in origin, and after the national humiliation of the Franco-Prussian war in 1870, Charcot reduced his contacts with the "outre-Rhine"(5). He nonetheless was keenly aware of Friedreich's description of ataxia and likely would have been aware of the same author's work on myoclonus (12,13). Charcot's personal library, now housed at the Salpêtrière hospital in Paris (Bibliothèque Charcot) has the Virchow's Archive volume where the description of paramyoclonus multiplex was published, although no personal markings of Charcot's hand grace the manuscript. Unverricht's monograph on epileptic myoclonus is catalogued in the library's collections of *tirés à part,* suggesting that Charcot received the individual reprint from the author himself (14). Myoclonus as a term, however, has not been not found by this author in any reference to Parkinson's disease in either Charcot's *Oeuvres Complètes* (2) or the transcripts of the *Leçons du mardt* (3).

Charcot studied tremor extensively and drew attention to its typical features in Parkinson's disease. He conducted his tremor examination with patients at rest and during activity. In addition to clinical observation, he used tremor oscillometers and small portable lamps that he attached to the shaking extremities in order to record the trajectory movements on light-sensitive paper (15). To accentuate an appreciation of very mild tremor, he attached feathers or other lightweight objects to the shaking body part to magnify the oscillations. He held strongly that titubation was not part of Parkinson's disease, but lip and tongue tremors could occur. Discussing the typical tremor he emphasized:

> Thus in some patients, the thumb moves over the fingers, as when a pencil or small wad of paper is rolled between them; in others, the movements are more complicated and resemble what takes place in crumbling a piece of bread. I have shown you some examples of this kind. These are, if I am not mistaken, peculiarities that belong specifically to the tremor of paralysis agitans; I do not believe that they are to be found in any other condition (2).

In their studies of tremor and Parkinson's disease, Charcot and his colleagues described several cases of Parkinsonian patients who never suffered with either prominent resting or postural tremor. His student Bourneville published two cases in 1876 (16), and later French students chose this subclass of patients for special clinical emphasis (17). In his thesis on atypical forms of

Parkinson's disease, Compin specifically noted that Parkinsonian cases without tremor showed especially marked rigidity (17). His first case history documented several additional features, including early age of onset, prominent gait and balance difficulty within the first years of illness, and midline dysfunction such as marked and early speech impairment.

Importantly, in Charcot's descriptive nosology, these atypical tremor variants still were considered as subdivisions of Parkinson's disease itself. As such, Charcot deplored the term "paralysis agitans" coined by Parkinson, first, because patients with Parkinsonism were not weak until very late in their disease, and second, because tremor was not always present (2,3).

Parkinsonism with Atypical Posture

Charcot drew strong attention to the phenomenon of rigidity in Parkinson's disease, and he fundamentally contributed to the distinction between this form of hypertonicity and spasticity (2). In studying rigidity, he identified the typical flexed posture of the patient with Parkinson's disease and, in his own medical drawings as well as his descriptions (Fig. 1), he noted that the neck, arms, and legs flexed in highly typical fashion. In contrast, he found a small number of Parkinsonian patients who were bradykinetic, unstable in their stance and gait, and yet showed a very different posture. These subjects, collectively termed "Parkinson's disease with extended posture" were of particular interest to Charcot. In his Tuesday teaching sessions, he presented a man named Bachère on several occasions. Commenting on June 12, 1888, Charcot mentioned that Bachère did not have marked tremor, but then turned to the issue of extension posture:

> There is something else unusual here worth noting. Look how he stands. I present him in profile so you can see the inclination of the head and trunk, well described by Parkinson. All this is typical. What is atypical, however, is that Bachère's forearms and legs are extended, making the extremities like rigid bars, whereas in the ordinary case, the same body parts are partly flexed. One can say then that in the typical case of Parkinson's disease, flexion is the predominant feature, whereas here, extension predominates and accounts for this unusual presentation. The difference is even more evident when the patient walks (3) (Fig. 1).

In addition to extended posture, this patient had particular facial bradykinesia and contracted forehead muscles (Fig. 2). Charcot commented that the patient had a perpetual look of surprise, because his

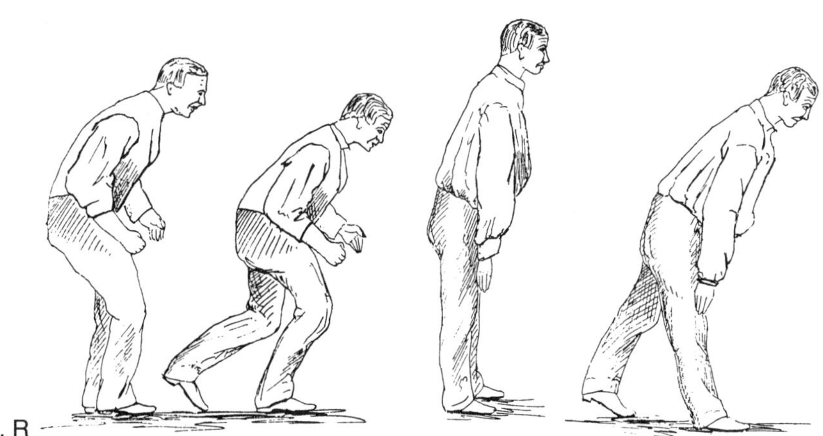

FIG. 1. Drawing from Charcot's original lesson, given on June 12, 1888, where he presented a typical case of Parkinson's disease (**L**) and his patient, Bachère (**R**), whose Parkinsonian variant included the absence of tremor and the extended posture. Charcot regularly taught his students by comparing and contrasting cases of patients from the Salpêtrière inpatient and outpatient services (3).

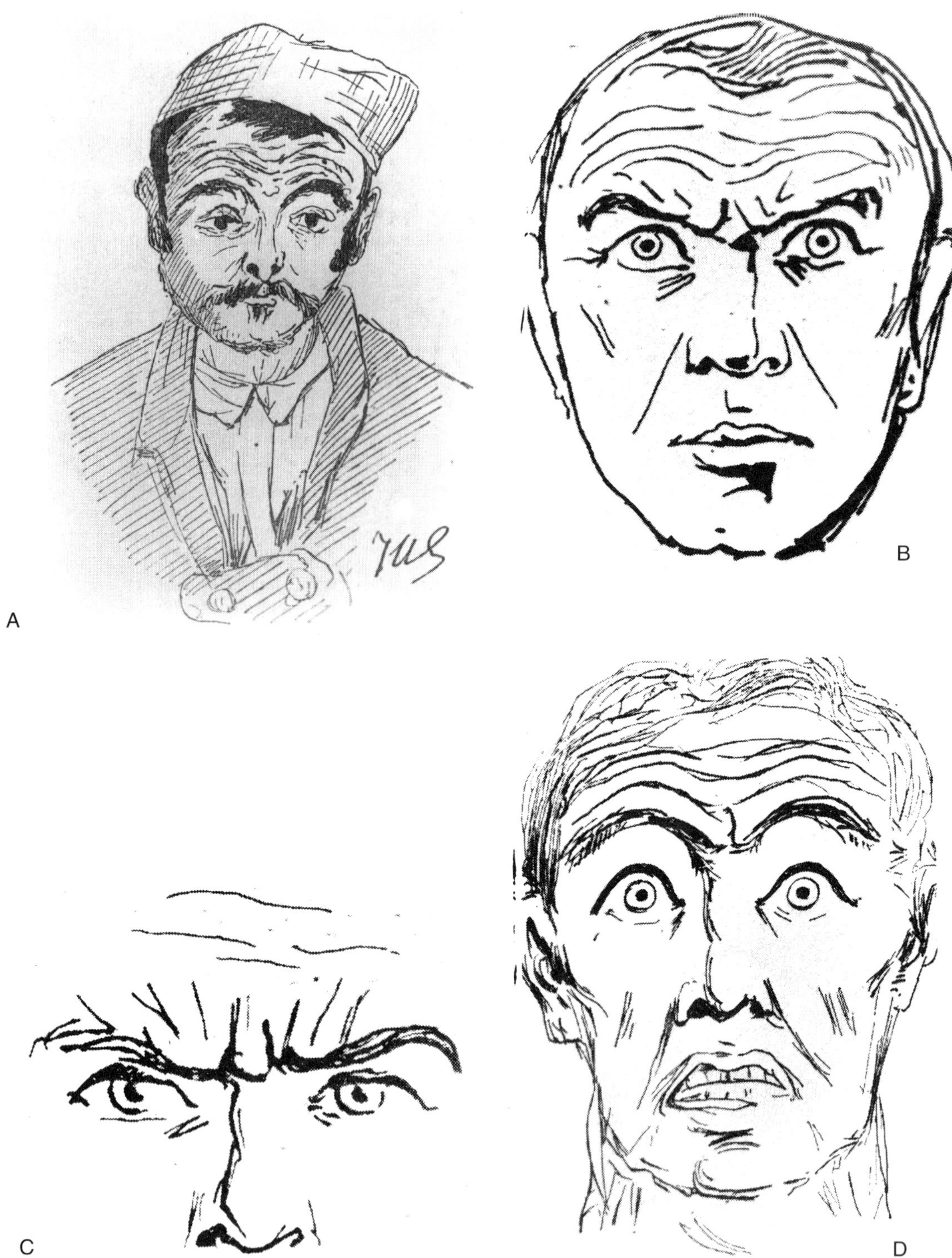

FIG. 2. Four drawings from the Charcot lesson on atypical Parkinson's disease, dated June 12, 1888, showing the distinctive facial features of these patients. (**A**) A portrait of Bachère, drawn by Charcot. (**B**) Forehead muscles and superior orbicularis in simultaneous contraction. (**C**) Combined activation of frontalis superior portion of the orbicularis and platysma, giving a frightened expression in contrast to the placid, blank stare of typical Parkinson's disease patients (3). (**D**) Activation of the palpebral portion of the orbicularis.

eyes remained widely opened and his forehead was continually wrinkled (3). In a modern setting, Jankovic has detailed similar facial morphology in atypical Parkinsonian syndromes, specifically in patients with PSP (18). The extended truncal posture of this patient would be compatible with the posture of PSP, although no specific supranuclear eye movement abnormalities were described. Another Salpêtrière patient with "Parkinson's disease in extension" was described by Dutil in 1889 and eye movement abnormalities are mentioned, although a supranuclear lesion is not documented clinically (19,20). This case also had highly asymmetric rigidity of the extremities (Fig. 3), a feature more reminiscent of CBD than PSP. In this case, the extended neck posture was graphically emphasized:

> The face is masked, the forehead wrinkled, the eyebrows raised, the eyes immobile. . . . This facies, associated with the extended posture of the head and trunk, gives the patient a singularly majestic air (19).

With clinical features reminiscent of both PSP and CBD, this patient was mentioned in several articles from the Salpêtrière school, although no autopsy was apparently performed (Fig. 3).

"Hemiplegic" Parkinsonism

One of the hallmarks of CBD is its asymmetry of clinical presentation and the contracted, dystonic deformity of one upper extremity (21). Charcot's descriptions of Parkinson's disease variants include some instances of highly asymmetric disease with prominent disability in the involved upper extremity beyond that expected with bradykinesia alone (2). Collectively termed "Hemiplegic Parkinson's disease," these cases form a large series in the French neurological literature of the late nineteenth century and include cases of abrupt stroke-like onset as well as slowly progressive disability (22). In the thesis by Béchet (23), one patient (case VIII) developed tremor and progressive contracture of the right upper extremity. Gradually, the trunk and neck developed extreme rigidity as well. The remarkable posture of the right upper extremity dominated the atypical picture:

> The right upper extremity is held alongside the body, extended and stiff, the elbow held straight, the wrist flexed, the hand pronated and held in front of the thigh. The hand is markedly contorted . . . the fingers completely flexed, especially the last three digits to the point that the finger nails sometimes leave impressions on the palm. The flexion of the index finger is less marked and the adducted thumb is held over the palmar surface of the middle finger. This contracture of the flexor muscles, however is only one of appearance, for the examiner can (with some effort, admittedly) extend the hand and fingers completely, and afterwards, they can hold this position briefly (23).

Further discussing the poor functional utility of the involved right upper extremity and the asymmetry of the case, he continued:

> Spontaneous movements of the upper extremity are practically impossible, very limited and extremely slow. The upper left extremity is only mildly flexed and the hand has no notable deformity (23).

Similarly, the case presented by Dutil (19,20) (Fig. 3), with its contracted upper extremity, was published, not only as a case of extended posture but also as a hemiplegic variant.

Apraxia and Alien Limb

Charcot and his school did not describe or appreciate the distinctive features of apraxia or alien limb. Liepmann was the first to systematically study limb apraxia, but his publication, which set up the working models of apraxia, dated from the turn of the century, after Charcot's death (24). Alien limb phenomenon likewise was not distinctly described by the French school, although Charcot was very interested in athetosis, and the involuntary floating postures of alien limb phenomenon could have been categorized in this nosology (25,26). Most of his cases of athetosis, however, were posthemiplegic in origin and no patient specifically was Parkinsonian.

"Atypical Parkinson's Disease" after Charcot

After Charcot died in 1893, the French school's influence waned and Germanic, British, and American schools of neurology shared the focus

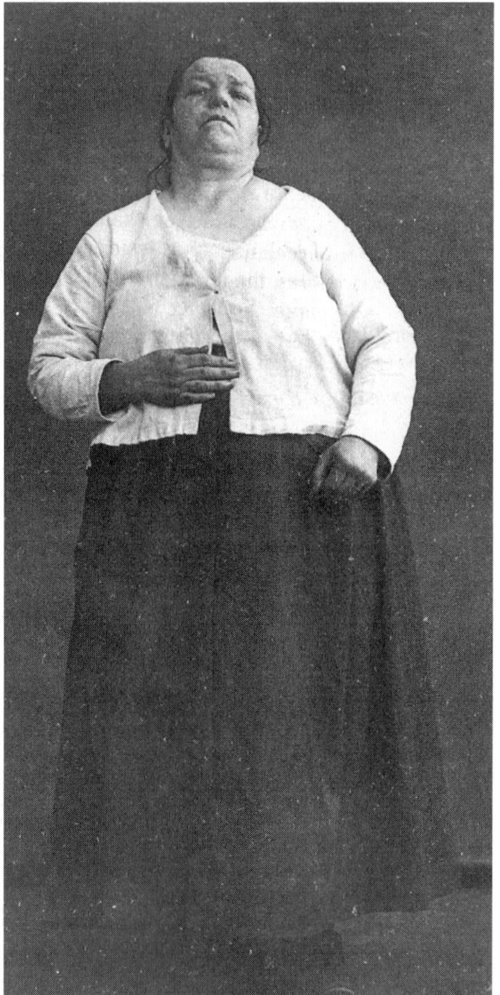

A

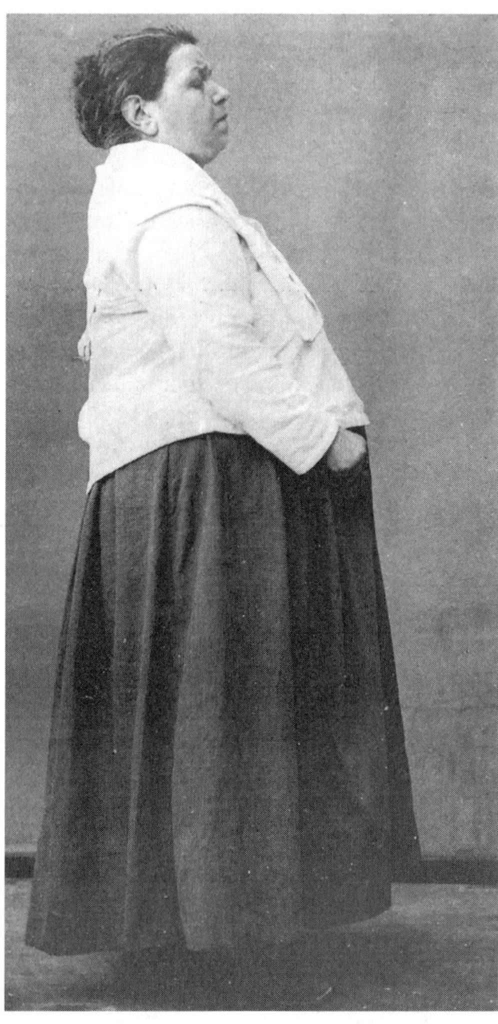

B

FIG. 3. Patient presented by A Dutil (19) as an atypical case of Parkinson's disease for two reasons, first she presented as a highly asymmetric case with hemiplegic features, and second because of her extended posture. This case has been reviewed and published recently as a possible case of PSP (20), but the asymmetry of motor features and the flexed elbow and wrist suggest that CBD is another possibility. No autopsy information is available. (**A**) Shows frontal view and asymmetry of arm posture. (**B**) Shows profile view with truncal extension.

of international neurology. Tretiakoff's identification of degeneration of the substantia nigra in Parkinson's disease brought renewed attention to the French anatomoclinical method, but the pathological distinction between Parkinson's disease and the other atypical Parkinsonian syndromes awaited the mid-twentieth century. The introduction of L-dopa helped to separate patients with clear-cut benefit from those who experienced less marked or minimal improvement. Whereas a definite improvement to L-dopa has been posited as suggestive of Parkinson's disease, many patients with atypical Parkinsonian syndromes and alternative pathological diagnoses (including CBD), are known to have beneficial responses to L-dopa during at least part of their illness. The clear delineation of CBD today raises the obvious clinical questions, where were these patients, and how were they classified, prior to the first well-established description in the 1960s (7)? Without a strong environmental hypothesis for CBD, it is difficult to accept that such cases were not available among the very large hospitalized population of the Salpêtrière in the nineteenth century. Whereas Charcot and his well-trained group did not specifically identify a prototypic case of CBD, his approach to the nosography of "atypical Parkinson's disease" provided the primary basis on which the later definition of this syndrome would be built.

Charcot died in 1893, nearly 75 years before Rabeiz and colleagues described the three cases of CBD that have become the archetypes of the syndrome. These cases showed unilateral or highly asymmetrical motor impairment that developed over several weeks or months. A useless, rigid, and dystonic arm that was flexed at the elbow and wrist predominated the syndrome and resulted in marked physical and functional impairment. Tremulous and jerking movements could be characteristic in the early phases and primary gait dysfunction and dyspraxia added to functional disability. Dementia and aphasia could likewise be present.

Following the tradition of Charcot, Rebeiz's report provided the descriptive details of a small series of prototypic cases. Later investigators built on this base, adding variants or *formes frustes* to the literature. Charcot described this process (3):

> Studying archetypes is a fundamental task in nosography. Duchenne de Boulogne practiced it instinctively, and many others have done it before and after him. It is indispensable and the only way to extract from the chaos of imprecision a specific pathologic state. The history of medicine, which is long and grand, shows this truth well. But once the archetype is established, the second nosographic operation begins: dissect the archetype and analyze its parts. One must, in other words, learn how to recognize the imperfect cases, the formes frustes, or examples where only one feature occurs in isolation. Using this second method, the physician will see the archetypical illness in an entirely new light. One's scope enlarges, and the illness becomes much more important in the doctor's daily practice. To the patient's benefit, the doctor becomes attentive and sensitive to recognizing a disease, even when it is in its earliest developmental stages.

REFERENCES

1. Parkinson J. *The shaking palsy.* London: Whittingham and Rowland, 1817.
2. Charcot J-M. De la paralysie agitante. In: *Oeuvres complètes. Vol. 1. Paris: Bureaux du Progrès Médical, 1892: 155–189. [In English: On paralysis agitans. In: Sigerson G., trans.* Lectures on diseases of the nervous system, Philadelphia: HC Lea and Co., 1879:105–127.
3. Charcot J-M. *Leçons du mardi: Policlinique de la Salpêtrière.* Paris: Bureaux du Progrès Médical, 1887–1888.
4. Charcot J-M, Vulpian A. De la paralysie agitante. Gazette Hebdomadaire de Médecine et de Chirurgie 1861–1862;8:765–767, 8:816–820, 9:54–59.
5. Goetz CG, Bonduelle M, Gelfand T. *Charcot: Constructing neurology.* New York: Oxford University Press, 1995.
6. Litvan I, Agid Y, Goetz C, Jankovic J. Accuracy of the clinical diagnosis of corticobasal degeneration: a clinicopathological study. *Neurology* 1997;48:119–125.
7. Rebeiz JJ, Kolodny EH, Richardson EP Jr. Corticodentatonigral degeneration with neuronal achromasia. *Trans Amer Neurolog Assoc* 1967;92:23–26.
8. von Braunmühl A. Über Stammganlienveränderungen bei Picksher Krankheit. *A gesamte Neurol Psychiatrie* 1930,124.214–223.
9. van Husen T. Über ein Fall von Pick'scher Krankheit. *Allg Z Pshciatrie* 1934;101:381–396.
10. Tretiakoff C. Contribution à l'étude de l'anatomie pathologique du locus niger de Sommering. Paris: Thèse de Médecine, 1919. Bureaux du Progrès Médical.
11. Laplane D. Charcot and the neurological examination. In: Goetz CG, ed. Charcot Centenary Symposium. Minneapolis, MN: American Academy of Neurology Publications, 1993.
12. Friedreich N. Über denerative Atrophie der spinalen Hinterstränge. *Virchow Arch Pathol Anat* 1877;70:140–148.
13. Friedreich N. Neuropathologische Beobachtung beim Paramyoklonus mutiplex. *Virchow Arch Pathol Anat* 1881;86:421–434.
14. Unverricht H. Die Myoclonie. Franz Deuticke (no publication city given), 189.
15. Goetz CG. Visual art in the neurological career of Jean-Martin Charcot. *Arch Neurol* 1991;48:421–425.
16. Bourneville D-M. Deux cas de la maladie de Parkinson sans tremblement. Paris: Progrès Médical, Sept 17, 1876.
17. Compin P. Etude clinique des formes anormales de la maladie de Parkinson. Lyon: Thèse de Médecine, 1902.
18. Jankovic J. Progressive supranuclear palsy. *Neurol Clin* 1984;2:473–486.
19. Dutil A. Sur un cas de paralysie agitante à forme hemiplégique avec attitude anormale de la tête et du tronc (extension). *Nouvelle Iconographie de la Salpêtrière 1889;2:165–169.*
20. Goetz CG. An early photographic case of probable progressive supranuclear palsy. *Move Dis* 1996;11(6): 617–618.
21. LeWitt PA. The movement disorders of corticobasal degeneration. In: Kertesz A, Munoz DG, eds. *Pick's disease and Pick complexes.* New York: Wiley-Liss, 1998, 105–119.
22. Marie P. Hémiplégie chez les parkinsoniens. In: Brouardel P, Gilbert JP, eds. *Traité de Médecine et de Thérapeut.* Paris: Masson, 1911.

23. Béchet A. Etude clinique des formes de la maladie de Parkinson. Thèse de Médecine, Paris: Bureaux du Progrès Médical, 1892.
24. Liepmann H, Moss O. Fall von linksseitiger Agraphia und Apraxie bei rechsseitiger Lahmng. *Z Psychol Neurol* 1907;10:214–227.
25. Charcot JM. De l'athétose. In: *Oeuvres complètes.* Vol. 2. Paris: Bureaux du Progrès Médical, 1886, 491–494. [In English: On athethosis. In: Sigerson G, trans. *Lectures on Diseases of the Nervous System.* London: New Sydenham Society, 1887, 390–394.
26. Charcot JM. De l'hemichorée post-hémiplégique. In: *Oeuvres complètes, Vol. 2. Paris: Bureaux du Progrès Médical, 1886, 358–371. In English: On athethosis. In: Sigerson G, trans.,* Lectures on diseases of the nervous system. London: New Sydenham Society, 1887, 275–286.

Corticobasal Degeneration.
Advances in Neurology, Vol. 82,
edited by I. Litvan, C. G. Goetz, and A. E. Lang.
Lippincott Williams & Wilkins, Philadelphia © 2000.

2

Neuropathologic and Molecular Considerations

Dennis W. Dickson,* Wan-Kyng Liu,† Hanna Ksiezak-Reding,‡ and Shu-Hui Yen†

*Departments of *Pathology and †Pharmacology, Mayo Clinic, Jacksonville, Florida, 32224; ‡Department of Pathology, Albert Einstein College of Medicine, Bronx, New York 10461*

INTRODUCTION

Historical Considerations and Terminology

The first report of pathologic findings in corticobasal degeneration (CBD) was by Rebeiz and coworkers (1), who referred to the disorder as "corticodentatonigral degeneration with neuronal achromasia." Subsequent reports referred to the disorder as corticonigral degeneration (2–6), and Gibb and coworkers coined the term "corticobasal degeneration" (7). Some groups have also used the term "corticobasal ganglionic degeneration" for CBD (8–10). All names emphasize the predominant distribution of pathology to cortex and deep gray matter structures. The advantage of the term corticobasal over the others is that it is the most generic and encompasses degenerative changes in deep gray matter areas other than the basal ganglia, substantia nigra, and cerebellar dentate.

NEUROPATHOLOGY

Gross Findings

Focal Cortical Atrophy

On external examination the brain usually shows narrowing of cortical gyri that is most marked in parasagittal regions (Fig. 1). The superior frontal gyrus is often more affected than middle and inferior frontal gyri in cases with a typical progressive asymmetrical rigidity and apraxia syndrome. The pre- and postcentral regions are also affected to varying degrees. The temporal and occipital lobes are usually spared. In cases presenting with dementia or progressive aphasia the distribution of the atrophy is often more generalized and involves the inferior frontal and temporal lobes as well (11–13). The atrophy is often asymmetric, but the side-to-side differences can be subtle (Fig. 1) and only obvious by weighing both hemispheres separately. Given that most research brain banks have protocols that call for fixation of at most half the brain, it is often impossible to assess asymmetry. Nevertheless, the biochemical and genetic information gained by having frozen tissue far outweighs the value of any structural information that could be obtained from histopathologic examination of both hemispheres. Despite asymmetry of pathology, fixation of the entire brain to document this fact is strongly discouraged in the evaluation of CBD.

On sectioning the brain, cortical atrophy is often obvious in the dorsal half of the frontal lobe, with sometimes striking preservation of the frontal opercular region and the temporal lobe (Fig. 2). The cingulate gyrus is not consistently affected. The brainstem and cerebellum are not consistently reduced in size.

White Matter Pathology: Frontobulbar Degeneration

The cerebral white matter in affected areas is often attenuated (Fig. 2), and may have a gray and gelatinous consistency in severe cases. The

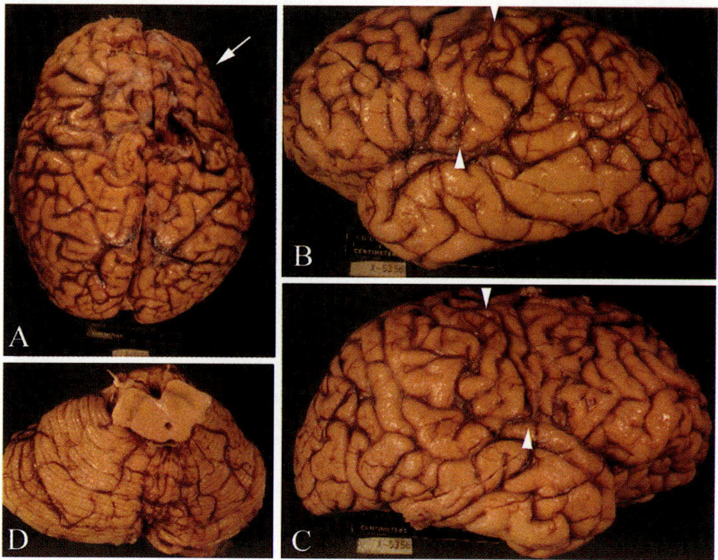

FIG. 1. Gross findings of brain in CBD. The cerebral hemispheres are asymmetrical, with widening of the sulcal spaces in the superior frontal parasagittal region (**A**). The right hemisphere is smaller than the left, especially in the frontal region (**A**, *arrow*). Both left (**B**) and right (**C**) hemispheres have peri-Rolandic atrophy (*between arrowheads*) that is clearly worse on the right. The brainstem and cerebellum (**D**) show slight loss of pigment in the substantia nigra and a dilated aqueduct.

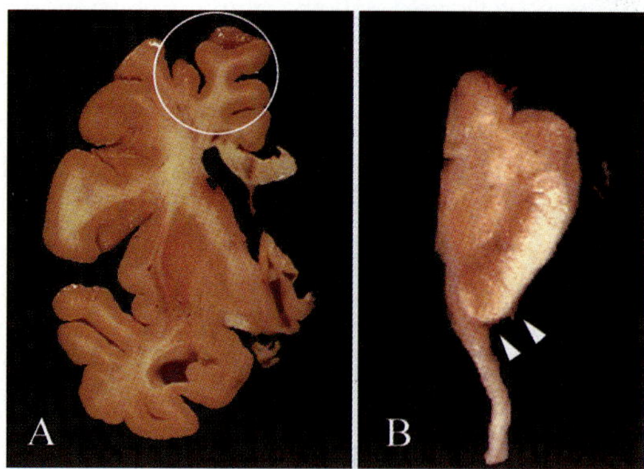

FIG. 2. Gross findings of brain in CBD. On coronal sections of the cerebrum (**A**) the superior frontal gyrus is disproportionately small (*circle*) compared to adjacent middle frontal and cingulate gyri. The white matter also has gray discoloration. The basal ganglia have minimal rust color in the globus pallidus. The transverse section of midbrain (**B**) shows loss of neuromelanin pigment in the substantia nigra and slight attenuation and gray discoloration of the corticopontine fibers in the medial cerebral peduncle (*arrowheads*).

anterior corpus callosum is sometimes thinned, and corpus callosum thinning has been confirmed as a useful diagnostic feature of CBD in recent clinical imaging studies (14). The anterior limb of the internal capsule may show attenuation, as well, but other white matter tracts, such as the optic tract, anterior commissure, and fornix, are preserved.

Basal Ganglia and Brainstem Pathology

There may be flattening of the head of the caudate, and in many cases the thalamus is smaller than expected. In some cases there is a rust-like color of the globus pallidus, red nucleus, and pars reticularis of the substantia nigra. Transverse sections of the brainstem invariably show loss of neuromelanin pigment in the substantia nigra, usually atrophy of the midbrain tegmentum and associated dilation of the aqueduct (Fig. 2). The neuromelanin pigment in the locus ceruleus may be grossly preserved. The cerebral peduncles may show attenuation of the medial third, representing degeneration of corticobulbar fibers. It is unusual to detect gross atrophy of the pons and medulla, and significant degeneration of the cerebellar dentate nucleus, with demyelination of the superior cerebellar peduncle, should raise the possibility of progressive supranuclear palsy (PSP) rather than CBD.

Microscopic Findings

Nonspecific Changes (Superficial Spongiosis and White Matter Gliosis)

In affected cortical areas the cortical ribbon is usually thinner than expected and rarefied because of neuronal loss and gliosis. Superficial spongiosis is a common finding in atrophic cortical regions (Fig. 3). There is also astrocytic gliosis that is prominent in the superficial cortical layers and at the gray–white junction (Fig. 3). The cerebral white matter shows mild loss of myelin and gliosis that follows the topographic distribution of the cortical atrophy, as well as the corticostriatal and corticobulbar fiber systems. Most cases do not have obvious senile plaques or neurofibrillary tangles (NFT) on thioflavin fluorescent microscopy or diagnostic silver stains, such as the Bielschowsky stain, but some elderly individuals, particularly those with apolipoprotein E ε 4 genotype (15), may have coexistent Alzheimer's disease (AD) type pathology. Combined AD and CBD occurs, but is much less common than some other dementia disorders, most notably Lewy body dementia. In the latter condition, AD-type pathology is found in nearly two-thirds of cases. In some elderly cases of CBD Lewy bodies restricted to the substantia nigra may be a coincidental finding (Fig. 4).

Cellular Alterations Revealed with Immunocytochemistry

Although certain silver impregnation methods have great utility in evaluating neurodegenerative diseases, their specificity is not comparable to that obtained with antibody-based methods. Furthermore, silver stains such as the Gallyas stain are less adaptable to widespread use and have been the stock of specialized neurohistology research laboratories, often with particular laboratory procedural modifications. In contrast, antibody methods

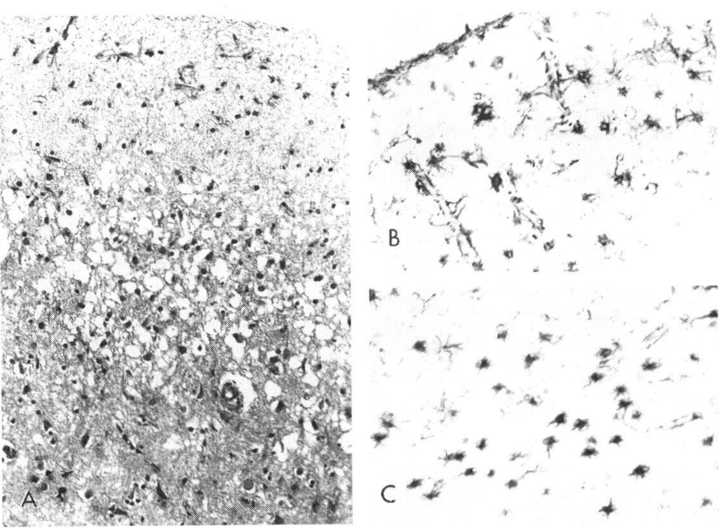

FIG. 3. The superficial cortex has microvacuolation or spongiosis (**A**). With immunostaining for glial fibrillary acidic protein, reactive astrocytes are prominent in the superficial cortex (**B**) and at the gray–white junction (**C**).

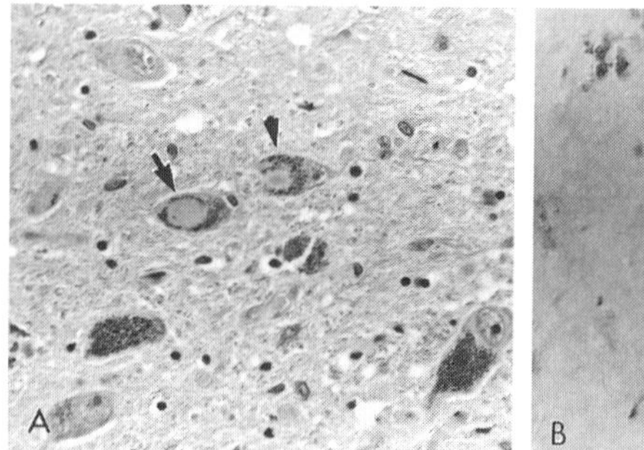

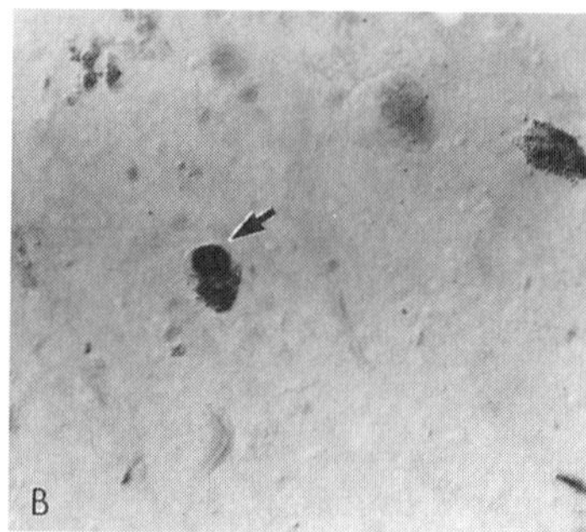

FIG. 4. Sections of the substantia nigra stained with H&E (**A**) and immunostained with a monoclonal antibody specific to NFT (**B**). Pale staining inclusion (*arrow*) in a pigmented neuron, a so-called corticobasal body, is intensely immunostained with the NFT antibody (**B**, *arrow*). An incidental Lewy body (**A**, *arrowhead*) is present in the cytoplasm of a pigmented neuron of the substantia nigra.

have gained widespread acceptance and are routinely used in virtually every modern diagnostic pathology laboratory, partly because of the ease of automating immunocytochemistry. Moreover, antibodies are exquisitely specific, whereas the chemical basis for specificity of silver stains, such as Bodian's method for neurofilaments and the Gallyas method for pathological tau, is largely unknown. Of all the silver stains used in diagnostic neuropathology, the latter has been advocated as the most sensitive and useful (16). Although the Gallyas silver stain may produce nearly comparable results to immunocytochemistry, the focus of this presentation is on antibody methods.

Neurofilament Antibodies and Ballooned Neurons

In affected areas swollen cortical neurons are scattered in the third, fifth, and sixth cortical layers (Fig. 5). These swollen neurons are the histological hallmark of CBD and have been likened to "chromatolysis" (17), which is a descriptive term for the series of changes that occur in a neuronal cell body in response to axonal injury. Chromatolysis is characterized by loss of Nissl substance, either in the central part of the cytoplasm (central chromatolysis) or in the periphery (peripheral chromatolysis). Given that there is no direct evidence to support the hypothesis that

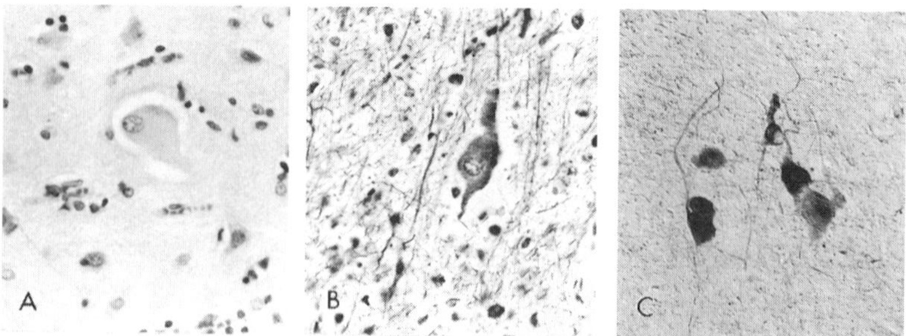

FIG. 5. Ballooned neurons from affected cortical regions are pale staining on H&E (**A**) and often surrounded by an artifactual space. On silver stains, such as a Bodian stain (**B**) the BN has weak and granular cytoplasmic staining. The most sensitive means of detecting BN is immunostaining for neurofilament (**C**), where a cluster of five BN is detected. Note the bizarre shape of the BN and staining of some of their apical dendrites.

axonal damage is the cause of swollen cortical neurons in CBD, many authors have preferred to use more descriptive terms such as "achromatic neurons" or "ballooned neurons" (BN) to describe swollen neurons (2,18–23) (Fig. 4). The latter term has gained wide acceptance and has largely replaced the term "achromasia" and "chromatolysis." In Pick's disease (PiD) swollen neurons analogous to BN are sometimes referred to as "Pick cells" (24,25).

The most common locations for detecting BN are anterior cingulate gyrus, amygdala, insular cortex, and claustrum, but this limbic and paralimbic distribution should not be considered specific. It is not uncommon to find BN limited to the limbic and paralimbic gray matter in a host of other disorders, including aging, AD, Creutzfeldt-Jakob disease, Braak's argyrophilic grain dementia, and PSP (2,18,19,22,23,26–28). Of much more diagnostic significance is the presence of BN in the affected convexity cortical areas, such as the superior frontal gyrus. They are much less frequently found in neostriatum and brainstem. On routine histological stains BN are eosinophilic to amphophilic and are often vacuolated (Fig. 4a). They may be weakly argyrophilic, but they are not stained well with routine silver stains such as Bodian or Bielschowsky stains (Fig. 3). They are also not stained with thioflavin S fluorescence microscopy. They lack apparent Nissl substance on a cresyl violet stain, hence the term "achromasia." Useful cytologic features of BN are swelling of proximal dendrites and cytoplasmic vacuolation. In some cases BN contain granulovacuolar bodies similar to those detected in pyramidal neurons of the hippocampus in aging and AD.

BN are strongly immunoreactive for phosphorylated neurofilaments (2,6,22) (Fig. 5). The reaction with antibodies to phosphoepitopes is diminished or eliminated if the sections are pretreated with alkaline phosphatase (2). This distinguishes Pick bodies and neurofibrillary tangles (NFT) from BN, since the phosphoepitopes in Pick bodies and NFT are partially or totally resistant to the effects of phosphatase for reasons that remain unclear. The pronounced reaction of BN for phosphorylated neurofilaments has been suggested to distinguish BN from lower motor neurons undergoing axotomy response (6). Experimental studies, however, indicate that phosphorylated neurofilaments also accumulate in neuronal perikarya following axotomy (29).

BN also show reactivity for αB-crystallin (18,19), heat shock protein 27 (16), and sometimes for ubiquitin (22,30,31), but not for epitopes specific to Alzheimer NFT (2). BN also show immunoreactivity for markers of oxidative stress, such as heme oxidase (32). Ballooned neurons are also negative for α-synuclein, a sensitive and specific marker for cortical Lewy bodies (33).

Tau Pathology: Neurofibrillary Lesions

As is sometimes the case with silver stains, where focal argyrophilia is sometimes detected in the cytoplasm of BN (2), focal tau immunoreactivity is also sometimes detected in BN, most often at the cell margins (30). In addition to BN, scattered neurons in atrophic cortical areas have tau immunoreactivity. The tau-immunoreactive neuronal lesions are structurally pleomorphic (Fig. 6). In some neurons the immunoreactivity is densely packed into a small inclusion body somewhat reminiscent of Pick bodies or small NFT (Fig. 6). In other neurons the filamentous inclusions are more dispersed and disorderly. These skein-like neurofibrillary lesions are perhaps the most characteristic tau-immunoreactive neurofibrillary lesions in CBD.

Neuronal tau-positive inclusions were not included in the original descriptions of CBD since these methods were not available. Furthermore, the neuronal inclusions have inconsistent staining with most silver stains. The Gallyas stain is a clear exception to this rule (16) (Fig. 6). In contrast to NFT of AD where lesions are readily detected with a host of diagnostic silver stains and even with thioflavin fluorescent microscopy, the neuronal lesions in CBD are not easily seen and often completely negative. This points to the fact that tau pathology in CBD is different from that in aging and AD. Other differences in neurofibrillary pathology in CBD compared to AD include less ubiquitination and a restricted tau isoform composition (see the following).

Neurofibrillary lesions in brainstem monoaminergic nuclei, such as the locus ceruleus and substantia nigra, are common in CBD and are essentially identical to globose NFT found in AD and PSP (Fig. 4).

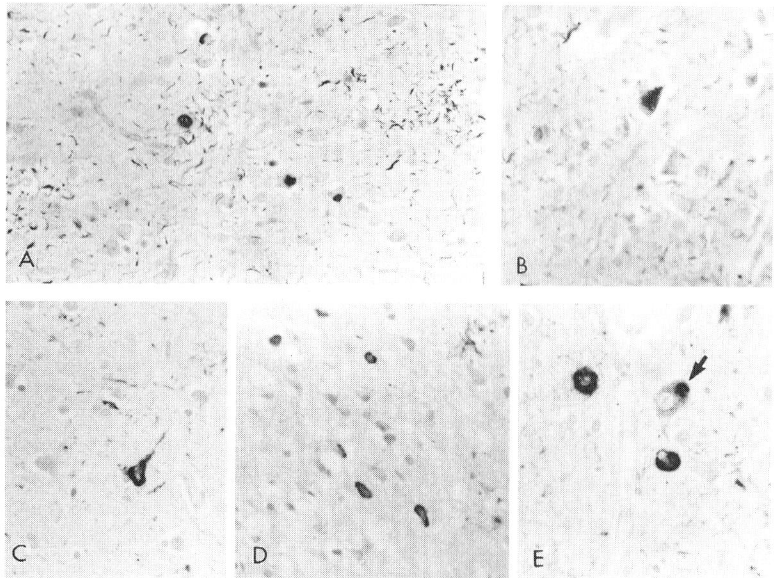

FIG. 6. Neuronal lesions are pleomorphic and best seen with silver stains such as the Gallyas stain (**A, B**) or immunostaining for tau (**C, D, E**). In addition to many grain and thread-like lesions, the Gallyas stains reveal small round (**A**) and irregular skein-like inclusions (**B**). Similar lesions are seen with tau, including NFT-like lesions (**C**), ring-like lesions (**D**), and Pick body-like (*arrow*) lesions (**E**).

Tau Pathology: Grains and Threads

In addition to fibrillary lesions in perikarya of neurons, the neuropil of CBD invariably contains an assortment of tau-immunoreactive cell processes (Fig. 7). Although these lesions are sometimes referred to as "neuropil threads" (34) after the lesions described in AD (35), it is strictly incorrect to use this term in CBD. In AD virtually all neuropil threads are neuronal in origin as demonstrated by immunoelectron microscopy (36,37). In contrast, in CBD only a small fraction of thread-like structures are double labeled with neurofilament antibodies (30), which indicates that many thread-like processes in CBD are probably from glial rather than neuronal cells. In CBD thread-like processes and shorter, stubbier tau-immunoreactive lesions are usually profuse in affected areas of gray and white matter (Fig. 7). The predominance of tau-immunoreactivity in cell processes is an important attribute of CBD and a useful feature in differentiating it from other disorders. In other disorders with which CBD can be confused, tau-related pathology is more often located in cell bodies (e.g., NFT and Pick bodies) and the proximal cell processes of neurons and glia.

Braak originally described argyrophilic grains in a form of neurodegenerative disease that had a predilection for the limbic lobe and certain hypothalamic nuclei (38). Subsequent studies have demonstrated that grains can be detected in a variety of neurodegenerative diseases, including CBD (28,39). In contrast to Braak's argyrophilic grain disease, the grain-like lesions in CBD are more widespread, including affected cortical and deep gray matter regions (Fig. 7). In some cases of CBD they are also located in the limbic lobe where they overlap with pathology of Braak's grain disease. It is interesting to note that BN are also present in some cases of Braak's grain disease (28), but BN in Braak's grain disease are usually limited to the limbic lobe.

Tau Pathology: Oligodendroglial Coiled Bodies

Tau-positive argyrophilic inclusions in oligodendroglia are increasingly recognized in several neurodegenerative diseases, including CBD,

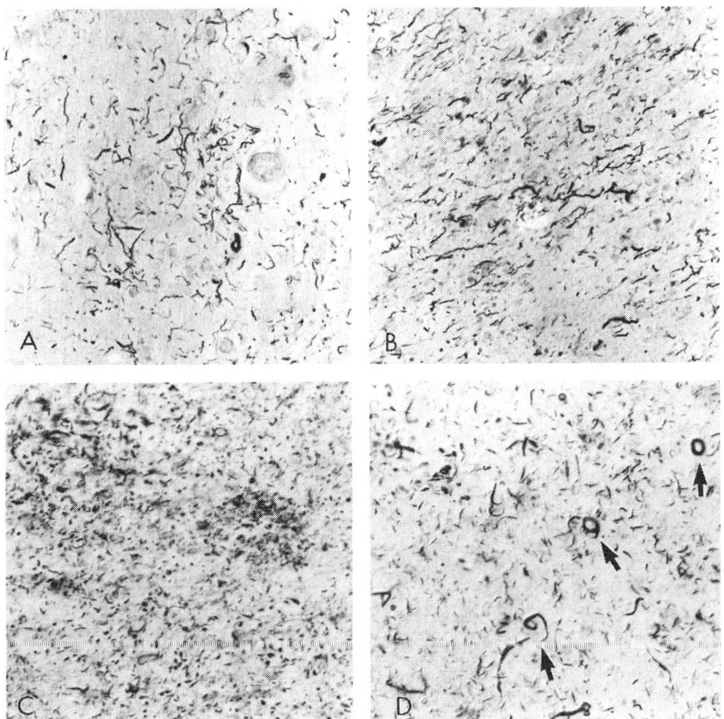

FIG. 7. A profusion of thread-like and grain-like lesions are found in the gray (**A, C**) and white matter (**B, D**) of CBD. The lesions are readily detected with the Gallyas stain (**A, B**) and tau immunostains (**C, D**). In the gray matter the grain-like lesions are clustered in astrocytic plaques. In white matter coiled bodies (*arrows*) are readily apparent. (Gallyas stain preparation from Dr. T. Komori.)

Braak's grain disease, and PSP (16,26,30, 38–52). The lesions have been given a variety of names, including "oligodendroglia microtubular masses" (45) and "coiled bodies" (38). Coiled body is descriptive of the most common appearance of the lesion, namely, a bundle of fibrils that coil around the nucleus and extend into proximal cell process (Figs. 7 and 8). The name has certain utility because it clearly distinguishes this tau-positive oligodendroglial lesion from the oligodendroglial inclusions that are the hallmark of multiple system atrophy. The latter lesions are usually referred to as "glial cytoplasmic inclusions" or GCI (53). There are a number of differences between GCI and coiled bodies. GCI are consistently immunoreactive for ubiquitin and α-synuclein, but usually negative for tau. In contrast, coiled bodies of CBD and other neurodegenerative disorders are consistently immunoreactive for tau and negative for synuclein. Coiled bodies are negative or inconsistently immunoreactive for ubiquitin. Like GCI (53), double labeling studies demonstrate that coiled bodies are in oligodendroglia since they can sometimes be labeled with oligodendroglial markers, such as Leu 7, myelin basic protein, and C4d (30,45,47,48,50,52). The lack of robust markers for mature oligodendroglia is a problem that plagues modern neuropathology. On the other hand, immunoelectron microscopic studies have shown unequivocally that coiled bodies are in oligodendroglia (54,55). The abnormal tau-immunoreactive filaments are detected in the cell bodies of small white matter glial cells as well as inner and outer myelin loops of myelinated fibers, but not in the axon (see the following).

Tau Pathology: Astrocytic Plaques

A host of tau-immunoreactive astrocytic lesions have been described in various neurodegenera-

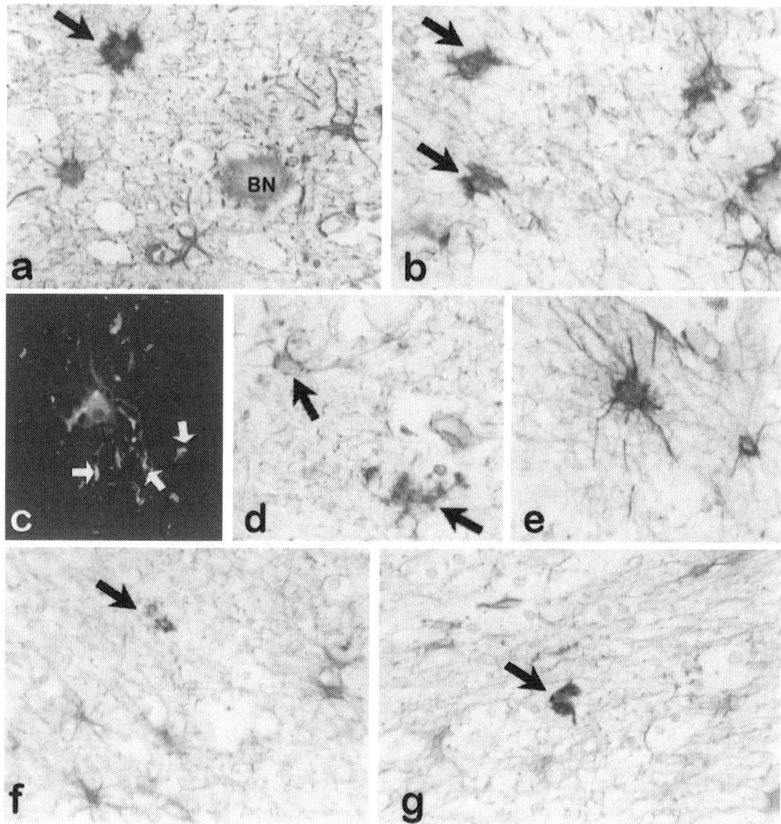

FIG. 8. Double immunostaining for GFAP (brown color in **A**, **B**, **D**, **E**, **F**, and **G**; green color in **C**) and tau (blue color in **A**, **B**, **D**, **E**, **F**, and **G**; and red color in **C**). A variety of tau-positive astrocytes are found in the cortex in CBD, including astrocytes in the cortex (**A**, **B**, and **D**) and adjacent to blood vessels (**E**). (Note tau immunostaining in some BN [**A**].) Astrocytic plaques (**C** and **D**) have centrally placed astrocyte cell bodies and short tau-positive inclusions in glial processes. (Note the double staining—yellow color—in **C** [*arrow*].) Tau immunoreactive glia in the white matter (**F** and **G**) are negative with GFAP and consistent with oligodendroglial coiled bodies. (**C**—fluorescent stain and confocal microscopy; from Dr. M. Feany.)

tive diseases, including CBD. Astrocytic tau-immunoreactive lesions have been referred to as "tufted astrocytes," "star-like tufts," "spider-like radiating fibers," "thorn-shaped astrocytes," and "gliofibrillary tangles" (52). The terminology is not standardized, and it is likely that the different morphologies and terms for the lesions reflect methodologic as much as biologic differences. In particular, the morphology of the lesions varies dramatically depending on the thickness of the tissue section. In routine 5–7 micron thick sections only a small cross-sectional sample of the lesion is included, whereas in thicker (40–100 micron) sections the lesions are visible in their entirety (Fig. 9). The different morphologies of tau-immunoreactive astrocytic lesions may also be a function of which type of astrocyte (protoplasmic vs. fibrous, subpial vs. parenchymal) is affected.

The most characteristic tau-immunoreactive astrocytic lesion in CBD, particularly in the neocortex, is an annular cluster of grain-like processes that may be highly suggestive of an Alzheimer type neuritic plaque. (Figs. 7, 8, and 9). These lesions, in contrast to Alzheimer plaques, do not contain amyloid based on histochemical, fluorescent, and immunocytochemical methods for detecting amyloid. The only exception is in rare cases of coexistent CBD and AD. In further con-

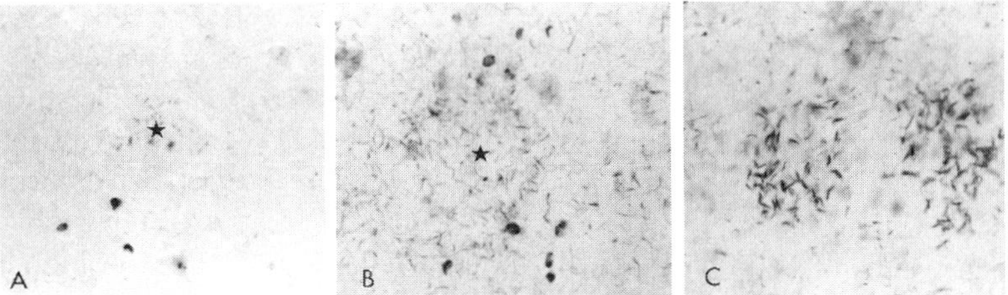

FIG. 9. The appearance of astrocytic plaques (*stars*) with tau immunostaining varies dramatically depending on the section thickness. They are barely visible in 5-micron paraffin sections (**A**), but are much better defined in 40-micron thick Vibratome sections (**B**). The appearance also varies from case to case and with different antibodies (**B**—Alz-50, **C**—PHF-1, both antibodies from Dr. P. Davies).

tradistinction with neuritic plaques in AD, most of the tau immunoreactivity is not within dystrophic neuronal processes, but rather processes of glial cells. Double immunostaining for tau and glial fibrillary acid protein, vimentin, or CD44, which are all markers with varying degrees of specificity for astrocytes, demonstrates that the tau-positive cell processes in these lesions are derived from astrocytes (30). These lesions are called "astrocytic plaques" (30). Somewhat similar lesions can be seen in some cases of PSP, but the classic astrocytic plaque with its distinct annular array of tau-immunoreactive processes should suggest a diagnosis of CBD (Fig. 10). Some investigators (30,51,52,56,57) have argued that the astrocytic plaque may be the most specific histopathologic feature of CBD. Other less distinctive tau-immunoreactive astrocytic lesions are also seen in CBD, and the latter, in particular, may have overlapping morphological features with tau-positive astrocytes of PSP and PiD.

Neuroanatomical Distribution of Lesions

The brunt of the cortical pathology is in the superior frontal and pre- and postcentral gyri. Given the focal nature of the degeneration, it is important that the most severely affected areas be sampled, since BN, in particular, may not be detected in other areas. This can lead to a mis-

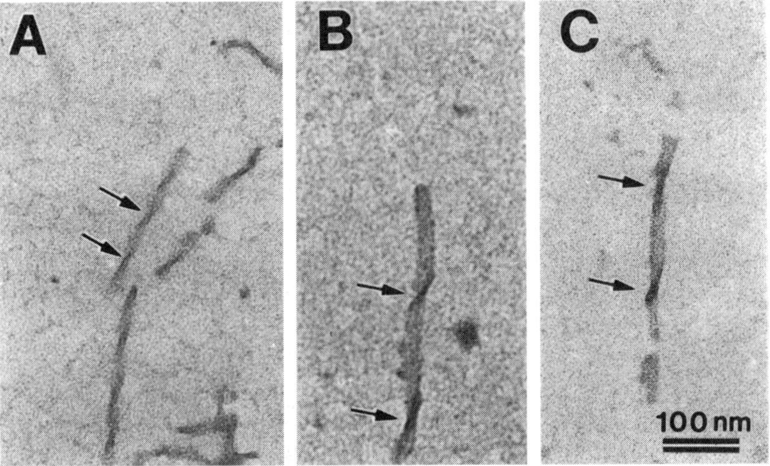

FIG. 10. The ultrastructural appearance of PHF differs between AD (**A**) and CBD (**B** and **C**). In AD the filaments are approximately 20 nm wide and twisted at 60–70 nm intervals, whereas those in CBD are wider (27 nm) and twisted at longer intervals (approximately 140 nm). Uranyl acetate staining of isolated filaments.

taken perception that the disorder does not have BN. Although tau-immunoreactive lesions also have a relatively restricted distribution, in most cases a few lesions can be found in areas with less severe atrophy. White matter in areas not directly contiguous with focal atrophy may show tau-immunoreactive thread-like lesions and coiled bodies.

In most cases the hippocampus and parahippocampus show normal neuronal content and organization without gliosis. Although a few pyramidal neurons may contain NFT and granulovacuolar degeneration, this is usually not greater than expected for the age of the individual. Tau-immunoreactive grains may be detected in some cases.

The caudate nucleus and putamen invariably have tau-immunoreactive lesions, and these often have a predilection for the striatal fiber bundles. Scattered neurons may have NFT, and there may be a few astrocytic plaques in the striatum. The globus pallidus and inner putamen show nerve cell depletion with gliosis and occasional NFT. There may be granular axonal spheroids and hemosiderin-like pigmentary degeneration in the globus pallidus and pars reticularis of the substantia nigra that is more than expected for age. The basal nucleus of Meynert is usually well populated, but may have a few NFT.

The substantia nigra usually has moderate to marked neuronal loss with extraneuronal neuromelanin in phagocytes. Residual neurons often contain ill-defined neurofibrillary inclusions that may have a spooled or whorled morphology consistent with globose NFT. These lesions have been referred to as "corticobasal bodies" (Fig. 4), but there are no demonstrable differences between corticobasal bodies and NFT. Of more use in the differential diagnosis is the presence of ill-defined skein-like neurofibrillary lesions, numerous tau-immunoreactive cell processes, and abundance of tau-immunoreactive glial lesions in the same regions. The locus ceruleus, raphe nuclei, and tegmental gray have similar neurofibrillary lesions.

The red nucleus and subthalamic nucleus may have mild neuronal loss, gliosis, and tau-immunoreactive neurofibrillary lesions. Thalamic nuclei may also be affected, particularly the ventrolateral nucleus. Mild neuronal depletion and gliosis of the dentate nucleus occurs even though Rebeiz and coworkers emphasized this finding in the original reports. In contrast to PSP, where it may be found in the majority of cases, dentate nucleus grumose degeneration is uncommon in CBD. The cerebellar cortex is relatively unaffected, but scattered Purkinje cell axonal torpedoes and mild Bergmann gliosis are not uncommon.

ULTRASTRUCTURAL FINDINGS

There are only a limited number of published reports on the fine structural alterations in CBD (6,30,41,42,48), with much of the research focused on morphology of isolated filaments (44,58,59) where the cell of origin is not known. Given that abnormal cytoskeletal lesions are found in neurons and glia in CBD, additional descriptive studies are warranted.

Neuronal Lesions

Ultrastructurally, the cytoplasm of abnormal cortical neurons in CBD contain increased filaments. Although typical ballooned neurons and tau-positive neurofibrillary lesions are different structures at the light microscopic level, there have been no reports that clearly differentiate the two lesions at the ultrastructural level. Murayama and coworkers have reported such a study in PiD (60). In this study BN appeared to share features with Pick bodies, with both types of lesions containing similar types of filaments. In other disorders, BN usually contain a disorderly array of filaments about 10 nm in diameter, interspersed with other cytoplasmic elements (5,17). In contrast, the filaments in tau-positive lesions tend to have a wider diameter (20–24 nm) paired helical filament-like structure. These wider filaments are also the predominant and most characteristic finding in isolated preparations. They have been referred to as "twisted tubules" or "twisted ribbons" (Fig. 10). Although they appear somewhat similar to paired helical filaments of AD, they have several differences, including physical dimensions, mass per unit length, and ultrastructural stability. The twisted ribbons of CBD are wider, have a longer periodicity of the twists, less mass per unit length, and greater instability as assessed by increased tendency to dissociate into protofilaments (44,58,59). They are also less phosphorylated and less ubiquitinated than filaments in AD (61) (Fig. 10).

Fine structural analysis of grains has not been reported in CBD, but these lesions have been described in other disorders, where they appear to be composed of 15–18 nm diameter straight filaments and granular material (62). Ultrastructural analysis of neuropil threads and thread-like structures in CBD is complicated by the fact that they undoubtedly have multiple cellular origins, including neurons, astrocytes, and oligodendroglia. Threads in AD contain paired helical filaments and 18 nm straight filaments (36,37), whereas those in CBD contain 15–18 nm diameter straight filaments or 20–24 nm diameter twisted filaments (47).

Glial Lesions

The ultrastructure of oligodendroglial coiled bodies has not been reported in CBD, but has been described in immunoelectron microscopic studies in PSP (55). These are non–membrane bound tubular structures with a diameter of 13–15 nm and a fuzzy outer contour. They are located in the cytoplasm of oligodendrocytes and also in the inner and outer loops of myelin sheaths. Ultrastructural studies of astrocytic plaques have yet to be reported. Given that astrocytic plaques are large lesions with inclusions in distal processes, it has proven difficult differentiating processes of astrocytic plaques form other thread- and grain-like lesions in the cortical neuropil. The proximal cell bodies of astrocytes in CBD cortex contain accumulations of intermediate-sized (18–20 nm diameter) straight filaments (30).

BIOCHEMICAL FINDINGS

There are very few studies of postmortem neurochemical changes in CBD. In one of the first studies Clark and coworkers showed that cortical choline acetyl transferase, a marker for cholinergic neurons, was not decreased (17), which demonstrated a significant difference between CBD and AD. These findings are similar to those in PiD and other frontotemporal dementias, where the basal forebrain cholinergic neurons, if affected at all, are not one of the major targets of the disease process, as in AD and Lewy body disease.

Given the marked loss of pigmented neurons in the pars compacta of the substantia nigra, a population of neurons know to be the major dopaminergic innervation of the basal ganglia, it is not surprising that decreases in dopamine in the basal ganglia have been found in postmortem studies of CBD (63,64). Other neurotransmitter abnormalities have not been documented in CBD. It is unknown, for example, if the involvement of cortical neurons has any selectivity with respect to neurotransmitter.

By far most of the biochemical studies that have been conducted on CBD have focused on cytoskeletal proteins, and most of these have compared changes in tau protein in CBD to tau from normal control brains and AD (44,65–67).

Tau protein is a microtubule-associated phosphoprotein that promotes tubulin polymerization and stabilization of microtubules (66,68). It is present in neurons, preferentially in axons, and until recently was felt to be specific to neurons (69). More recent immunochemical evidence as described in the preceding suggests that tau protein is also expressed in glial cells, especially in pathologic conditions. It undergoes extensive posttranslational modification, including phosphorylation, which controls its functional state (68). Phosphorylated tau is less efficient in promoting tubulin polymerization. The tau gene is located on chromosome 17, and it has 15 exons, three of which are alternatively spliced (70). In the amino-terminal half of the molecule are conserved 30-amino acid tandem repeats, that along with flanking regions, are essential for interaction of tau with microtubules. One of the repeat domains is the product of exon 10 and is alternatively spliced. The various spliced combinations generate six proteins, but additional microheterogeneity is produced by posttranslational modifications (68).

In normal brain tissue tau is a natively unfolded, soluble protein that is heat-stable. Pathological tau protein has altered solubility properties, being soluble in detergents, and it forms abnormal filamentous structures. Western blots of normal brain tissue homogenates show six bands in a range of 50–62 kDa. Homogenates of detergent soluble tau protein from CBD migrates at a higher molecular weight because of increased phosphorylation. In addition, the immunoblotting pattern is reduced to two major bands at about 64 and 68 kDa (44,65) (Fig. 11). The conflicting reports about whether exon 10 is expressed in pathological tau protein of CBD (44,65) are owing to the fact that the amino acid sequences in the repeat regions are very similar. Antibodies raised to exon 10 often crossreact with sequences in the other repeat regions, especially exons 9 and 11. The weight of the current evidence, however, would suggest that pathological tau protein in CBD is generated preferentially from transcripts that contain exon 10. This is based on analysis not only with exon 10 specific antibodies, but also by immunoblotting tau preparations after extensive dephosphorylation. Analysis with antibodies specific to exon 3, another alternatively spliced exon, suggest that exon 3, in contrast to exon 10, is underrepresented in pathological tau protein of CBD (46,50).

Given the abundance of tau pathology in glial cells in CBD, an unanswered question is how much the observed difference in tau isoform composition in CBD reflects tau derived from glial cells compared with tau from neurons. Interestingly, nonneuronal cells appear to express exclusively 4-repeat tau (71), and there is also more 4-repeat tau in white matter than gray matter (72). These observations may suggest that glial cells also express predominantly 4-repeat tau and this has been confirmed in preliminary studies (unpublished observations, HK-R). Other disorders with neuronal and glial tau pathology share immunoblotting patterns with CBD. For example, Western blots of detergent soluble tau protein from PSP, FTDP-17, and PiD all have predominantly two bands (44,65–79). Interestingly, the two bands in PiD appear to be different from those in CBD, PSP, and FTDP-17 (77). In PiD the proteins migrate at an estimated molecular weight of 55 and 64 kDa. Recent evidence suggests that in PiD pathological tau protein isoforms lack exon 10 (77,78), whereas those in CBD, PSP, and FTDP-17 preferentially contain exon 10 (79). This supports the concept that CBD, PSP, and FTDP-17 may have common pathogenesis, despite differences in clinical and pathologic features.

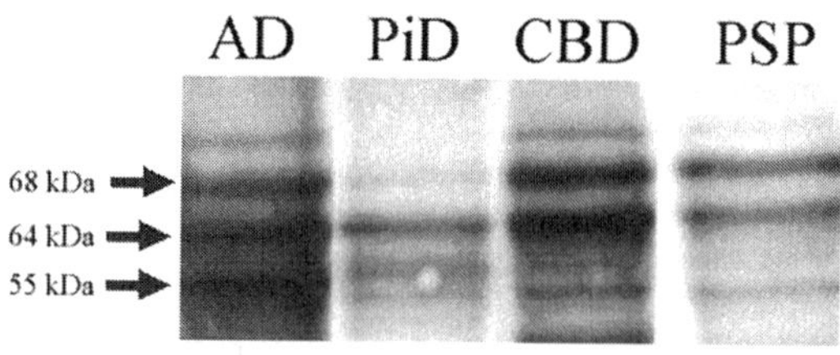

FIG. 11. Western blots of sarcosyl-insoluble proteins from AD, PiD, CBD, and PSP are immunostained with tau antibodies (PHF-1). Note that in AD there are three prominent bands at 68, 64, and 55 kDa, with a minor band at a higher molecular weight. In PiD, CBD, and PSP there are two major bands and less abundant minor bands. In PiD the two bands migrate at 64 and 55 kDa, whereas those in CBD and PSP migrate at 68 and 64 kDa.

DIFFERENTIAL DIAGNOSIS

The major neuropathological differential diagnosis of CBD is limited to those disorders associated with cortical and deep gray matter pathology associated with tau-immunoreactive inclusions in neurons and glia (57). The major disorders in this category are PSP, PiD, and FTDP-17. Tables 1 and 2 summarize neuropathologic and molecular features that are useful to consider in differential diagnosis. FTDP-17 can be differentiated from CBD by clinical history since it is an autosomal dominant disorder and CBD is almost always sporadic (80). Although there are reports of rare families with pathologic features suggestive of CBD (81), it is imperative that such cases be tested for mutations in the tau gene before they are accepted as examples of true familial CBD. One might argue that CBD is a sporadic form of FTDP-17 analogous to sporadic and familial forms of AD. Until definitive molecular markers are established for the various disorders, this issue will remain unresolved. At present, however, mutations in the tau gene, a common defining feature of FTDP-17, are not found in CBD.

From a morphological perspective, the differential diagnosis of CBD from PSP and PiD is not so clearly based on the appearance, but more the neuroanatomical distribution of lesions (26). For example, PSP has far more pathology in the deep

TABLE 1. *Neuropathologic differential diagnosis of CBD, PSP, and PD*

	CBD	PSP	Pick's disease
Gross findings			
Cortical atrophy	Mild to moderate, focal (often asymmetric, superior frontoparietal, or parasagittal)	Mild (usually symmetric, frontal, parasagittal, or paracentral)	Marked, lobar (often asymmetric, frontotemporal and limbic lobe; paracentral spared)
White matter pathology	Frontal (corticostriate fibers in anterior internal capsule and corticobulbar fibers in cerebral peduncle)	Central and cerebellar outflow (corticospinal in posterior internal capsule and cerebral peduncle; superior cerebellar peduncle)	Frontotemporal (Papez circuit; anterior commissure; corticostriatal fibers in anterior internal capsule)
Basal ganglia	Caudate atrophy Pallidonigral pigment-spheroid degeneration	Pallidonigral pigment-spheroid degeneration; subthalamic nucleus atrophy	Caudate atrophy
Microscopic findings			
Nonspecific cortical changes	Superficial spongiosis	Minimal cortical changes	Severe status spongiosis
Ballooned neurons	Present in affected cortical areas	Rare (or none)	Present in affected cortical areas, especially limbic lobe
Neuronal tau-pathology	Corticobasal bodies (i.e., globose NFT) and other neurofibrillary lesions: Cortex Basal ganglia Substantia nigra Locus ceruleus	Globose NFT: Basal ganglia Subthalamic nucleus Substantia nigra Oculomotor nuclei Raphe nuclei Locus ceruleus Pontine nucleus Tegmental gray Inferior olive Cerebellar dentate	Pick bodies: Cortex Dentate fascia Amygdala External pallidum Substantia nigra Locus ceruleus Pontine nuclei
Neuropil threads	Usually numerous: Cerebral cortex Cerebral white matter Internal capsule Pencil fibers in striatum Thalamic fasciculus Cerebral peduncle (corticobulbar) Tegmental fibers Pontine base Inferior olive Cerebellar dentate nucleus	Usually sparse: Basal ganglia Internal capsule Thalamic fasciculus Cerebral peduncle (corticospinal)	Variable amount: Cortex Limbic lobe
Astrocytic tau pathology	Many astrocytic plaques: Cortex	Many tufted astrocytes: Motor cortex Corpus striatum	Variable number of thorn-shaped astrocytes: Cortex
Oligodendroglial tau pathology (coiled bodies)	Numerous: Cerebral white matter Basal ganglia fibers Internal capsule Thalamic fasciculus	Many: Central white matter Basal ganglia fibers Thalamic fasciculus	Variables: Cerebral white matter

gray matter and brainstem than the cerebral cortex. The reverse is true for PiD, where the cortex, especially in the limbic lobe, bears the brunt of the pathology. This is not to say that deep gray matter and brainstem are not affected in PiD, since they consistently are affected, but only that cortical pathology is predominant. Neuroanatomically, CBD overlaps both PSP and PiD in that CBD has abundant pathology in both cortex and deep gray matter.

TABLE 2. *Molecular pathology of CBD, PSP, PD, and FTDP-17*

	Pick's disease	PSP	CBD	FTDP-17 (exon 10 and splice site mutations)	FTDP-17 (non–exon 10 mutations)
Ultrastructure of major abnormal filaments	15-nm Straight filaments and wide twisted ribbons	15-nm Straight filaments	15-nm Straight filaments and wide twisted ribbons	15-nm Straight filaments and wide twisted ribbons	22-nm Paired helical filaments (Alzheimer-like)
Predominant insoluble tau Western blot	Two bands (64 and 55 kDa)	Two bands (68 and 64 kDa)	Two bands (68 and 64 kDa)	Two bands (68 and 64 kDa)	Three bands (68, 64, and 55 kDa) (Alzheimer-like)
Tau exon 10 expression	Absent	Present	Variable reports, but probably present	Present	Present
Tau exon 3 expression	Not assessed	Not assessed	Absent	Not assessed	Present

Although initial studies frequently suggest that biomarkers are disease-specific, as further studies are conducted, these claims almost always need to be qualified. So it is with the cytopathologic lesions. Of the neuronal lesions that carry the most specificity, the Pick body comes closest to being a biomarker for PiD. Although tau-positive neuronal lesions that bear close resemblance to Pick bodies may be found in a variety of disorders, even AD, sharply circumscribed, spherical densely argyrophilic Pick bodies, when found in vulnerable neurons (e.g., dentate fascia), are structures that have proven diagnostic utility (82).

Although ballooned neurons are an attribute of the cortical degeneration of CBD, they are not limited to CBD. As previously mentioned, when they are numerous and distributed in the convexity gray matter, they are highly significant lesions and found in few other disorders except PiD. Glial lesions have been given a whole host of names, and it is not entirely clear if any of these lesions carry disease specificity, except for GCI in multiple system atrophy. There are numerous transitional and atypical forms of the glial lesions and ill-defined structural parameters for so-called "tufted astrocytes," "thorn shaped astrocytes," "gliofibrillary tangles," and "astrocytic plaques" (52).

Progressive Supranuclear Palsy (PSP)

Features that are most useful for differentiating PSP from CBD include the limited cortical pathology and rarity of BN in PSP (26). Extensive white matter pathology is also much more common in CBD than PSP. The distribution of tract degeneration is also different; in PSP degeneration more often affects the corticospinal tract, whereas in CBD the corticostriatal and corticobulbar tracts are affected. In PSP tau-immunoreactive lesions tend to be located in cell bodies, whereas they are in cell processes in CBD. A good example is the presence of globose NFT and tufted astrocytes in PSP compared with neuropil threads and astrocytic plaques in CBD. Examination of tau-related pathology in the pontine base has proven useful in the differential diagnosis of these disorders (83) (Figs. 12 and 13). In CBD the most abundant pathology is thread-like and glial, whereas in PSP NFT are much more abundant than threads and glial lesions. Similarly, the subthalamic nucleus has many NFT in PSP, but thread-like and glial pathology in CBD.

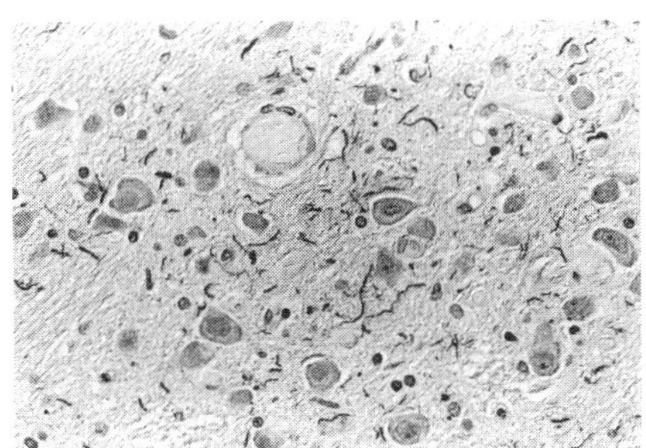

FIG. 12. Evaluation of pontine nuclei is helpful in differential diagnosis of CBD from PSP and PiD. In CBD the most characteristic appearance is a plethora of thread-like processes and weak granular immunoreactivity, if any, in neurons and a few glia.

Pick's Disease (PiD)

One of the major differences between CBD and PiD is the distribution of the cortical pathology (84–86). In typical cases of CBD, the limbic lobe is spared, but in PiD the limbic lobe bears the brunt of the pathology. The hippocampus and amygdala often show very severe neuronal loss and gliosis in PiD, along with numerous Pick bodies in pyramidal neurons in Ammon's horn and in small granular neurons of the dentate fascia (Fig. 13). These areas may be almost normal in CBD. Although basal ganglia, thalamus, and brainstem lesions are definitely found in all cases of PiD (87) (Fig. 13), such pathology is less marked than in most cases of CBD. As in PSP the neurons in pontine nuclei of PiD have inclusions, namely Pick bodies, whereas thread-like lesions predominate in CBD. Glial pathology occurs in PiD, but it is morphologically closer to that seen in PSP, with tufted and thorn-shaped appearance, than astrocytic plaques of CBD. Thread-like structures are found, and in some cases of PiD in great numbers, but numerous thread-like

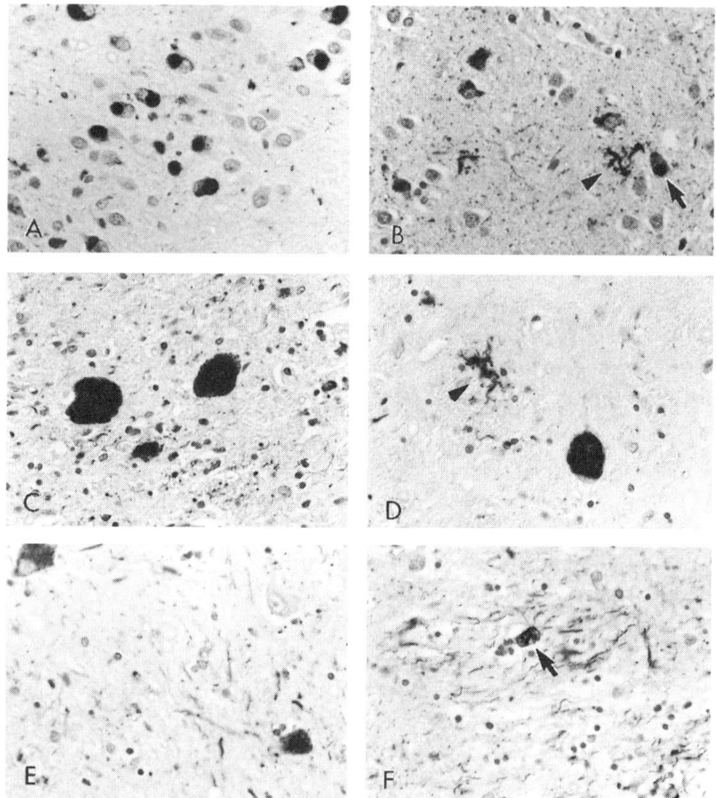

FIG. 13. The major differential diagnosis of CBD (**E, F**) is with PiD (**A, B**) and PSP (**C, D**). With tau immunostaining the dentate fascia neurons are unusually susceptible to Pick bodies in PiD. In the basal ganglia of PiD (**B**) Pick bodies are detected (*arrow*) as are tau-positive glia (*arrowhead*). Similar glia are detected in the basal ganglia in PSP (**D**, *arrowhead*), but neuronal lesions in PSP are larger globose NFT (**C**—substantia nigra and **D**—basal ganglia). In CBD brainstem tegmentum has neurons with skein-like and granular immunoreactivity accompanied by threads and grains. In the basal ganglia in CBD many thread-like lesion and tau-positive neuronal inclusions (*arrow*) are detected (**F**).

lesions are generally restricted to cortical and limbic areas in PiD, whereas they are widespread in gray and white matter of cortex and deep gray matter in CBD. The subthalamic nucleus is minimally affected in PiD as in CBD.

Frontotemporal Dementia and Parkinsonism Linked to Chromosome 17 (FTDP-17)

This is a recently recognized group of disorders with variable clinical and pathological phenotypes, but sharing linkage to a gene on chromosome 17 (88). In most cases examined there is a mutation in the tau gene (89–92), but there may be some families that show linkage to other genes on chromosome 17 other than tau. Recent genetic, clinical, and pathological studies have provided insight into the relationship of the mutations to the phenotype. Mutations in the tau gene that are located in exon 10 or the 5′-exon splice site of exon 10 have a phenotype that is similar to CBD, whereas those with tau mutations outside the microtubule binding domain show either nonspecific pathology or Alzheimer-type pathology without plaques.

Cases of FTDP-17 with mutations in or about exon 10, in which adequate pathological descriptions are available, have had cortical BN, although possibly not as numerous as in CBD. Tau-immunoreactive lesions are also found in both neuronal and glial cells in FTDP-17. Most cases have lesions in gray and white matter and also basal ganglia, thalamus, brainstem, and cerebellum. Furthermore, biochemical and ultrastructural features show a number of similarities to CBD (Table 2). In particular, detergent-soluble tau has two major bands on Western blots (68 and 64 kDa), which contain predominantly exon 10-positive, 4-repeat tau as in CBD (91). The filaments in detergent extracts are twisted ribbons like those in CBD, with wide-diameter and a longer periodicity of the twist than AD paired helical filaments.

Atypical Cases

There are reports of cases of CBD without BN (93) and also cases without either BN or tau-positive neuronal or glial lesions (94). Given the lack of specificity of the clinical phenotype (95), at this time it is reasonable to consider such cases separate pathological entities. Obviously, a specific molecular marker would facilitate understanding of CBD and its relationship to frontotemporal dementias that lack distinctive histopathology and the major sporadic tauopathies, namely, PSP and PiD. Until these become available, the pragmatic approach is to define the disorders based on the classical clinical and pathological phenotype, understanding that variability in this phenotype may not necessarily negate the concept of CBD as a distinct neurodegenerative disorder.

REFERENCES

1. Rebeiz JJ, Kolodny EH, Richardson EP Jr. Corticodentatonigral degeneration with neuronal achromasia: a progressive disorder of late adult life. *Trans Am Neurol Assoc* 1967;92:23–26.
2. Dickson DW, Yen SH, Suzuki KI, Davies P, Garcia JH, Hirano A. Ballooned neurons in select neurodegenerative diseases contain phosphorylated neurofilament epitopes. *Acta Neuropathol* 1986;71:216–223.
3. Paulus W, Selim M. Corticonigral degeneration with neuronal achromasia and basal neurofibrillary tangles. *Acta Neuropathol* 1990;81:89–94.
4. Wang LN, Kowall NW, Richardson EP Jr. Phosphorylated neurofilament epitopes in the achromasic neurons of corticonigral degeneration. *Chin Med J* 1991; 104:1011–1017.
5. Lippa CF, Smith TW, Fontneau N. Corticonigral degeneration with neuronal achromasia. A clinicopathologic study of two cases. *J Neurol Sci* 1990;98:301–310.
6. Arima K, Uesugi H, Fujita I, Sakurai Y, Oyanagi S, Andoh S, Izumiyama Y, Inose T. Corticonigral degeneration with neuronal achromasia presenting with primary progressive aphasia: ultrastructural and immunocytochemical studies. *J Neurol Sci* 1994;127:186–197.
7. Gibb WR, Luthert PJ, Marsden CD. Corticobasal degeneration. *Brain* 1989;112:1171–1192.
8. Bergeron C, Pollanen MS, Weyer L, Black SE, Lang AE. Unusual clinical presentations of cortical-basal ganglionic degeneration. *Ann Neurol* 1996;40:893–900.
9. Bergeron C, Pollanen MS, Weyer L, Lang AE. Cortical degeneration in progressive supranuclear palsy. A comparison with cortical-basal ganglionic degeneration. *J Neuropathol Exp Neurol* 1997;56:726–734.
10. Bergeron C, Davis A, Lang AE. Corticobasal ganglionic degeneration and progressive supranuclear palsy presenting with cognitive decline. *Brain Pathol* 1998;8:355–365.
11. Kertesz A, Hudson L, Mackenzie IR, Munoz DG. The pathology and nosology of primary progressive aphasia. *Neurology* 1994;44:2065–2072.
12. Black SE. Focal cortical atrophy syndromes. *Brain Cognition* 1996;31:188–229.
13. Ikeda K, Akiyama H, Iritani S, et al. Corticobasal degeneration with primary progressive aphasia and accentuated cortical lesion in superior temporal gyrus: case report and review. *Acta Neuropathol* 1996;92:534–539.
14. Yamauchi H, Fukuyama H, Nagahama Y, et al. Atrophy of the corpus callosum, cortical hypometabolism, and cognitive impairment in corticobasal degeneration. *Arch Neurol* 1998; 55:609–614.
15. Schneider JA, Gearing M, Robbins RS, de l'Aune W, Mirra SS. Apolipoprotein E genotype in diverse neurodegenerative disorders. *Ann Neurol* 1995;38:131–135.
16. Horoupian DS, Chu PL. Unusual case of corticobasal degeneration with tau/Gallyas-positive neuronal and glial tangles. *Acta Neuropathol* 1994;88:592–598.
17. Clark AW, Manz HJ, White CL 3d, Lehmann J, Miller D, Coyle JT. Cortical degeneration with swollen chromatolytic neurons: its relationship to Pick's disease. *J Neuropathol Exp Neurol* 1986;45:268–224.
18. Kato S, Hirano A, Umahara T, Llena JF, Herz F, Ohama E. Ultrastructural and immunohistochemical studies on ballooned cortical neurons in Creutzfeldt-Jakob disease: expression of alpha B-crystallin ubiquitin and stress-response protein 27. *Acta Neuropathol* 1992;84:443–448.
19. Lowe J, Errington DR, Lennox G, et al. Ballooned neurons in several neurodegenerative diseases and stroke contain alpha B crystallin *Neuropathol Appl Neurobiol* 1992;18:341–350.
20. Mori H, Oda M, Mizuno Y. Cortical ballooned neurons in progressive supranuclear palsy. *Neurosci Lett* 1996; 209:109–112.
21. Mizutani T, Inose T, Nakajima S, et al. Familial parkinsonism and dementia with ballooned neurons, argyrophilic neuronal inclusions, atypical neurofibrillary tangles, tau-negative astrocytic fibrillary tangles, and Lewy bodies. *Acta Neuropathol* 1998;95:15–27.
22. Smith TW, Lippa CF, de Girolami U. Immunocytochemical study of ballooned neurons in cortical degeneration with neuronal achromasia. *Clin Neuropathol* 1992;11:28–35.
23. Mori H, Oda M. Ballooned neurons in corticobasal degeneration and progressive supranuclear palsy. *Neuropathology* 1997;17:248–252.
24. Constantinidis J, Richard J, Tissot R. Pick's disease: histological and clinical correlations *Eur Neurol* 1974; 11:208–217.
25. Dickson DW. Pick's disease, a modern definition. *Brain Pathol* 1998;8:339–354.
26. Feany MB, Mattiace LA, Dickson DW. Neuropathologic overlap of progressive supranuclear palsy, Pick's disease and corticobasal degeneration. *J Neuropathol Exp Neurol* 1996;55:53–67.
27. Mackenzie IR, Hudson LP. Achromatic neurons in the cortex of progressive supranuclear palsy. *Acta Neuropathol* 1995;90:615–619.

28. Martinez-Lage P, Munoz DG. Prevalence and disease associations of argyrophilic grains of Braak. *J Neuropathol Exp Neurol* 1997;56:157–164.
29. Koliatsos VE, Price WL, Pardo CA, Price DL. Ventral root avulsion: an experimental model of death of adult motor neurons. *J Comp Neurol* 1994;342:35–44.
30. Feany MB, Dickson DW. Widespread cytoskeletal pathology characterizes corticobasal degeneration. *Am J Pathol* 1995;146:1388–1396.
31. Halliday GM, Davies L, McRitchie DA, Cartwright H, Pamphlett R, Morris JG. Ubiquitin-positive achromatic neurons in corticobasal degeneration. *Acta Neuropathol* 1995;90:68–75.
32. Castellani R, Smith MA, Richey PL, Kalaria R, Gambetti P, Perry G. Evidence for oxidative stress in Pick disease and corticobasal degeneration. *Brain Res* 1995;696: 268–271.
33. Dickson DW, Farrer MJ, Mehta ND, Perez-Tur J, Tiseo P, Yen S-H, Hardy J. Antibodies to non-amyloid component of plaques (NACP) specifically label Lewy bodies and Lewy neurites, but not other inclusions in neurodegenerative diseases. *J Neuropathol Exp Neurol* 1998;57:516.
34. Komori T, Arai N, Oda M, et al. Morphologic difference of neuropil threads in Alzheimer's disease, corticobasal degeneration and progressive supranuclear palsy: a morphometric study. *Neurosci Lett* 1997;233:89–92.
35. Braak H, Braak E, Grundke-Iqbal I, Iqbal K. Occurrence of neuropil threads in the senile human brain and in Alzheimer's disease: a third location of paired helical filaments outside of neurofibrillary tangles and neuritic plaques. *Neurosci Lett* 1986:65:351–355.
36. Perry G, Kawai M, Tabaton M, et al. Neuropil threads of Alzheimer's disease show a marked alteration of the normal cytoskeleton. *J Neurosci* 1991;11:1748–1755.
37. Yamaguchi H, Nakazato Y, Shoji M, Ihara Y, Hirai S. Ultrastructure of the neuropil threads in the Alzheimer brain: their dendritic origin and accumulation in the senile plaques. *Acta Neuropathol* 1990;80:368–374.
38. Braak H, Braak E. Cortical and subcortical argyrophilic grains characterize a disease associated with adult onset dementia. *Neuropathol Appl Neurobiol* 1989;15:13–26.
39. Jellinger K.A. Dementia with grains (argyrophilic grain disease). *Brain Pathol* 1998;8:377–386.
40. Iwatsubo T, Hasegawa M, Ihara Y. Neuronal and glial tau-positive inclusions in diverse neurologic diseases share common phosphorylation characteristics. *Acta Neuropathol* 1994;88:129–136.
41. Mori H, Nishimura M, Namba Y, Oda M. Corticobasal degeneration: a disease with widespread appearance of abnormal tau and neurofibrillary tangles, and its relation to progressive supranuclear palsy. *Acta Neuropathol* 1994;88:113–121.
42. Wakabayashi K, Oyanagi K, Makifuchi T, et al. Corticobasal degeneration: etiopathological significance of the cytoskeletal alterations. *Acta Neuropathol* 1994; 87:545–553.
43. Uchihara T, Mitani K, Mori H, Kondo H, Yamada M, Ikeda K. Abnormal cytoskeletal pathology peculiar to corticobasal degeneration is different from that of Alzheimer's disease or progressive supranuclear palsy. *Acta Neuropathol* 1994;88:379–383.
44. Ksiezak-Reding H, Morgan K, Mattiace LA, et al. Ultrastructure and biochemical composition of paired helical filaments in corticobasal degeneration. *Am J Pathol* 1994;145:1496–1508.
45. Yamada T, McGeer PL. Oligodendroglial microtubular massess: an abnormality observed in some human neurodegenerative diseases. *Neurosci Lett* 1995;120:163–166.
46. Feany MB, Ksiezak-Reding H, Liu WK, Vincent I, Yen SH, Dickson DW. Epitope expression and hyperphosphorylation of tau protein in corticobasal degeneration: differentiation from progressive supranuclear palsy. *Acta Neuropathol* 1995;90:37–43.
47. Nishimura T, Ikeda K, Akiyama H, et al. Immunohistochemical investigation of tau-positive structures in the cerebral cortex of patients with progressive supranuclear palsy. *Neurosci Lett* 1995;201:123–126.
48. Takahashi T, Amano N, Hanihara T, et al. Corticobasal degeneration: widespread argentophilic threads and glia in addition to neurofibrillary tangles. Similarities of cytoskeletal abnormalities in corticobasal degeneration and progressive supranuclear palsy. *J Neurol Sci* 1996;138: 66–77.
49. Matsumoto S, Udaka F, Kameyama M, Kusaka H, Ito H, Imai T. Subcortical neurofibrillary tangles, neuropil threads, and argentophilic glial inclusions in corticobasal degeneration. *Clin Neuropathol* 1996;15:209–214.
50. Nishimura T, Ikeda K, Akiyama H, et al. Glial tau-positive structures lack the sequence encoded by exon 3 of the tau protein gene. *Neurosci Lett* 1997;224:169–172.
51. Komori T, Arai N, Oda M, et al. Astrocytic plaques and tufts of abnormal fibers do not coexist in corticobasal degeneration and progressive supranuclear palsy. *Acta Neuropathol* 1998; 96:401–408.
52. Chin SSM, Goldman JE. Glial inclusions in CNS degenerative diseases. *J Neuropathol Exp Neurol* 1996;55: 499–508.
53. Lantos PL. The definition of multiple system atrophy: a review of recent developments. *J Neuropathol Exp Neurol* 1998;57:1099–1111.
54. Ikeda K, Akiyama H, Haga C, Kondo H, Arima K, Oda T. Argyrophilic thread-like structure in corticobasal degeneration and supranuclear palsy. *Neurosci Lett* 1994; 174;157–159.
55. Arima K, Nakamura M, Sunohara N, et al. Ultrastructural characterization of the tau-immunoreactive tubules in the oligodendroglial perikarya and their inner loop processes in progressive supranuclear palsy. *Acta Neuropathol* 1997;93:558–566.
56. Dickson DW, Feany MB, Yen SH, Mattiace LA, Davies P. Cytoskeletal pathology in non-Alzheimer degenerative dementia: new lesions in diffuse Lewy body disease, Pick's disease, and corticobasal degeneration. *J Neural Transm Suppl* 1996;47:31–46.
57. Feany MB, Dickson DW. Neurodegenerative disorders with extensive tau pathology: a comparative study and review. *Ann Neurol* 1996;40:139–148.
58. Ksiezak-Reding H, Tracz E, Yang LS, Dickson DW, Simon M, Wall JS. Ultrastructural instability of paired helical filaments from corticobasal degeneration as examined by scanning transmission electron microscopy. *Am J Pathol* 1996; 149:639–651.
59. Tracz E, Dickson DW, Hainfeld JF, Ksiezak-Reding H. Paired helical filaments in corticobasal degeneration: the fine fibrillary structure with NanoVan. *Brain Res* 1997; 773:33–44.
60. Murayama S, Mori H, Ihara Y, Tomonaga M. Immunocytochemical and ultrastructural studies of Pick's disease. *Ann Neurol* 1990;27:394–405.

61. Yan L-S, Ksiezak-Reding H. Ubiquitin immunoreactivity of paired helical filaments differs in Alzheimer's disease and corticobasal degeneration. *Acta Neuropathol* 1998;96:520–526.
62. Ikeda K, Akiyama H, Kondo H, Haga C. A study of dementia with argyrophilic grains. Possible cytoskeletal abnormality in dendrospinal portion of neurons and oligodendroglia. *Acta Neuropathol* 1995;89:409–414.
63. Riley DE, Lang AE, Lewis A, Resch L, Ashby P, Hornykiewcz, Black S. Cortical-basal ganglionic degeneration. *Neurology* 1990;40:1203–1212.
64. Marshall EF, Perry RH, Perry EK, Piggott MA, Thompson P, Jaros E, Burn DJ. Striatal dopaminergic loss without parkinsonism in a case of corticobasal degeneration. *Acta Neurol Scand* 1997;95:287–292.
65. Buee-Scherrer V, Hof PR, Buee L, et al. Hyperphosphorylated tau proteins differentiate corticobasal degeneration and Pick's disease. *Acta Neuropathol* 1996;91: 351–359.
66. Delacourte A, Buee L. Normal and pathological Tau proteins as factors for microtubule assembly. *Int Rev Cytol* 1997;171:167–224.
67. Mailliot C, Sergeant N, Bussiere T, Caillet-Boudin ML, Delacourte A, Buee L. Phosphorylation of specific sets of tau isoforms reflects different neurofibrillary degeneration processes. *FEBS Lett* 1998;433:201–204.
68. Mandelkow EM, Biernat J, Drewes G, Steiner B, Lichtenberg-Kraag B, Wille H, et al. Microtubule-associated protein tau, paired helical filaments, and phosphorylation. *Ann NY Acad Sci* 1993;695:209–216.
69. Binder LI, Frankfurter A, Rebum LI. The distribution of tau in the mammalian central nervous system. *J Cell Biol* 1985;101:1371–1378.
70. Andreadis A, Brown WM, Kosik KS. Structure and novel exons of the human tau gene. *Biochemistry* 1992; 31:10626–10633.
71. Vanier MT, Neuville P, Michalik L, Launay JF. Expression of specific tau exons in normal and tumoral pancreatic acinar cells. *J Cell Sci* 1998; 111:1419–1432.
72. Janke C, Holzer M, Klose J, Arendt T. Distribution of isoforms of the microtubule-associated protein tau in grey and white matter areas of human brain: a two-dimensional gel electrophoretic analysis. *FEBS Lett* 1996; 379:222–226.
73. Flament S, Delacourte A, Verny M, Hauw J-J, Javoy-Agid F. Abnormal tau proteins in progressive supranuclear palsy. *Acta Neuropathol* 1991;81:591–596.
74. Reed LA, Schmidt ML, Wszolek ZK, et al. The neuropathology of a chromosome 17-linked autosomal dominant parkinsonism and dementia ("pallido-ponto-nigral degeneration"). *J Neuropathol Exp Neurol* 1998;57: 588–601.
75. Spillantini MG, Bird TD, Ghetti B. Frontotemporal dementia and Parkinsonism linked to chromosome 17: a new group of tauopathies. *Brain Pathol* 1998;8:387–402.
76. Hong M, Zhukareva V, Vogelsberg-Ragaglia V, Miller BI, Mckeel D, Morris JC, et al. Mutation-specific functional impairments in distinct tau isoforms of hereditary FTDP-17. *Science* 1998;282:1914–1917.
77. Delacourte A, Robitaille Y, Sergeant N, et al. Specific pathological Tau protein variants characterize Pick's disease. *J Neuropathol Exp Neurol* 1996;55:159–168.
78. Sergeant N, David JP, Lefranc D, Vermersch P, Wattez A, Delacourte A. Different distribution of phosphorylated tau protein isoforms in Alzheimer's and Pick's diseases. *FEBS Lett* 1997;412:578–582.
79. Spillantini MG, Goedert M. Tau protein pathology in neurodegenerative diseases. *Trends Neurosci* 1998; 21: 428–433.
80. Caselli RJ, Reiman EM, Timmann D, et al. Progressive apraxia in clinically discordant monozygotic twins. *Arch Neurol* 1995;52:1004–1010.
81. Brown J, Lantos PL, Roques P, Fidani L, Rossor MN. Familial dementia with swollen achromatic neurons and corticobasal inclusion bodies: a clinical and pathological study. *J Neurol Sci* 1996;135:21–30.
82. Litvan I, Hauw JJ, Bartko JJ, et al. Validity and reliability of the preliminary NINDS neuropathologic criteria for progressive supranuclear palsy and related disorders. *J Neuropathol Exp Neurol* 1996;55:97–105.
83. Dickson DW, D'Aversa T. Pontine cytoskeletal pathology in the differential diagnosis of non-Alzheimer dementias. *J Neuropathol Exp Neurol* 1997;56:592.
84. Jendroska K, Rossor MN, Mathias CJ, Daniel SE. Morphological overlap between corticobasal degeneration and Pick's disease: a clinicopathological report. *Mov Disord* 1995;10:111–114.
85. Lang AE, Bergeron C, Pollanen MS, Ashby P. Parietal Pick's disease mimicking cortical-basal ganglionic degeneration *Neurology* 1994;44:1436–1440.
86. Tsuchiya K, Ikeda K, Uchihara T, Oda T, Shimada H. Distribution of cerebral cortical lesions in corticobasal degeneration: a clinicopathological study of five autopsy cases in Japan. *Acta Neuropathol* 1997; 94:416–424.
87. Yoshimura N. Topography of Pick body distribution in Pick's disease: a contribution to understanding the relationship between Pick's and Alzheimer's diseases. *Clin Neuropathol* 1989;8:1–6.
88. Foster NL, Wilhelmsen K, Sima AAF, et al. Frontotemporal dementia and parkinsonism linked to chromosome 17: a consensus conference. *Ann Neurol* 1997;41: 706–715.
89. Poorkaj P, Bird TD, Wijsman E, et al. Tau is a candidate gene for chromosome 17 frontotemporal dementia. *Ann Neurol* 1998;43:815–825.
90. Hutton M, Lendon CL, Rizzu P, Baker M, Froelich S, Houlden H, et al. Association of missense and 5′-splice-site mutations in tau with the inherited dementia (FTDP-17). *Nature* 1998;393:702–705.
91. Spillantini MG, Murrell JR, Goedert M, Farlow MR, Klug A, Ghetti B. Mutation in the tau gene in familial multisystem tauopathy with presenile dementia. *Proc Natl Acad Sci USA* 1998;95:7737–7741.
92. Spillantini MG, Bird TD, Ghetti B. Frontotemporal dementia and Parkinsonism linked to chromosome 17: a new group of tauopathies. *Brain Pathol* 1998;8:387–402.
93. Schneider JA, Watts RL, Gearing M, Brewer RP, Mina SS. Corticobasal degeneration: neuropathologic and clinical heterogeneity. *Neurology* 1997;48:959–969.
94. Kawasaki K, Iwanaga K, Wakabayashi K, et al. Corticobasal degeneration with neither argyrophilic inclusions nor tau abnormalities: a new subgroup? *Acta Neuropathol* 1996;91:140–144.
95. Boeve BF, Parisi JE, Maraganore DM, et al. Pathologic findings in 11 cases of clinically suspected cortical-basal ganglionic degeneration. *Brain Pathol* 1997;7:1177.

Corticobasal Degeneration.
Advances in Neurology, Vol. 82,
edited by I. Litvan, C. G. Goetz, and A. E. Lang.
Lippincott Williams & Wilkins, Philadelphia © 2000.

3

Clinical Diagnostic Criteria

David E. Riley* and Anthony E. Lang†

**Department of Neurology, University Hospitals of Cleveland, Cleveland, Ohio 44106; and †Division of Neurology, Toronto Western Hospital, Toronto, Ontario M5T 2S8, Canada*

INTRODUCTION

A report of three cases of a newly recognized degenerative disease of the nervous system, then called "corticodentatonigral degeneration with neuronal achromasia," appeared in 1968 (1). The authors described a seemingly unique constellation of clinical findings, and recognized almost all of the major features by which we make a clinical diagnosis today. Only focal reflex myoclonus was not noted in the original report but later identified as a common sign. It is a testament to the distinctiveness of the clinical presentation of the original corticobasal degeneration (CBD) cases, as well as the observational and descriptive skills of Rebeiz and colleagues (1), that the authors of the second series (2) felt confident enough to presume that a diagnosis could be made on the basis of the clinical findings alone. Time and experience have since tempered our self-assurance, but the notion persists that we can recognize many cases of CBD before death, and often early in the course of the illness.

CLINICAL DIAGNOSIS OF CBD

Based on personal clinical experience with 15 patients (two confirmed by autopsy) and a literature review of the 12 previous cases (seven with autopsy confirmation), Riley and Lang (3,4) first outlined criteria by which a diagnosis of CBD should be made. These consisted of (1) a unilateral onset and asymmetric course (2), an insidious onset and gradual progression, and (3) clinical manifestations reflecting dysfunction in both the cerebral cortex and the basal ganglia. Signs of a basal ganglia disorder (akinesia, rigidity, limb dystonia, postural instability) and evidence of cerebral cortical dysfunction (cortical sensory loss, apraxia, alien limb phenomenon, frontal lobe reflexes) accorded well with the main sites of pathologic involvement. There were additional findings that did not clearly localize to either of these areas (action tremor, hyperreflexia, Babinski signs, oculomotor impairment, dysarthria, dysphagia). This organization of clinical findings into three categories (Table 1) (5) remains a useful conceptual framework for the clinical diagnosis of CBD. In this series of patients (3), movement disorders and cortical dysfunction produced the initial symptoms equally frequently; the most common were a postural-action tremor, apraxia, dystonia, and cortical sensory loss. Riley and colleagues (3,4) also described a characteristic "stiff, dystonic, jerky, useless hand" as the cumulative result of multiple motor problems. Importantly, these publications emphasized that a definitive diagnosis of CBD required a combination of an appropriate clinical history and typical pathologic changes at autopsy, since neither the clinical nor the pathologic picture appeared to be specific.

These guidelines for clinical diagnosis have been modified somewhat by subsequent authors, but still form the essential elements of diagnostic recognition of CBD. Watts and colleagues (6,7) have stated that the core feature of CBD is an asymmetric, insidiously progressive akinetic-rigid syndrome, with signs of cortical impairment developing within 1 to 3 years of onset. In

TABLE 1. *Clinical manifestations of CBD**

Basal ganglia signs	Cerebral cortical signs	Other manifestations
Akinesia, rigidity	Cortical sensory loss	Postural-action tremor
Limb dystonia	Alien limb phenomenon	Hyperreflexia
Athetosis	Dementia	Impaired ocular motility
Postural instability, falls	Apraxia	Dysarthria
Orolingual dyskinesia	Frontal lobe reflexes	Focal reflex myoclonus
	Dysphasia	Babinski signs
		Impaired eyelid motion
		Dysphagia

* (From ref. 5, with permission.)

our experience, the clinical presentation may begin with either basal ganglia or cortical problems, and only rarely is there an early akinetic-rigid syndrome free of clues that one is not dealing with Parkinson's disease. Watts and colleagues divided the clinical manifestations of CBD into major and minor categories (Table 2). The qualifications for listing as "major" features of CBD were not cited, but this group includes the more common manifestations encountered in CBD patients (3,8). Unlike similar lists of diagnostic features where a certain number or combination of major and minor criteria must be met, no required criteria for clinical diagnosis of CBD were specified.

Maraganore and colleagues devised a scheme of clinical criteria for CBD progressively graded as "possible," "probable," and "definite" diagnoses (Table 3). These investigators added lack of L-dopa response and the presence of mirror movements to the list of clinical features of CBD. The nearly universal absence of sustained improvement with L-dopa had been commented on by previous authors, and was corroborated by subsequent study (9). No publication on CBD, however, has documented mirror movements as a clinical feature. The authors sought to use their diagnostic scheme as a predictive tool (10), but found too much contamination from false positive diagnoses. In fact, of nine patients clinically suspected of having CBD, only one showed the characteristic cortical pathology (11). Even if one discards the nebulous "possible" category, whose criteria could be met by most people with Parkinson's disease, two of the three patients with "probable," and both with "definite," clinical CBD had other diagnoses at autopsy.

In the largest series of CBD patients published to date, Rinne and colleagues (8) followed the scheme of three categories of clinical manifestations (movement disorders, cerebral cortical signs, other) established by Riley and Lang (3,4). In addition, they outlined five types of initial clinical presentation they had encountered in their 36 cases. The majority of their patients presented with a "useless arm," which could be due to combined rigidity, dystonia, akinesia, and apraxia, or to rigidity and myoclonus. Other initial problems included a gait disorder (due to leg rigidity and apraxia, disequilibrium, or both), a sensory

TABLE 2. *Clinical manifestations of CBD**

Major	Minor
Akinesia, rigidity, postural/gait disturbance	Choreoathetosis
Action/postural tremor	Dementia
Alien limb phenomenon	Cerebellar signs
Cortical signs (apraxia, cortical sensory loss, dysphasia, corticospinal tract signs)	Supranuclear gaze abnormalities
Dystonia	Frontal "release" signs
Myoclonus	Blepharospasm

* (From refs. 6 and 7, with permission.)

TABLE 3. *Diagnostic classification scheme of Maraganore et al.**

Clinically possible CBD	Clinically probable CBD	Clinically definite CBD
At least three of the four following criteria, in the absence of identifiable causes	All four of the clinically possible criteria, no identifiable cause, and at least two of the following	Same as for clinically probable, with at least one of the following
Chronic, progressive course	Focal or asymmetric appendicular dystonia	Alien limb phenomenon
Asymmetric distribution	Focal or asymmetric appendicular myoclonus	Cortical sensory loss
Limb rigidity	Focal or asymmetric appendicular postural/action tremor	Mirror movements
Limb apraxia	Lack of L-dopa response	

* (Personal Communication.)

disturbance with "clumsiness," and a speech disturbance. A single patient presented with behavioral changes and disequilibrium.

Lang and colleagues (12) set out formal diagnostic criteria designed for research purposes (Table 4). They subscribed to the concept of requiring evidence of cerebral cortical and basal ganglia signs, but specified that the basal ganglia manifestations must include rigidity, and that the cortical signs include at least one of apraxia, cortical sensory loss, or the alien limb phenomenon. An alternative presentation of asymmetric rigidity, dystonia, and stimulus-sensitive myoclonus was acceptable. This publication highlighted clinical findings inconsistent with CBD, and listed them as exclusion criteria for research purposes (admitting that the rate of false positive diagnoses would increase excessively if such features as early dementia or the presence of a vertical gaze palsy early in the course of the disorder were permitted). Another useful aspect of this review was to set out a hierarchy of the clinical manifestations of CBD according to the frequency with which they occurred. Both the frequency estimates and the research diagnostic criteria were refined in a later publication (13). Here the authors estimated the frequency of occurrence of each of the clinical manifestations of CBD (see Table 1, this chapter) at three stages of the illness: onset, the first 3 years and later in the course. Akinesia/rigidity and apraxia were considered "universal" findings in CBD, each occurring in over 90% of cases within the first 3 years. No other individual finding occurred in

TABLE 4. *Proposed diagnostic criteria of Lang et al.**

Inclusion criteria	Qualifications of clinical features	Exclusion criteria
Rigidity plus one cortical sign (apraxia, cortical sensory loss, or alien limb phenomenon); *or*	Rigidity: easily detectable without reinforcement	Early dementia (This will exclude some patients who have CBD, but whose illness cannot clinically be distinguished from other primary dementing diseases.)
	Apraxia: more than simple use of limb as object; clear absence of cognitive or motor deficit sufficient to explain disturbance	
Asymmetric rigidity, dystonia, and focal reflex myoclonus	Cortical sensory loss: preserved primary sensation; asymmetric	Early vertical gaze palsy
		Rest tremor
	Alien limb phenomenon: more than simple *levitation*	Severe autonomic disturbances
	Dystonia: focal in limb; present at rest at onset	Sustained responsiveness to levodopa
	Myoclonus: reflex myoclonus spreads beyond stimulated digits	Lesions on imaging studies indicating another pathologic process is responsible

* (From ref. 12, with permission.)

even half of patients until later disease stages. However, the following were considered "common" (30% to 50% of cases) within the first 3 years and "frequent" (51% to 90% of cases) after 3 years of illness: limb dystonia, focal reflex myoclonus, postural instability, corticospinal tract signs, (apraxic) oculomotor dysfunction, and dysarthria. The research criteria for clinical diagnosis of CBD set forth by Kumar and colleagues (13) (Table 5) reverted to the original scheme of Riley and colleagues (3). The three major characteristics of the evolution of the illness were the chronic progressive course, the asymmetry at onset and the combination of movement disorders and "higher" cortical dysfunction. This last group consisted of apraxia, cortical sensory loss, or the alien limb phenomenon. The movement disorders had to include an akinetic-rigid syndrome unresponsive to L-dopa, and limb dystonia or focal myoclonus. The exclusions were the same as proposed earlier (12).

ALTERNATIVE PRESENTATIONS

The clinical syndrome discussed to this point may be referred to as the "classical" motor form of CBD, although our notions of what constitutes a "variant" presentation have been shaped by the delineation of "typical" CBD by those whose main interest is movement disorders, and not dementia. Kumar and colleagues (13) drew attention to the fact that a growing number of case reports have established that patients presenting with progressive cognitive disturbances could show pathologic abnormalities identical to those of CBD at autopsy. These nonmotor syndromes usually take one of two forms, either an aphasia or a frontal lobe dementia. Recent pathologic series record that the majority of patients with the pathologic findings of CBD have dementia as the presenting syndrome (14,15). Other, rarer presenting manifestations of CBD include speech apraxia, behavioral disturbances, a gait disorder, and a sensory disturbance (8). At present, it is not possible to predict the pathology on the basis of these nonclassical presentations of CBD (see Chapter 17).

TABLE 5. *Proposed research criteria of Kumar et al.**

Chronic progressive course
Asymmetric at onset (includes speech dyspraxia, dysphasia)
Presence of:
- "Higher" cortical dysfunction (apraxia, cortical sensory loss, or alien limb) and
- Movement disorders (akinetic-rigid syndrome resistant to L-dopa, and limb dystonia or spontaneous and reflex focal myoclonus)

Qualifications of clinical features: same as Table 4
Exclusion criteria: same as Table 4

* (From ref. 13, with permission.)

CONCLUSION

The whole notion of the clinical diagnosis of CBD must be evaluated in the light of emerging information about the pathologic findings. From the beginning it has been difficult to draw a clear demarcation between CBD and Pick's disease. More recently, the finding of similar tau pathology in CBD and progressive supranuclear palsy brings into question the duality of these diseases.

The diagnostic accuracy will vary with the distribution. The closer the pathologic findings to the original descriptions of Rebeiz and colleagues (1), the more likely they are to produce a classical syndrome (sometimes referred to as the "CBD syndrome"). Conversely, cases with "atypical" clinical presentations that do not suggest a diagnosis of classical CBD antemortem are often associated with pathology in differing cortical distributions (e.g., more anterior frontotemporal than posterior frontoparietal).

None of the above schemes of diagnostic criteria has been subjected to statistical analysis. The only work that even approaches this goal was that of Litvan and colleagues (16). Their study of clinical diagnostic accuracy involving 10 cases of autopsy-verified CBD found that specificity of the clinical features used was high, but sensitivity was very low even after 3 years, and remained low throughout the course (median 8 years) (16). In part, this was owing to the inclusion of several "atypical" cases. Unfortunately, as noted, we are discovering that an increasingly substantial proportion of CBD patients present with symptoms and signs that are distinct from the "classical" syndrome. Nevertheless, this study indicates that CBD is underdiagnosed; and there is ample room for increasing premortem recognition, although it is not clear how this can be achieved without producing a high number of false positive diagnoses. A second report, based on the same pathologic material plus four additional cases (17), sheds further light on the difficulty inherent in formulating clinical criteria for diagnosis. Although the first paper concluded that "late onset" of gait or balance disturbances was one of the best predictors used by clinicians for the diagnosis of CBD, the second pointed out that postural imbalance was detected in 5 of 11 patients at the first encounter with a neurologist. This discrepancy can be partially resolved if one accepts that the qualification of "late" used by Litvan and colleagues (16) was meant relative to progressive supranuclear palsy (PSP), which features postural instability as its most common initial symptom and was the main source of false negative diagnoses in their study. It also helps if one realizes that the first encounter with a neurologist recorded in these two studies did not occur until an average of 3 years after onset, at which time the majority of patients still had normal postural stability. Thus, the absence of postural instability was helpful in distinguishing CBD patients from those with PSP, but disequilibrium is clearly an earlier manifestation of CBD than of Parkinson's disease. In assessing the usefulness of criteria for differential diagnosis of disorders with such frequently overlapping clinical features, context is critical.

The work of Litvan and colleagues (16) measured the reliability and validity of using clinical features to arrive at a diagnosis of CBD according to the level of agreement among six neurologists. No specific criteria for diagnosis were provided, and each diagnostician was free to apply his or her own reasoning to the exercise. Indeed, no set of diagnostic criteria has ever been formally studied for CBD. It remains a challenge for the future to study any of the existing criteria, or develop new ones, that will withstand such scrutiny and be accepted as an established standard for clinical diagnosis of CBD.

Lacking any further understanding of the pathogenesis of CBD, and mindful of the difficulty of differential diagnosis, we believe that there should be a hierarchy of diagnostic certainty varying with the intended goal of clinical classification. For the purposes of routine clinical practice, it is reasonable to make a diagnosis of probable CBD on the basis of the criteria originally proposed by Riley and colleagues (3). The minimum features required for diagnosis under this scheme would include an asymmetric presentation and course, gradual progression, and at least one each of the basal ganglia and cerebral cortical signs listed in Table 1. For research studies, however, the criteria must be more stringent, limiting patients to those with a very specific syndrome, as outlined in Table 5. Only by maximizing clinical diagnostic accuracy by using strict criteria will we be able to identify biologic markers that can certify an early diagnosis. Ironically, identification of a biologic marker would subsequently allow us to expand the spectrum of clinical presentations of CBD.

Even within the research field, however, different diagnostic criteria may be needed for different purposes. Using criteria such as outlined in Table 5 may assure us of the highest possible accuracy, but at the cost of excluding many CBD patients with alternative clinical findings. A high rate of false negative diagnosis is not a major obstacle to the search for biological markers of disease, but it is a problem for large-scale epidemiologic studies. Incidentally, imaging studies do not appear to satisfy the criteria of "biological markers," since the abnormalities found (e.g. on FDG PET scanning), reflect only the distribution of pathologic changes and not the nature of the pathology itself. Population studies and searches for predisposing factors, depend on maximizing both sensitivity and specificity. This is a much more difficult prospect than when one can be sacrificed for the other. Unfortunately, it is likely that no accurate epidemiologic study will be made until a suitable biological marker is found.

REFERENCES

1. Rebeiz JJ, Kolodny EH, Richardson EP. Corticodentatonigral degeneration with neuronal achromasia. *Arch Neurol* 1968;18:20–33.
2. Watts RL, Williams RS, Growdon JD, Young RR, Haley EC, Beal MF. Corticobasal ganglionic degeneration [abstract]. *Neurology* 1985;35(suppl 1):178.

3. Riley DE, Lang AE, Lewis A, Resch L, Ashby P, Hornykiewicz O, Black S. Cortical-basal ganglionic degeneration. *Neurology* 1990;40:1203–1212.
4. Riley DE, Lang AE. Cortical-basal ganglionic degeneration. In: Appel SH, ed. *Current Neurology,* Vol. 12. St. Louis: Mosby, 1992;155–171.
5. Riley DE, Lang AE. Cortical-basal ganglionic degeneration. In: Stern MB, Koller WC, eds. *Parkinsonian Syndromes.* New York: Dekker, 1993;379–392.
6. Watts RL, Mirra SS, Richardson EP. Corticobasal ganglionic degeneration. In: Marsden CD, Fahn S, eds. *Movement Disorders 3.* London: Butterworth, 1994;282–299.
7. Watts RL, Brewer RP, Schneider JA, Mirra SS. Corticobasal degeneration. In: Watts RL, Koller WC, eds. *Movement Disorders: Neurologic Principles and Practice.* New York: McGraw-Hill, 1997;611–621.
8. Rinne JO, Lee MS, Thompson PD, Marsden CD. Corticobasal degeneration: a clinical study of 36 cases. *Brain* 1994;117:1183–1196.
9. Kompoliti K, Goetz CG, Boeve BF, et al. Clinical presentation and pharmacological therapy in corticobasal degeneration. *Arch Neurol* 1998;55:957–961.
10. Maraganore DM, Ahlskog JE, Petersen RC. Progressive asymmetric rigidity with apraxia: a distinctive clinical entity (abstract). *Mov Disord* 1992;7(suppl 1):80.
11. Boeve BF, Maraganore DM, Parisi JE, et al. Disorders mimicking the "classical" clinical syndrome of cortical-basal ganglionic degeneration: report of nine cases (abstract). *Mov Disord* 1996;11:351.
12. Lang AE, Riley DE, Bergeron C. Cortical-basal ganglionic degeneration. In: Calne DB, ed. *Neurodegenerative Diseases.* Philadelphia: WB Saunders, 1994;877–894.
13. Kumar R, Bergeron C, Pollanen MS, Lang AE. Cortical-basal ganglionic degeneration. In: Jankovic J, Tolosa E, eds. *Parkinson's Disease and Movement Disorders,* 3rd, ed. Baltimore: Williams & Wilkins, 1998;297–316.
14. Feany MB, Dickson DW. Widespread cytoskeletal pathology characterizes corticobasal degeneration. *Am J Pathol* 1995;146:1388–1396.
15. Grimes DA, Lang AE, Bergeron C. Dementia is the most common presentation of cortical-basal ganglionic degeneration (abstract). *Neurology* 1998;50(suppl 4):A96.
16. Litvan I, Agid Y, Goetz C, Jankovic J, Wenning GK, Brandel JP, et al. Accuracy of the clinical diagnosis of corticobasal degeneration: a clinicopathologic study. *Neurology* 1997;48:119–125.
17. Wenning GK, Litvan I, Jankovic J, et al. Natural history and survival of 14 patients with corticobasal degeneration confirmed at postmortem examination. *J Neurol Neurosurg Psychiatry* 1998;64:184–189.

Corticobasal Degeneration.
Advances in Neurology, Vol. 82,
edited by I. Litvan, C. G. Goetz, and A. E. Lang.
Lippincott Williams & Wilkins, Philadelphia © 2000.

4

Focal and Asymmetric Cortical Degenerative Syndromes

Richard J. Caselli

Department of Neurology, Mayo Clinic, Scottsdale, Arizona 85259

INTRODUCTION

Corticobasal degeneration (CBD) is a clinically striking disorder, in particular because of its focal somatic features. Yet CBD's uniqueness in regard to its focality is shared by a family of other degenerative syndromes, inspiring the terms focal and "asymmetric cortical degeneration syndromes" (ACDS) (1–3). All ACDSs present with slowly progressive, focal cortical symptomatology early in their course (Table 1). There is clinical and pathological overlap between member diseases of the ACDS group so that no single clinical syndrome is invariably characterized by a single histopathology, and no single histopathology is invariably characterized by a single clinical syndrome. Rather, the topographic distribution of the responsible neurodegenerative process rather than the histopathology determines the clinical presentation.

Current interest in focal cortical degenerative syndromes was rekindled in 1982 when Mesulam described six patients with slowly progressive aphasia (without apparent accompanying dementia) caused by focal degeneration of left perisylvian cortices (4). There are, however, much earlier descriptions of patients with progressive aphasia and other focal cortical degenerative syndromes (5,6). Since Mesulam's 1982 report, many more patients have been described with progressive aphasia, and autopsy studies have shown that underlying histopathology varies from case to case (7–14). Longitudinal neuropsychological studies generally have demonstrated that the greatest cognitive deterioration occurs in language-related skills, but milder decline also occurs in nonverbal cognitive domains (1,2,15,16).

Aphasia is not the only cortical syndrome that has been recognized to present in a slowly progressive, degenerative fashion. Many permutations of the focal cortical degeneration theme have been observed, including various frontal, parietal, temporal, occipital, and mixed (concurrent involvement of contiguous cortical regions) syndromes (1,2). As with other neuropathologic processes, the clinical manifestations of these degenerative diseases are determined by their neuroanatomical location. The nosologic status of CBD, therefore, is most properly considered within the broader category of ACDSs. The four broad ACDS categories to be considered are progressive aphasia, frontal lobe or frontotemporal syndromes, perceptual-motor syndromes, and bitemporal syndromes. CBD typically falls into the perceptual-motor syndrome category, but occasionally into the progressive aphasia (nonfluent) category.

EPIDEMIOLOGY AND GENETIC RISK FACTORS

There are no incidence and prevalence studies of this group of disorders, but clinical experience suggests they are, as a group, perhaps one-tenth as common as Alzheimer's disease. There has been modest published evidence of a familial ten-

TABLE 1. *ACDS: clinical classification*

Syndrome	Major topography	Main pathology	Other pathology/ disease
Progressive aphasia			
Nonfluent	Dominant frontal operculum	Nonspecific	CBD, ALS
Fluent	Dominant temporal	Nonspecific	CJD, Alzheimer's
Anomic	Dominant anterior temporal	Pick's	Alzheimer's?
Mixed	Dominant perisylvian	Nonspecific	Alzheimer's
Frontal lobe			
Neuropsychiatric	Asymmetric bilateral prefrontal/ temporal	Pick's, nonspecific (FTD)	ALS
Spasticity	Asymmetric bilateral precentral gyrus	Nonspecific (PLS)	ALS
Mixed	Asymmetric bilateral frontal	Unknown	ALS?
Perceptual-motor			
Visual	Asymmetric bilateral parietal/ temporal/occipital	Alzheimer's	Nonspecific, CJD
Motor	Asymmetric parietofrontal	CBD	Alzheimer's, Pick's
Mixed	Asymmetric parietofrontal and parieto-occipital	CBD	
Bitemporal			
Amnesia	Bilateral mesial temporal	Alzheimer's	Nonspecific, microvascular
Prosopagnosia	Nondominant greater than dominant temporal	Unknown	Alzheimer's?
Neuropsychiatric	Bilateral anterior temporal	Unknown	Pick's?

ALS, amyotrophic lateral sclerosis; CBD, Corticobasal degeneration; CJD, Creutzfeldt-Jakob disease; FTD, frontotemporal dementia; PLS, primary lateral sclerosis.

dency in patients with CBD (17,18). One reported set of identical twins remains clinically discordant for CBD 8 years after onset in the proband, although PET (positron emission topography) disclosed metabolic abnormalities in relevant cortical substrates in the clinically unaffected twin, arguing for a genetic contribution with incomplete penetrance (19). Further evidence of a genetic link came from a study of a family with overlap features of various degenerative syndromes, including frontal lobe dementia, parkinsonism, and motor neuron disease (disinhibition-dementia-parkinsonism-amyotrophy-complex, or DDPAC), which mapped to a specific region of chromosome 17 (20,21). It has subsequently been shown that other types of atypical cortical dementia, including progressive subcortical gliosis characterized by its nonspecific histologic appearance, and a familial form of aphasic dementia with more variable histopathology also mapped to the same region of chromosome 17 (22,23). This region is of interest in particular because it contains the genes for low affinity nerve growth factor receptor, the microtubule associated protein tau, and the homeobox B gene cluster. Most recently, mutations in the tau gene have been described for familial frontotemporal dementia (24). Whether this ultimately will prove to have relevance for the remaining ACDSs is under study.

ASYMMETRIC CORTICAL DEGENERATION SYNDROMES

General Considerations

Despite the semiologic and pathologic diversity of the ACDS group, there is a common clinicopathologic theme to all members of this group: clinical presentation is dictated by the topographic distribution. In most cases there is a diffuse component in addition to the more severe degenerative focus. Nonspecific degenerative histopathology is common in all clinical subtypes, and consists of neuronal loss, gliosis, and vacuolation of neuropil predominantly effecting superficial cortical laminae. Nonspecific histology has been reported in progressive frontal/frontotemporal dementia syndrome (25,26), progressive aphasia syndrome (14,27–35), and progressive perceptual-motor syndrome (36). Several familial neurodegenerative disorders with variable combinations of dementia, parkinsonism, and motor neuron disease also have nonspecific changes (20), including patients with ALS-dementia complex (37–49).

Progressive Aphasia

Although Arnold Pick deserves the original credit for correlating lobar atrophy with aphasic dementia (and the entire concept of focal cerebral degenerative syndromes) (5), Mesulam's 1982 report of progressive aphasia (4) essentially refocused modern neurology on the relationship of focal cortical degeneration to a progressive cortical syndrome. Because most patients are left-hemisphere dominant for language, most patients with progressive aphasia have left-sided asymmetric cortical atrophy. However, occasional patients are found who are left-handed and who have right hemisphere asymmetric atrophy (or less apparent asymmetry) accompanying progressive aphasia. Nonfluent, fluent, anomic, and mixed varieties of progressive aphasia can be distinguished.

Nonfluent Progressive Aphasia

Nonfluent progressive aphasia generally reflects anterior perisylvian cortical degeneration (Fig. 1). It should be readily distinguished from typical Alzheimer's disease. Mesulam's 1982 article included a patient with anomic speech that was "labored, diminished in quantity, and dysarthric" (4). Since then, many more patients with a progressive nonfluent aphasia characterized by effortful, halting, and sometimes dysarthric speech have

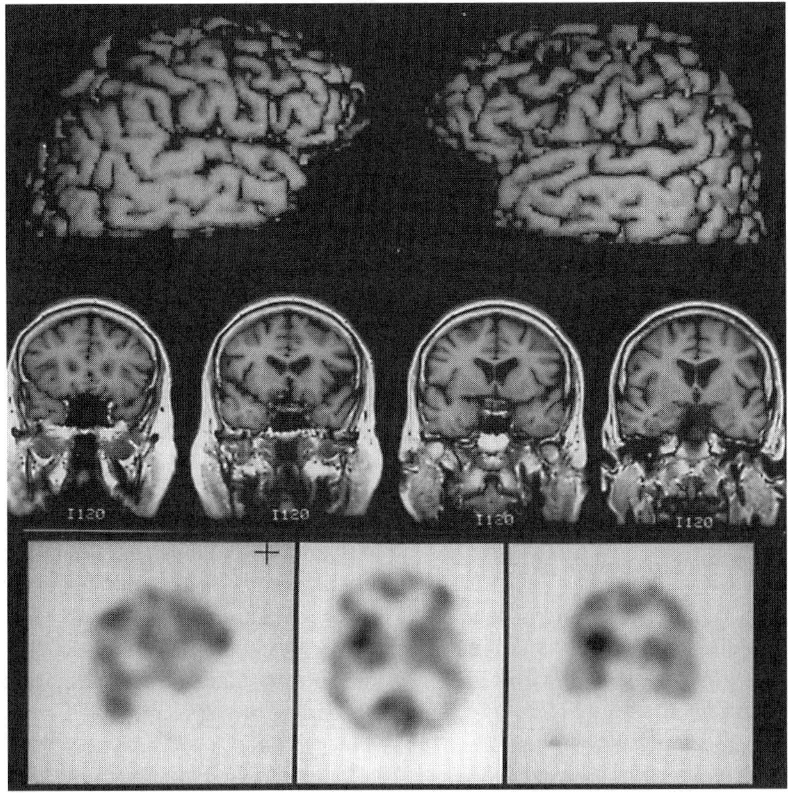

FIG. 1. Progressive nonfluent aphasia. Surface rendered MRI (*top row*), coronal MRI (*middle row*), and HMPAO-SPECT (*bottom row*) demonstrating left frontal opercular atrophy and hypoperfusion in a 73-year-old woman with a 5-year history of progressive nonfluent aphasia. (From Caselli RJ and Jack CR. *Neurology* 1992;42:1462–1468. Used with permission from Lippincott-Raven Publishers.)

been described (1,2,14,27,32,50–55). Naming ability in these patients is marked by phonemic paraphasic errors. That is, the target name is apparent, but its production is flawed: for example, "calicopter" for helicopter. Repetition is generally severely impaired. Writing is sometimes easier than speaking, but is usually abnormal. Aural and reading comprehension are less impaired in mild to moderate stages, deteriorate in most patients with disease progression, and should be formally assessed. Some patients have orofacial apraxia, but not gestural or limb apraxia. Verbal memory tests are difficult to administer, but verbal memory is typically impaired.

Other associated clinical abnormalities are found less consistently, which include right-sided hyperreflexia, constructional apraxia, and impaired visual memory. Nonfluent aphasia may also occur within the context of a severe frontal lobe syndrome or motor neuron disease (see the following).

Neuropathologic findings have included: (a) nonspecific degenerative changes with increased neuronal lipofuscin (28), neuronal loss, astrocytosis, and perineuronal microvacuolation in superficial laminae with or without occasional amyloid plaques (27,14); (b) CBD with focal accumulations of achromatic neurons (50); and (c) unusual combinations of Alzheimer, Pick, and Lewy body disease type pathology (32). Additional pathologic findings include asymmetric atrophy of perisylvian language cortices, and loss of pigmented midbrain neurons (27,14,50,51). The hippocampal formation is involved by the asymmetric degeneration, but the nucleus basalis is spared (14).

Fluent Progressive Aphasia

Fluent progressive aphasia involves degeneration of temporal and posterior perisylvian cortices. Contiguous involvement of neighboring cortices may complicate the clinical picture, making it difficult to distinguish a focal left temporoparietal syndrome (with aphasia, amnesia, apraxia, and acalculia) from a "diffuse" cognitive disorder, or Alzheimer's dementia. The nonlanguage impairments, however, are much less disabling than the language impairment in progressive fluent aphasia. Fluency, articulation, and prosody are normal, but comprehension and naming are impaired (1,14,56–58). Sentence repetition appears to be impaired less consistently (1). The characteristic naming errors are semantic paraphasias, but phonemic paraphasias occur as well. Typically, a patient may recognize and describe the object or action they cannot name (e.g., "something that flies" for a helicopter). Alternatively, they may give a generic descriptor (e.g., "plant" for a flower) or select the wrong member of the generic family to which the object or action belongs (e.g., "sofa" for a bench). Spelling errors are also frequent in these patients.

Additional clinical abnormalities that are more variable include verbal and visual memory loss, acalculia, constructional apraxia, and apraxic agraphia.

The perisylvian degenerative focus includes Wernicke's area, although often the entire left temporal lobe appears atrophic (56). Neuropathologic findings have included nonspecific degenerative changes (14), Alzheimer's disease (59), and Creutzfeldt-Jakob disease (60).

Anomic Aphasia

Anomic aphasia involves degeneration of anterior temporal cortices. Patients are fluent, comprehend well, and can repeat, read, and write with minimal difficulty (28,61–65). However, their speech lacks semantic precision. They substitute generic terms for specific words (e.g., "machine" for computer), and make semantic paraphasias (e.g., "staple" for paperclip). Anomia is also a feature of Alzheimer's dementia. In progressive anomia as well as in more typical cases of Alzheimer's dementia, verbal memory is usually impaired owing to concurrent mesial temporal degeneration.

Additional clinical abnormalities relate to progressive anomia's relationship to Pick's disease, which also has a predilection for the frontal lobe. Hence, frontal lobe signs may occur as well.

In addition to patients with anomic aphasia occurring within the context of Alzheimer's disease, neuropathological findings in cases of pure progressive anomic aphasia have disclosed Pick's disease. Pick's disease may cause frontotemporal atrophy that is most severe in the left anterior temporal lobe and insula, with relative sparing of the nucleus basalis of Meynert (61).

Mixed Progressive Aphasia

Mixed progressive aphasia is a more nonspecific pattern involving degeneration of left temporal and perisylvian cortices. These patients have impairment of all aspects of language, making classification into a single taxonomic category impossible (14,29,64,66–68). They are nonfluent with impaired comprehension, naming, repetition, writing, and reading.

If additional disabling abnormalities include other features of a dementia syndrome, such patients are better described as having an aphasic dementia rather than progressive aphasia.

Once again pathologically, the degenerative focus appears to involve the left perisylvian cortices, particularly the left temporal lobe. Neuropathological findings have included nonspecific degenerative changes (29), and Alzheimer's disease (66,67).

Progressive Frontal/Frontotemporal Syndromes

The three main frontal lobe syndromes are a progressive neuropsychiatric syndrome (frontal lobe or frontotemporal dementia, FLD), a progressive spastic syndrome, and a mixture of these two.

Progressive Neuropsychiatric Syndrome

The progressive neuropsychiatric syndrome is the best known example of this group, and has been referred to as frontal lobe (and frontotemporal [37]) dementia (Fig. 2). Pick's disease is prominently represented in this group (5,69). More recently, Brun (25) and Gustafson (70) described a similar clinical syndrome in the absence of Pick bodies. Although the clinical picture is characteristic (1,2,43,71), many clinicians have difficulty distinguishing these patients from patients with Alzheimer's type dementia. Another common misdiagnosis is depression. The errors of these patients tend to be omissions rather than commissions, and the term that describes this is abulia. They fail to change their clothes, brush their teeth, pursue their former interests, initiate many activities that constitute a normal day. They are typically less talkative, and walk more slowly but without a frankly shuffling gait. Just as they fail to start something new, they may fail to stop what they are doing, and perseveratively fixate, in a seemingly idiosyncratic fashion, on some particular activity, such as going to the bathroom or sorting through their wallet or watching television. Some patients have greater disinhibition and emotional lability, crying at the least provocation or laughing loud and long. They may complain that they are hungry, yet be unmoved to fix themselves a snack. Some may perseveratively want to eat over and over. Memory and language (especially naming) are typically impaired. Despite their sometimes reduced temporal latency in responding to the examiner (they may start answering a question before the physician has finished asking it), their answers are brief, and often consist of "I don't know." FLD patients may stick close to their caregiver, and generally cause fewer disruptions than Alzheimer's patients, particularly in mild to moderate stages (although there are notable exceptions).

Associated clinical abnormalities reflect dysfunction of other frontal lobe functions, including spasticity and nonfluent aphasia. Because Pick's disease has a predilection for the temporal as well as the frontal lobe, some patients also develop signs referable to the temporal lobe, particularly anomia (1,2). One patient with right greater than left frontotemporal degeneration developed severe aprosodia and inability to sing (72).

Neuropathologically, Pick's disease and nonspecific degeneration are most often found. Arnold Pick introduced the concept of a focal cortical degenerative syndrome in his description of a patient with progressive aphasic dementia owing to atrophy of the left temporal lobe (5). Over the following decades three related patterns of pathology have been assumed under the Pick's disease designation: lobar atrophy with swollen chromatolytic neurons (SCN) and Pick bodies (Pick's-Type A), lobar atrophy with SCN but not Pick bodies (Pick's-Type B), and lobar atrophy without SCN or Pick bodies (Pick's-Type C, or nonspecific degeneration) (73). Some recent

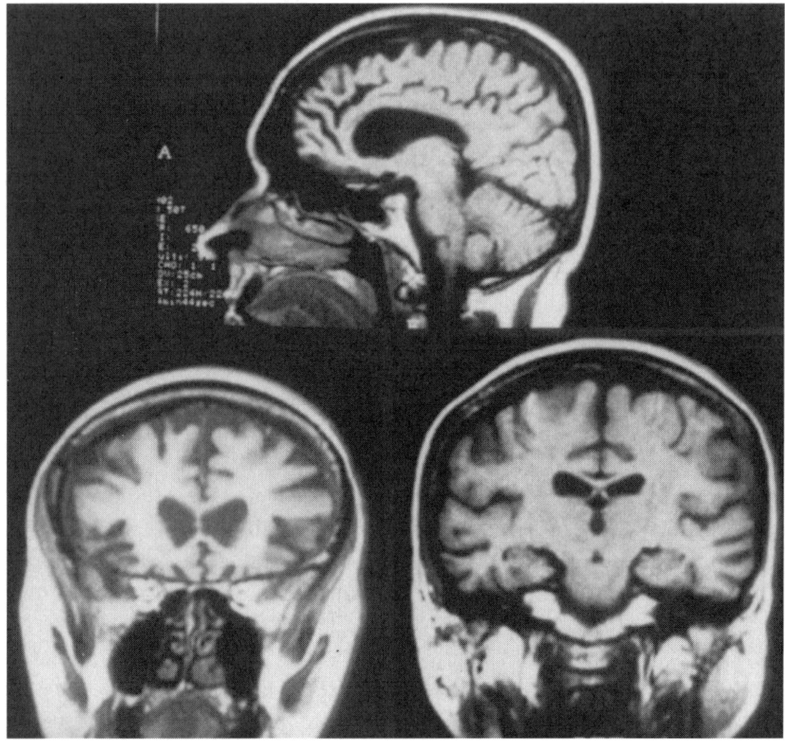

FIG. 2. Frontal lobe neuropsychiatric syndrome (frontotemporal dementia). Sagittal (*top*) and coronal (*bottom*) MRI demonstrating severe bifrontal atrophy in a 70-year-old woman with a 3-year history of a progressive neuropsychiatric syndrome.

reviews question whether the findings in Pick's-Type B and C are indeed variants of Pick's disease or different disease processes (74). Pick's-Type B is thought by some to represent CBD, and Pick's-Type C is often regarded simply as nonspecific degeneration (74). Variable degrees of coexisting subcortical gliosis and degeneration of other subcortical nuclei can occur as well, although the basal forebrain tends to be spared (25,75).

Pick's disease usually involves the frontal and anterior temporal lobes, but rare cases with preferential parietal lobe atrophy and have also been described (76,77). Although most patients with Pick's pathology have exhibited frontal lobe/frontotemporal dementia, there are less common presentations reflecting atypical topography, including progressive aphasia (51,61,78), and progressive perceptual-motor syndrome (CBD) (76).

Syndrome of Progressive Spasticity

The syndrome of progressive spasticity has been termed primary lateral sclerosis (PLS), and historically, the nosologic focus has been on its relationship to amyotrophic lateral sclerosis rather than other frontal lobe degenerations. PLS reflects degeneration of the precentral gyrus/primary motor cortex. PLS has a long and controversial past, but only relatively recently have clinico/pathological studies confirmed its nosologic status (78–80). By definition, these are patients with no cognitive impairment except sometimes for emotional lability. However, formal neuropsychological testing discloses mild frontal lobe-related cognitive deficits and mild memory impairment (81). The syndrome is that of progressive generalized spasticity, typically asymmetric in onset and progression. It starts most commonly in the legs, but can start in the arms, or with speech, in the form of a progressive spastic dysarthria. All patients eventually develop a severe spastic dysarthria and may progress to anarthria. Patients become wheelchair bound after several years, but the rate of progression is variable (80). Additional clinical abnormalities include other frontal lobe features, such as saccadic breakdown of smooth pursuit eye movements (in most), and urinary incontinence (in about half) (80).

Neuropathologically, there is highly circumscribed atrophy of the precentral gyrus with loss of Betz cells, decreased numbers of pyramidal neurons, and laminar gliosis in the external and internal pyramidal cell cortical layers (78–80). No lower motor neuron abnormalities are typically found in hypoglossal or spinal gray nuclei, and the substantia nigra is generally unaffected (80). Occasionally, patients develop mild lower motor neuron features who otherwise follow the slower course of PLS rather than the more rapid course of ALS (82).

Mixed Syndromes

In addition to patients with either a cognitive or a motor frontal lobe syndrome, some patients present early in their course with a combination of both (1). Conceivably, these patients have Pick's disease, as it is known that Pick's disease will produce spasticity late in the course of the illness. Alzheimer's disease has also been reported to present with progressive spasticity (83).

Progressive Perceptual-Motor Syndromes

Although most patients have a mixed sensory (including visual and somatosensory-motor) syndrome, there are a few patients who have a pure sensory (typically visual) or motor syndrome (typically, a hemiakinetic rigid syndrome). Progressive spasticity is considered elsewhere in this chapter.

Progressive Visual Syndromes

Progressive visual syndromes involve degeneration of parietooccipital and parietotemporal visual association cortices. Visual association cortices can be broadly divided into dorsal (occipitoparietal) and ventral (occipitotemporal) pathways, and disorders of visual association cortices reflect this dichotomy. The occipitoparietal pathway is more concerned with localizing an object in space ("where"), and the occipitotemporal pathway is more concerned with object identification ("what"). The first description of a progressive complex visual disorder owing to posterior cortical degeneration may be that of Rosenfeld in 1909 (62), but the most detailed, colorful, and famous is certainly that of Oliver Sacks' *The Man Who Mistook His Wife for a Hat* (84). Two broad types of complex visual disturbance have been described with ACDS. The more commonly reported is progressive asimultanagnosia, reflecting dysfunction of the dorsal cortical visual pathway. Patients cannot integrate the numerous components of an ordinarily complex scene into a coherent whole. When viewing a street scene, for example, they might describe a car or a person or a lamppost, but overlook the fact that it is an innercity rush hour. Occasionally, such patients have ocular apraxia (the inability to voluntarily direct their gaze to a target of visual interest), and optic ataxia (the inability to benefit from visual guidance in reaching for an object). This triad of symptoms is Balint's syndrome (85). Associated problems that also reflect posterior parietal and temporal involvement include alexia, acalculia, right-left disorientation, and mild deficits of memory and language (fluent aphasia). Eventually, patients may be found to have an inferior quadrantanopia, although typically visual field testing produces inconsistent responses (86–89).

The second type of complex visual disorder resulting from ACD is visual agnosia, of which there are fewer reported examples (84,90–92). Visual agnosia results from dysfunction of the ventral cortical visual pathway. Some patients have been described with progressive prosopagnosia, a failure to recognize familiar faces (90,92). Rarely, patients may describe progressive atopographagnosia, the inability to recognize familiar places. In later stages, both ventral and dorsal visual pathways become involved, and a more globally encompassing visual agnosia results as illustrated best by Oliver Sacks' Professor P (84). Associated clinical abnormalities merge into the mixed sensorimotor syndromes discussed in the following, as well as impaired memory. Recognition deficits in somatosensory and auditory modalities may be present as well (84,91).

Neuropathological studies of patients with dorsal visual syndromes (asimultanagnosia) to date have generally shown senile plaques and neurofibrillary tangles, typical of Alzheimer's disease. The topographic distribution, however, differs from that seen in Alzheimer's dementia with heaviest involvement of primary and association visual cortices in the occipital lobes, and to a slightly lesser degree in the parietal lobes (93). The nucleus basalis is involved in these cases (93). Other causes include nonspecific degeneration and Creutzfeldt-Jakob disease (Haidenhain variant). Published neuropathological studies of patients with progressive ventral visual syndromes (progressive prosopagnosia and alexia) are lacking to date.

Progressive Motor Syndromes (including CBD)

Two major clinical characteristics, both slowly progressive in onset, make this disorder distinctive and easily recognized (1,2,87,94,95). The first are lateralized somatic deficits including hemispasticity, hemiparesis, hemisensory impairment (usually in the form of astereognosis or tactile agnosia with less consistent impairment of more basic somatosensory modalities), and myoclonic jerks. Some patients may have a hemirigid or hemidystonic syndrome with tremor. The second is severe and disabling apraxia, including limb apraxia (inability to use the limb in a meaningful way, such as to use a comb), gestural apraxia (inability to pantomime or imitate symbolic movements), dressing apraxia, constructional apraxia, and apraxic agraphia. If the lateralized limb defects reflect dominant hemispheric dysfunction, then a mild, fluent aphasia may be present that is milder than that seen in progressive fluent aphasia (1). When the lateralized limb defects reflect nondominant hemisphere dysfunction, it is uncommon (but possible) for a hemineglect syndrome to result.

Additional clinical abnormalities include acalculia in particular, and other parietal signs to a less frequent degree (1). Many patients are slow on tests of psychomotor speed that are not limited by impaired movement (e.g., the controlled oral word association test) (1). Eye movements become affected as the degenerative process ultimately invades more anterior regions of the frontal convexities, including the frontal eye fields (17,96). Although patients with severe apraxia, psychomotor slowing, and mild aphasia may appear demented by neuropsychological testing, they are usually rational, insightful, and quite upset by their condition. In late stages, patients can barely move or speak despite preserved consciousness (17,96). Contiguous involvement of visual association cortices leads to perceptual disorders as well (see the preceding).

Neuropathologically, many (perhaps most) patients have CBD. In addition to mild generalized atrophy, severe asymmetric atrophy affects the parietal lobe, medial and lateral frontal cortices, and sometimes other contiguous areas (such as Wernicke's area, which causes severe aphasia) (17,94,95) (see Chapter 2). Not all patients described with the motor syndrome, however, have had CBD. With a similar topographic distribution, other histological patterns have included Pick's disease (76,77), Alzheimer's disease (97), and progressive supranuclear palsy (98).

Mixed Syndromes

Many patients have both a sensorimotor and a visuospatial disorder (1,2,99), combining features of both of the preceding groups (Fig. 3). Possibly the first patient ever reported with this type of disorder was Maurice Ravel (100), who was described by Alajouanine to have "a cerebral atrophy with bilateral ventricular enlargement" (101). Ravel had a fluent aphasia with apraxic agraphia, and left upper limb apraxia. Note reading was impaired but recognition of scores was relatively preserved. His apraxic agraphia extended to music writing as well, and he was unable to express music either by writing or playing an instrument. Although his ability to name individual notes that he heard was impaired, his aural comprehension of music appeared intact (101). Most patients simply share the features described in the preceding for both perceptual and motor disorders.

One pair of identical twins was reported who were clinically discordant for this condition (19); this is particularly instructive (Fig. 4). Three properties of the atrophy topography were dis-

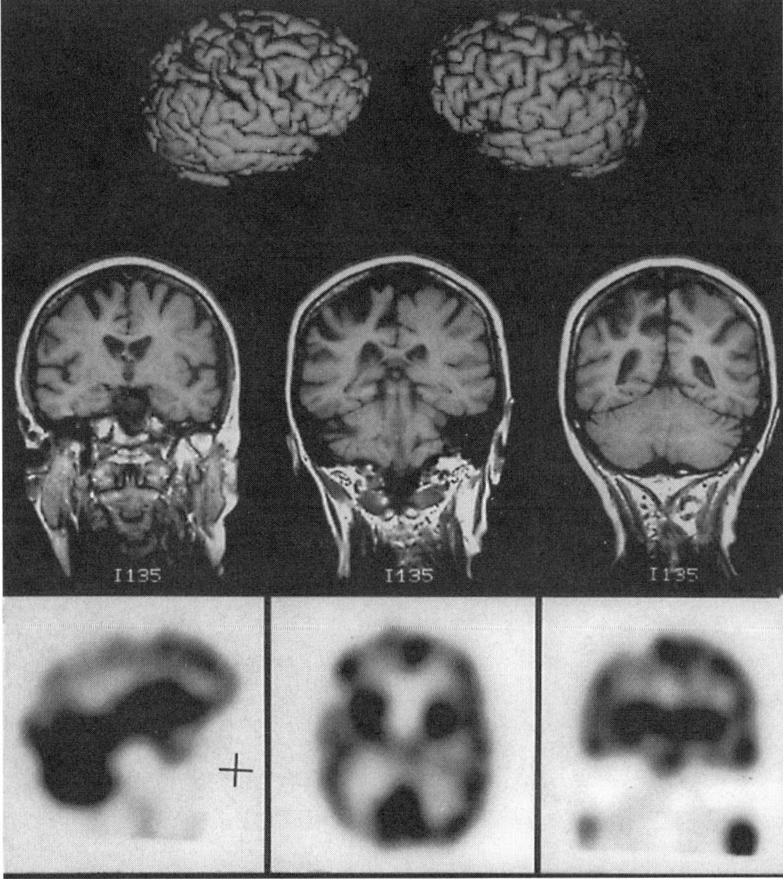

FIG. 3. Mixed perceptual-motor syndrome. Surface rendered MRI (*top row*), coronal MRI (*middle row*), and HMPAO-SPECT (*bottom row*) demonstrating right parietal atrophy in a 64-year-old woman with a 2-year history of progressive apraxis and visual-spatial impairment. (From Caselli RJ and Jack CR. *Neurology* 1992;42:1462–1468. Used with permission from Lippincott-Raven Publishers.)

cernible: (a) there is a lateralized major atrophic focus; (b) there is a contralateral area of focal atrophy that is less severe than the primary focus, in homologous cortices; and (c) there is milder generalized atrophy. Metabolic abnormalities reflect this pattern as well (19). Comparison of neuropsychologic test scores between these two brothers demonstrated that all scores were lower in the patient, including memory and verbal skills, despite normal absolute scores.

Neuropathologically, some CBD patients have severe decline in visuospatial skills before their death (98). One patient had Alzheimer-type pathology on frontal lobe biopsy (99).

Progressive Bitemporal Syndromes

The three syndromes in this category are progressive amnesia, progressive prosopagnosia, and progressive neuropsychiatric syndrome. Progressive amnesia is generally a *forme fruste* of Alzheimer's disease, but nonspecific degeneration and microvascular changes in the medial temporal lobe have also been described. Progressive prosopagnosia is discussed under progressive visual syndromes as this entity overlaps both categories of ACDS. Patients with a progressive neuropsychiatric syndrome owing to bitemporal degeneration (Fig. 5) are related to, but sufficiently

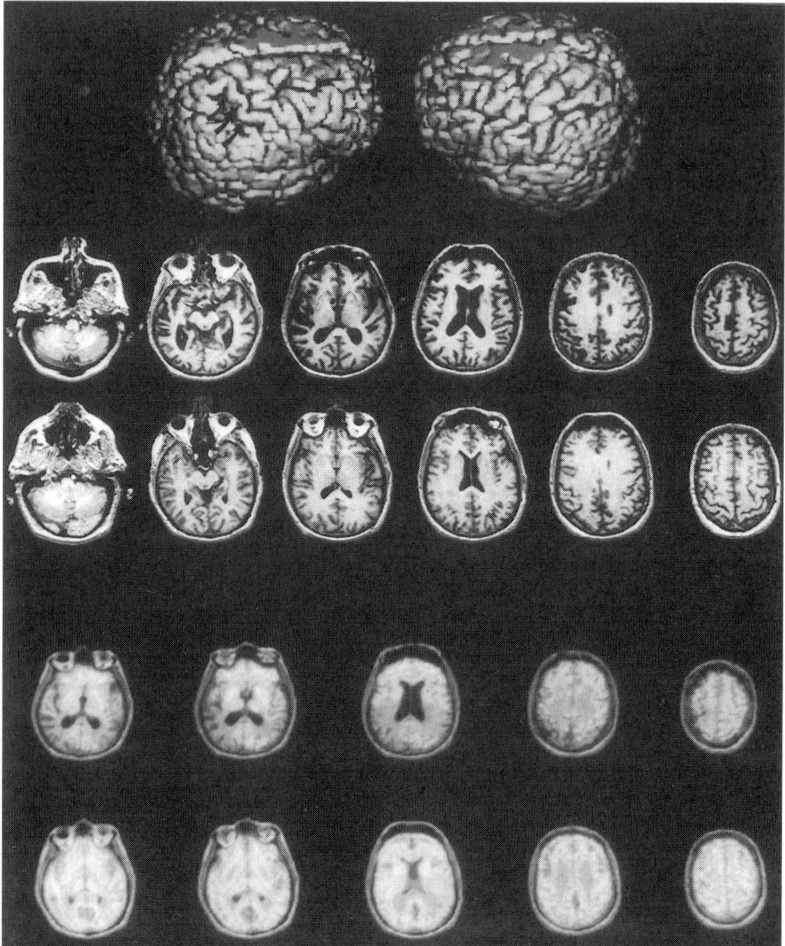

FIG. 4. Identical twins discordant for progressive apraxia. Surface rendered MRI of proband (*top row*), transverse MRI of proband and brother (*middle two rows, proband on top*), and fluorodeoxyglucose PET of proband and brother (*bottom two rows, proband on top*) of 63-year-old identical twin brothers discordant for the syndrome of progressive apraxia (see text). (From Caselli RJ, Reiman EM, Timmann D, et al. *Arch Neurol* 1995;52:1004–1010. Used with permission from American Medical Association Journals.)

distinct from frontotemporal dementia to warrant separate consideration. Anomia and amnesia are more prominent, but relative indifference to their own condition, and mild perseverative behaviors are shared with the frontal lobe group. Psychomotor speed is normal or only mildly impaired. Neuroimaging shows bilateral severe anterior temporal atrophy and hypoperfusion with relative sparing of the frontal lobes. Neuropathological study is lacking for progressive bitemporal neuropsychiatric syndromes, although on a clinical basis they probably have either Pick's or Alzheimer's disease.

ASSOCIATION OF ACDS WITH AMYOTROPHIC LATERAL SCLEROSIS

Several types of ACDS are associated with ALS (including progressive aphasia) (44,102) (Fig. 6), frontal lobe syndromes (including Pick's

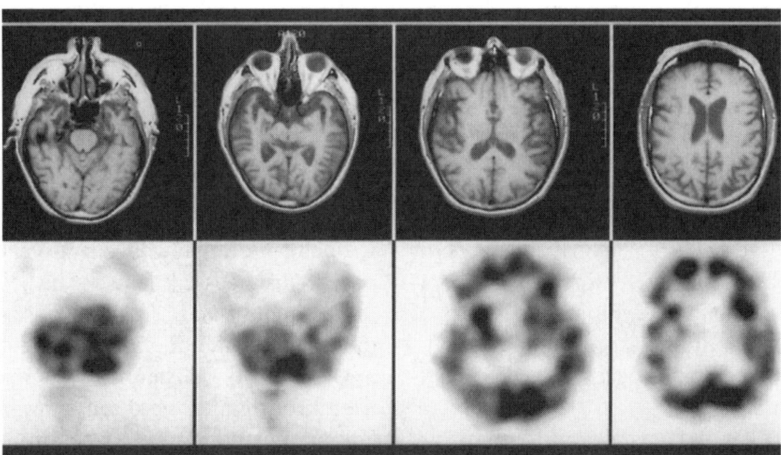

FIG. 5. Bitemporal neuropsychiatric syndrome. Transverse MRI (*top*) and HMPAO-SPECT (*bottom*) demonstrating right greater than left bilateral anterior temporal atrophy and hypoperfusion in a 71-year-old man with a 3-year history of a progressive neuropsychiatric syndrome. (From Caselli RJ *Neurologist* 1995;1:1–19. Used with permission from Williams & Wilkins.)

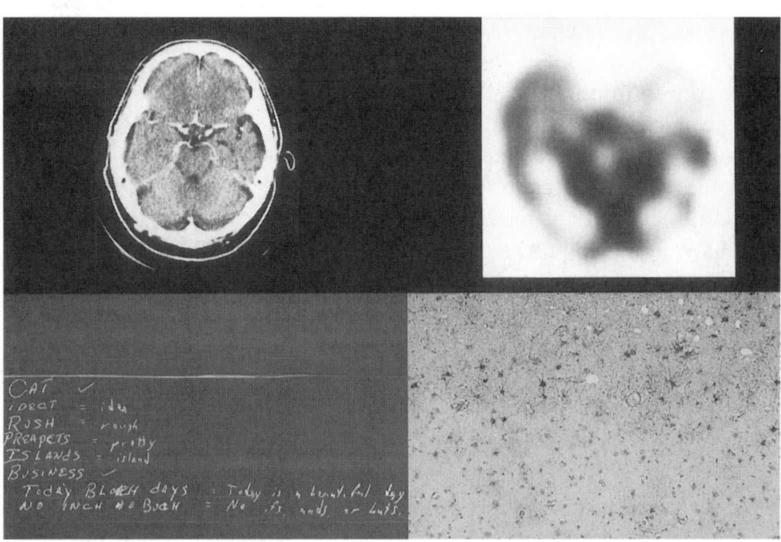

FIG. 6. ALS-dementia complex with aphasia. Transverse CT (*top left*), HMPAO-SPECT (*top right*) demonstrating left temporal atrophy and hypoperfusion in a 57-year-old man with a 10-month history of rapidly progressive aphasic dementia with motor neuron disease. Writing sample (*bottom left*) demonstrating aphasia, and neuropathological sample of left temporal cortex (*bottom right*, glial fibrillary astrocytic protein stain ×30 magnification) demonstrating nonspecific degenerative changes of gliosis and vacuolation of superficial cortical layers. (From Caselli RJ, Windebank AJ, Petersen RC, et al. *Ann Neurol* 1993;33: 200–207, 418. Used with permission from Lippincott-Raven Publishers.)

disease) (103,104), nonspecific frontal lobe degeneration (42,105), and bitemporal syndromes (106). In such cases, longevity is determined by the ALS component, and in the case of progressive aphasia with ALS, the disease course appears particularly rapid (44). Occasional patients with apparent PLS may have mild lower motor neuron abnormalities, and they appear to have a slower course than typical ALS (82). Patients with a bitemporal or frontotemporal syndrome and ALS may have a more severe neuropsychiatric syndrome with Kluver-Bucy features (106) compared to those without ALS. Finally, subtypes of ACDS may overlap in the same patient, such as progressive aphasia and progressive perceptual-motor syndrome.

Differential Diagnosis

The two broad categories to consider are nondegenerative structural focal brain lesions, such as a slowly growing tumor, and other degenerative conditions. Regarding the first, a slowly progressive neurologic syndrome that can be reasonably localized could be neoplastic, whether malignant or benign. Rarely, high-grade arterial stenoses will cause stuttering infarction mimicking a slowly progressive degenerative cortical syndrome, but this is very uncommon. Infection/abscess and demyelinating/vasculitic pathological processes also may occur focally. Other degenerative illnesses include Creutzfeldt-Jakob disease in rapidly progressive cases (60,88), and the wide variety of degenerative pathologies discussed previously. For example, a patient suspected of having CBD may prove to have had Alzheimer's disease at autopsy. Among the frontal lobe, aphasic, and bitemporal varieties of ACDS, association with ALS must also be considered.

Evaluation

The most important diagnostic test is adequate neuroimaging (2). Magnetic resonance imaging (MRI) is preferable to computed tomography (CT) but either will generally suffice to evaluate the possibility of a tumor. In addition to excluding nondegenerative structural abnormalities, an MRA (Magnetic Resonance Angiogram) could be included if available to search for a potentially relevant high-grade arterial stenosis. Patients with ACDS usually, but not invariably, have radiologically discernible focal atrophy in the symptomatic region. It is often subtle and of insufficient severity to permit blinded diagnosis of ACDS, but in a patient with progressive anomic aphasia, for example, focal left anterior temporal atrophy should be considered not only important because of the absence of a tumor, but important also because it shows the responsible lesion to be atrophic, presumably degenerative. Formal neuropsychological assessment can be helpful to further assess quality and severity of cognitive impairment, and usually demonstrates a pattern that is not typical for Alzheimer's dementia. It is also useful for monitoring disease progression. Other laboratory studies are less helpful because of the apparent focal nature of the ACDSs. Metabolic encephalopathies do not usually cause the syndrome of slowly progressive aphasia, which is difficult to confuse with a diffuse encephalopathy. Nonetheless, it is still reasonable to make certain that basic laboratory data are normal, as was discussed for Alzheimer's disease.

Management

Prevention

There is no known way to entirely protect against any degenerative brain disease, but Alzheimer's and Parkinson's disease-related research has led to some possible insights. Beneficial trends have been noted among people who take Vitamin E supplements (and possibly other antioxidants) (107), antiinflammatory drugs (108–110), and have a highly educated background, although plenty of college graduates and accomplished professionals who take antiinflammatory drugs for arthritis and Vitamin E to "stay young" still develop Alzheimer's disease. Some studies have suggested that among postmenopausal women, there is a moderate protective effect of estrogen replacement (111,112).

Cognitive Loss

In treating the ACDS patient, it is important to consider that, apart from frontotemporal dementia patients, they are usually quite aware of their limitations, and are not likely to unwittingly get themselves in trouble by wandering, refusing medications, and so forth. They require nursing home placement less often if a caregiver exists. There are few "memory tonics" available to patients and physicians, regardless of the underlying disease or dementia syndrome. Currently, the only class of drugs with possible cognitive enhancing effects in Alzheimer's disease and associated disorders are acetylcholinesterase inhibitors. Tacrine, a centrally acting acetylcholinesterase inhibitor, was the first described, although its usage has dropped off in favor of donepezil, a subsequently released less toxic and more easily administered agent. Both are thought to partially reverse the decline in cortically projected acetylcholine that results from degeneration of the cholinergic basal forebrain (113,114). The effects of both drugs are modest, and side effects, particularly of tacrine, are significant particularly at higher doses. Nonetheless, each has resulted in functionally important gains in some patients, and should be considered in patients with mild to moderate stages of the disease. Tacrine should either not be used, or used with great caution in patients with cardiac conduction defects, liver disease, or seizures. Sudden decline in cognitive status or other neurologic function (e.g., ambulation) in a patient with degenerative dementia generally implies a second disease process, often one that is nonneurologic (e.g., a urinary tract infection, pneumonia, and fluid and electrolyte disturbances). Medication side effects (particularly tricyclic antidepressants, benzodiazepines, and narcotic analgesics) or complications from improper medication administration should be sought, especially if the patient has continued to administer his or her own medications without adequate supervision. Common neurologic causes include subdural hematoma, stroke, and complex partial seizures. The differential diagnosis, of an acute encephalopathy, is extensive.

Psychotic Symptoms

Although disabling and characteristic of dementing illnesses, cognitive loss is not the only or even the greatest obstacle posed by patients to their caregivers. Paranoid delusions and other psychotic symptomatology are disruptive, pose extraordinary obstacles to effective caregiving, and are probably the most common reasons patients are sent to nursing homes. ACDS patients with frontotemporal predominance, including progressive aphasia, frontal and bitemporal neuropsychiatric syndromes, and ALS-dementia complex are particularly vulnerable. Small doses of neuroleptic medications may produce sufficient relief to permit the caregiver to continue to keep the patient at home, and should be part of the therapeutic armamentarium, but they must be used with great caution in patients with concurrent extrapyramidal problems (including CBD patients).

Haloperidol, at doses ranging from 0.5 milligram to 2 milligrams/day, is often sufficient, but sometimes higher doses are required. Extrapyramidal side effects, however, can become dose-limiting problems. Risperadone is a newer neuroleptic agent with greater dopamine receptor selectivity that generally results in fewer extrapyramidal side effects at equivalent dosage compared to haloperidol; however, extrapyramidal side effects still may occur. Most recently, olanzapine has been released with even fewer extrapyramidal effects, although it is more costly than risperadone.

Depression

Antidepressants with anticholinergic side effects (which includes all the tricyclic antidepressants), often exacerbate the confusion of these patients, and are generally not recommended. Rather, selective serotonin reuptake inhibitors (SSRIs) such as fluoxetine, sertraline, and paroxetine, can enhance energy levels (and possibly attentiveness as a result in some patients), and have antidepressant effects without the risk of anticholinergic side effects. They should not be used, however, in agitated patients, or in patients with psychotic symptomatology, as SSRIs can exacerbate such symptoms. For anxiety, buspirone, although generally less effective than benzodiazepines, has much less risk of paradoxical agitation, and should be tried first. Neuroleptic agents can also be considered for anxiety in some patients, especially if there is accompanying psychotic symptomatology.

Sleep

Sedative hypnotic agents can be used in patients in whom sleep-wake disturbances are disrupting their home care. Agents that have few side effects or risks of exacerbating confusion and agitation include diphenhydramine, chloral hydrate, and zolpidem. Many patients fall asleep without difficulty but waken at an early hour. In such instances, it is important that the sleeping aide be given when they waken. These medications help patients fall asleep, but they will not reliably keep them asleep for prolonged periods, which is in part why they are more advisable than longer-acting agents.

Motor Disturbances

Physical therapy is very important for patients with CBD and PLS, especially because of the complications resulting from altered muscle tone and gait unsteadiness. Occupational therapy is particularly important for ACDS patients with apraxia and spatial disorders to assist with dressing, eating, and other activities of daily living. Speech therapy is appropriate to consider for progressive aphasia, not only because of the aphasia, but also because of dysphagia, particularly in the later stages of nonfluent aphasia. Late-stage complications are similar for Alzheimer's disease, but perhaps are most severe for CBD. In this condition, as all avenues of communication are lost, including speech and praxis, and as muscle tone contorts patients into painful dystonic postures with contracture formation, there remains relative preservation of insight, perhaps compounding their suffering. Trials of Sinemet in CBD should be considered, even though it is usually of minimal efficacy. In CBD patients with severe myoclonus, small doses of clonazepam can also be considered (115). Finally, in cases with severe dystonic posturing (especially hand closure), selective botulinum toxin injection can be considered to accomplish limited goals, such as allowing the hand to be opened for maintenance of skin hygiene and to retard contracture formation.

REFERENCES

1. Caselli RJ, Jack CR Jr. Asymmetric cortical degenerative syndromes: a proposed clinical classification. *Arch Neurol* 1992;49:770–780.
2. Caselli RJ, Jack CR Jr, Petersen RC, Wahner HW, Yanagihara T. Asymmetric cortical degenerative syndromes: clinical and radiologic correlations. *Neurology* 1992;42:1462–1468.
3. Caselli RJ. Asymmetric cortical degeneration syndromes. *Curr Opinion Neurol* 1996;9:276–280.
4. Mesulam MM. Primary progressive aphasia-differentiation from Alzheimer's disease. *Ann Neurol* 1987;22: 533–534.
5. Pick A. On the relation between aphasia and senile atrophy of the brain. Schoene WC trans. In: Pick A. *Uber die Beziehungen der senilen Hirnatrophie zur Aphasie.* Prager Medicinische Wochenschrift 17,16(1892), 165–167. In: Rottenberg DA, Hochberg FH, eds. *Neurological classics in modern translation.* New York: Hafner Press, 1977:35–40.
6. Luzzati C, Poeck K. An early description of slowly progressive aphasia. *Arch Neurol* 1991;48:228–229.
7. Delay J, Neveu P, Desclaux P. Les dissolutions du langage dans la maladie de Pick. Diagnostic de l'atrophie cerebrale par l'encephalographie et la ventriculographie. *Rev Neurol* 1944;76:37–38.
8. Morris JC, Cole M, Banker BQ, Wright D. Hereditary dysphasic dementia and the Pick-Alzheimer spectrum. *Ann Neurol* 1984;16:455–466.
9. Kirshner HS, Tanridag O, Thurman L, Whetsell WO Jr. Progressive aphasia without dementia: two cases with focal spongiform degeneration. *Ann Neurol* 1987;22: 527–532.
10. Mandell AM, Alexander MP, Carpenter S. Creutzfeldt-Jakob disease presenting as isolated aphasia. *Neurology* 1989;39:55–58.
11. Graff-Radford NR, Damasio AR, Hyman BT, et al. Progressive aphasia in a patient with Pick's disease: a neuropsychologic, radiologic, and anatomic study. *Neurology* 1990;40:620–626.
12. Benson DF, Zaias BW. Progressive aphasia: a case with postmortem correlation. *Neuropsych Neuropsychol Behav Neurol* 1991;4:215–223.
13. Lippa CF, Cohen R, Smith TW, Drachman DA. Primary progressive aphasia with focal neuronal achromasia. *Neurology* 1991;41:882–886.
14. Snowden JS, Neary D, Mann DMA, Goulding PJ, Testa HJ. Progressive language disorder due to lobar atrophy. *Ann Neurol* 1992;31:174–183.
15. Green J, Morris JC, Sandson J, McKeel DW Jr, Miller JW. Progressive aphasia: a precursor of global dementia? *Neurology* 1990;40:423–429.
16. Weintraub S, Rubin NP, Mesulam MM. Primary progressive aphasia: longitudinal course, neuropsychological profile, and language features. *Arch Neurol* 1990;47:1329–1335.
17. Rebeiz JJ, Kolodny EH, Richardson EP Jr. Corticodentatonigral degeneration with neuronal achromasia. *Arch Neurol* 1968;18:20–33.
18. Lippa CF, Smith TW, Fontneau N. Corticonigral degeneration with neuronal achromasia: a clinicopathologic study of two cases. *J Neurol Sci* 1990;98:301–310.
19. Caselli RJ, Reiman EM, Timmann D, et al. Progressive apraxia in clinically discordant monozygotic twins. *Arch Neurol* 1995;52:1004–1010.
20. Wilhelmsen KC, Lynch T, Nygaard TG. Localization of disinhibition-dementia-parkinsonism-amyotrophy complex to 17q21–22. *Am J Hum Genet* 1994;55: 1159–1165.

21. Lynch T, Sano M, Marder KS, et al. Clinical characteristics of a family with chromosome 17-linked disinhibition-dementia-parkinsonism-amyotrophy complex. *Neurology* 1994; 44:1878–1884.
22. Petersen RB, Tabaton M, Chen SG, et al. Familial progressive subcortical gliosis: presence of prions and linkage to chromosome 17. *Neurology* 1995;45: 1062–1067.
23. Lendon CL, Lynch T, Norton J, et al. Hereditary dysphasic disinhibition dementia: a frontotemporal dementia linked to 17q21–22. *Neurology* 1998; 50: 1546–1555.
24. Hutton M, Lendon CL, Rizzu P, et al. Association of missense and 5′-splice-site mutations in tau with the inherited dementia FTDP-17. *Nature* 1998;393:702–705.
25. Brun A. Frontal lobe degeneration of non-Alzheimer type. 1. Neuropathology. *Arch Gerontol Geriatr* 1987; 6:193–208.
26. Brun A. Frontal lobe degeneration of non-Alzheimer type revisited. *Dementia* 1993;4:126–131.
27. Green J, Morris J, Sandson J, McKeel D, Miller J. Progressive aphasia: a precursor of global dementia? *Neurology* 1990;40:423–429.
28. Mesulam M. Primary progressive aphasia without generalized dementia. *Ann Neurol* 1982;11:592–598.
29. Kirshner HS, Tanridag O, Thurman L, Whetsell WO Jr. Progressive aphasia without dementia. two cases with focal spongiform degeneration. *Ann Neurol* 1987;22: 527–532.
30. Mehier M, Horoupian D, Davies P, Dickson D. Reduced somatostatin-like immunoreactivity in cerebral cortex in nonfamilial dysphasic dementia. *Neurology* 1987;37:1448–1453.
31. Scheltens P, Ravid R, Kamphorst W. Pathologic findings in a case of primary progressive aphasia. *Neurology* 1994;44:279–282.
32. Morris JC, Cole M, Banker BQ, Wright D. Hereditary dysphasic dementia and the Pick-Alzheimer spectrum. *Ann Neurol* 1984;16:455–466.
33. Cole M, Wright D, Banker B. Familial aphasia due to Pick's disease. *Ann Neurol* 1979;6:158.
34. Turner R, Kenyon L, Trojanowski J, Gonatas N, Grossman M. Clinical, neuroimaging, and pathologic features of progressive nonfluent aphasia. *Ann Neurol* 1996;39:166–173.
35. Harasty J, Halliday G, Code C, Brooks W. Quantification of cortical atrophy in a case of progressive fluent aphasia. *Brain* 1996;119:181–190.
36. Boeve B, Maraganore D, Parisi L Ahiskog J. A case presenting clinically as cortical-basal ganglionic degeneration without neuronal achromasia. *Mov Dis* 1996;11:356–357.
37. Brun A, Englund B, Gustafson L, et al. Clinical and neuropathological criteria for frontotemporal dementia. *J Neurol Neurosurg Psychiatry* 1994;57:416–418.
38. Neary D, Snowden J, Mann D. Familial progressive aphasia: its relationship to other forms of lobar atrophy. *J Neurol Neurosurg Psychiatry* 1993;56:1122–1125.
39. Neary D, Snowden J, Mann D. The clinical pathological correlates of lobar atrophy. *Dementia* 1993;4:154–159.
40. Mann D, South P. The topographic distribution of brain atrophy in frontal lobe dementia. *Acta Neuropathol* 1993;85:334–340.
41. Mann D, South P, Snowden J, Neary D. Dementia of frontal lobe type: neuropathology and immunohistochemistry. *J Neurol Neurosurg Psychiatry* 1993;56: 605–614.
42. Neary D, Snowden J, Mann D, Northen D, Goulding P, Macdermott N. Frontal lobe dementia and motor neuron disease. *J Neurol Neurosurg Psychiatry* 1990;53: 23–32.
43. Neary D, Snowden JS, Northen B, Goulding P. Dementia of the frontal lobe type. *J Neurol Neurosurg Psychiatry* 1988;51:353–361.
44. Caselli RJ, Windebank A J, Petersen RC, et al. Rapidly progressive aphasic dementia and motor neuron disease. *Ann Neurol* 1993;33:200–207.
45. Gunnarsson L-G, Dahlbom K, Strandman E. Motor neuron disease and dementia reported among 13 members of a single family. *Acta Neurol Scand* 1991;84: 429–433.
46. Horoupian D, Thai L, Katzman R, et al. Dementia and motor neuron disease: morphometric, biochemical, and Golgi studies. *Ann Neurol* 1984;16:305–313.
47. Mitsuyama Y, Takamiya S. Presenile dementia with motor neuron disease in Japan. A new entity? *Arch Neurol* 1979;36:592–593.
48. Mitsuyama Y, Kogoh H, Ata K. Progressive dementia with motor neuron disease. An additional case report and neuropathological review of twenty cases in Japan. *Eur Arch Psychiatr Neurol Sci* 1985;235:1–8.
49. Salazar AM, Masters CL, Gajdusek DC, Gibbs CJ. Syndromes of amyotrophic lateral sclerosis and dementia: relation to transmissible Creutzfeldt-Jakob disease. *Ann Neurol* 1983;14:17–26.
50. Lippa CF, Cohen R, Smith TW, Drachman DA. Primary progressive aphasia with focal neuronal achromasia. *Neurology* 1991;41:882–886.
51. Holland AL, McBurney DH, Moossy J, Reinmuth OM. The dissolution of language in Pick's disease with neurofibrillary tangles: a case study. *Brain Lang* 1985;24: 36–58.
52. Weintraub S, Rubin NP, Mesulam MM. Primary progressive aphasia: longitudinal course, neuropsychological profile, and language features. *Arch Neurol* 1990; 47:1329–1335.
53. Mesulam MM. Primary progressive aphasia-differentiation from Alzheimer's disease. *Ann Neurol* 1987;22: 533–534.
54. Tyrrell PJ, Warrington EK, Frackowiak RS J, Rossor MN. Heterogeneity in progressive aphasia due to focal cortical atrophy. *Brain* 1990;113:1321–1336.
55. Heath PD, Kennedy P, Kapur N. Slowly progressive aphasia without generalized dementia. *Ann Neurol* 1983;13:687–688 (letter).
56. Hodges JR, Patterson K, Oxbury S, Funnell E. Semantic dementia: progressive fluent aphasia with temporal lobe atrophy. *Brain* 1992;115:1783–1806.
57. Poeck K, Luzzati C. Slowly progressive aphasia in three patients. *Brain* 1988;111:151–168.
58. Wechsler AF. Presenile dementia presenting as aphasia. *J Neurol* 1977;40:303–305.
59. Popagar S, Williams R. Alzheimer's disease presenting as slowly progressive aphasia. *Rhode Island Med J* 1984;67:181–185.
60. Mandell AM, Alexander MP, Carpenter S. Creutzfeldt-Jakob disease presenting as isolated aphasia. *Neurology* 1989;39:55–58.
61. Graff-Radford NR, Damasio AR, Hyman BT, et al. Progressive aphasia in a patient with Pick's disease:

a neuropsychologic, radiologic, and anatomic study. *Neurology* 1990;40: 620–626. *Neurosurg Psychiatry* 1977;40:303–305.
62. Luzzati C, Poeck K. An early description of slowly progressive aphasia. *Arch Neurol* 1991;48:228–229.
63. Basso A, Capitani E, Laiacona M. Progressive language impairment without dementia: a case with isolated category specific semantic defect. *J Neurol Neurosurg Psychiatry* 1988;51:1201–1207.
64. Sapin LR, Anderson FH, Pulaski PD. Progressive aphasia without dementia: further documentation. *Ann Neurol* 1989;25:411–413.
65. Chawluk JB, Mesulam MM, Hurtig H, et al. Slowly progressive aphasia without generalized dementia: studies with postron emission tomography. *Ann Neurol* 1986;19:68–74.
66. Kempler D, Metter E, Riege W, Jackson C, Benson DF, Hanson W. Slowly progressive aphasia: three cases with language, memory, CT and PET data. *J Neurol Neurosurg Psychiary* 1990;53:987–993.
67. Benson D, Zaias B. Progressive aphasia: a case with postmortem correlation. *Neuropsychiatry, Neuropsychol, Behav Neurol* 1991;4:215–223.
68. Kirshner HS, Webb WG, Kelly MP, Wells CE. Language disturbance: an initial symptom of cortical degenerations and dementia. *Arch Neurol* 1984;41:491–496.
69. Knopman DS, Christensen KJ, Schut LJ, Harbaugh RE, Reeder T, Ngo T, Frey W II. The spectrum of imaging and neuropsychological findings in Pick's disease. *Neurology* 1989;39:362–368.
70. Gustafson L. Frontal lobe degeneration of non-Alzheimer type. II. Clinical picture and differential diagnosis. *Arch Gerontol Geriatr* 1987;6:209–223.
71. Miller BL, Cummings JL, Villanueva-Meyer J, Boone K, Mehringer CM, Lesser IM, Mena I. Frontal lobe degeneration: clinical, neuropsychological, and SPECT characteristics. *Neurology* 1991;41:1374–1382.
72. Confavreux C, Croisile B, Garassus P, Aimard G, Trillet M. Progressive amusia and aprosody. *Arch Neurol* 1992;49:971–976.
73. Tissot R, Constantinidis J, Richard J. Pick's disease. In: Vinken P, Bruyn G, Klawans H, eds. *Handbook of clinical Neurology,* Vol. 46. Amsterdam: Elsevier, 1985: 233–246.
74. Baldwin B, Forsti H. "Pick's disease"—101 years on still there, but in need of reform. *Br J Psych* 1993;163: 100–104.
75. Mizukami K, Kosaka K. Neuropathological study and the nucleus basalis of Meynert in Pick's disease. *Acta Neuropathol* 1989;78:52–56.
76. Cambier J, Masson M, Dairou R, Henin D. Etude anatomo-clinique d'une forme parietale de maladie de Pick. *Rev Neurol* 1981;137:33–38.
77. Lang A, Bergeron C, Pollanen M, Ashby P. Parietal Pick's disease mimicking cortical-basal ganglionic degeneration. *Neurology* 1994;44:1436–1440.
78. Fisher CM. Pure spastic paralysis of corticospinal origin. *Can J Neurol Sci* 1977;4:251–258.
79. Beal MF, Richardson EP. Primary lateral sclerosis: a case report. *Arch Neurol* 1981;38:630–633.
80. Pringle CE, Hudson AJ, Munoz DG, Kiernan JA, Brown WF, Ebers GC. Primary lateral sclerosis: clinical features, neuropathology, and diagnostic criteria. *Brain* 1992;115:495–520.
81. Caselli RJ, Smith BE, Osborne D. Primary lateral sclerosis: a neuropsychological study. *Neurology* 1995; 45:2005–2009.
82. Bruyn RPM, Koelman JHTM, Troost D, de Jong JMBV. Motor neuron disease (amyotrophic lateral sclerosis) arising from longstanding primary lateral sclerosis. *J Neurol Neurosurg Psychiatry* 1995;58: 742–744.
83. Sodeyama N, Shimada M, Uchihara T, et al. Spastic tatraplegia as an initial manifestation of Alzheimer's disease. *J Neurol Neurosurg Psychiatry* 1995;59: 395–399.
84. Sacks O. *The Man Who Mistook His Wife for a Hat, and Other Clinical Tales.* New York: Harper Perennial, 1970.
85. Balint R. Seelenlahmung des "Schauens," optische Ataxie, raumliche Storung der Aufmerksamkeit. *Monatsscher Psychiat Neurol* 1909;25:51–81.
86. Levine DN, Lee JM, Fisher CM. The visual variant of Alzheimer's disease: a clinicopathologic case study. *Neurology* 1993;43:305–313.
87. DeRenzi E. Slowly progressive visual agnosia or apraxia without dementia. *Cortex* 1986;22:171–180.
88. Benson DF, Davis RJ, Snyder BD. Posterior cortical atrophy. *Arch Neurol* 1988;45:789–793.
89. Graff-Radford NR, Bolling JP, Earnest F IV, Shuster EA, Caselli RJ, Brazis PW. Simultanagnosia as the initial sign of degenerative dementia. *Mayo Clin Proc* 1993;68:955–964.
90. Tyrrell PJ, Warrington EK, Frackowiak RSJ, Rossor MN. Progressive degeneration of the right temporal lobe studied with positron emission tomography. *J Neurol Neurosurg Psychiatry* 1990;53:1046–1050.
91. Taylor A, Warrington EK. Visual agnosia: a single case report. *Cortex* 1971;7:152–161.
92. Evans JJ, Heggs AJ, Antoun N, Hodges JR. Progressive prosopagnosia associated with selective right temporal lobe atrophy: a new syndrome? *Brain* 1995; 118:1–13.
93. Hof PR, Bouras C, Constantinidis J, Morrison JH. Balint's syndrome in Alzheimer's disease: specific disruption of the occipito-parietal visual pathway. *Brain Res* 1989;493:368–375.
94. Gibb W, Luthert P, Marsden CD. Corticobasal degeneration. *Brain* 1989;112:1171–1192.
95. Riley DE, Lane AE, Lewis A, et al. Cortical-basal ganglionic degeneration. *Neurology* 1990;40:1203–1212.
96. Rebeiz JJ, Kolodny EH, Richardson EP Jr. Corticodentatonigral degeneration with neuronal achromasia: a progressive disorder of late adult life. *Trans Am Neurol Assoc* 1967;92:23–26.
97. Jagust W, Davies P, Tiller-Borcich J, Reed B. Focal Alzheimer's disease. *Neurology* 1990;40:14–19.
98. Gibb W, Luthert P, Marsden C. Clinical and pathologic features of corticobasal degeneration. In: Streifler M, Korczyn A, Melamed E, Youdim M, eds. *Parkinson's disease: anatomy, pathology, and therapy,* Vol. 53. New York: Raven, 1990:51–54.
99. Crystal HA, Horoupian DS, Katzman R, Jotkowitz S. Biopsy-proved Alzheimer disease presenting as a right parietal syndrome. *Ann Neurol* 1982;12:186–188.
100. Caselli RJ. Memory disorders in degenerative neurological diseases. In: Yanagihara T, Petersen RC, eds.

Memory disorders: research and clinical practice. New York, Marcel-Dekker, 1991:369–396.

101. Alajouanine T. Aphasia and artistic realization. *Brain* 1948;71:229–241.
102. Doran M, Xuereb J, Hodges JR. Rapidly progressive aphasia with bulbar motor neurone disease: a clinical and neuropsychological study. *Behav Neurol* 1995;8: 169–180.
103. Brion S, Mikol J, Psimaras A. Recent findings in Pick's disease. *Prog Neuropathol* 1973;2:421–452.
104. Brion S, Psimaras A, Chevalier JF, Plas J, Masse G, Jatteau O. L'association maladie de Pick et sclerose laterale amyotrophique. *L'Encephale* 1980;6:259–286.
105. Ferrer I, Roig C, Espino A, Pelto G, Guiu XM. Dementia of the frontal lobe type and motor neuron disease. A Golgi study of the frontal cortex. *J Neurol Neurosurg Psychiatry* 1991;54:932–934.
106. Dickson DW, Horoupian DS, Thai LJ, Davies P, Walkley S, Terry RD. Kluver-Bucy syndrome and amyotrophic lateral sclerosis: a case report with biochemistry, morphometrics, and Golgi study. *Neurology* 1986;36:1323–1329.
107. Sano M, Ernesto C, Thomas RG, et al. A controlled trial of selegeline, alpha-tocopherol, or both as treatment for Alzheimer's disease. *N Engl J Med* 1997;336: 1216–1222.
108. McGeer PL, Rogers J. Anti-inflammatory agents as a therapeutic approach to Alzheimer's disease. *Neurology* 1992;42:447–449.
109. Rogers J, Kirby LC, Hempelman SR, et al. Clinical trial of indomethacin in Alzheimer's disease. *Neurology* 1993; 43:1609–1611.
110. Breitner JCS, Gau BA, Welsh KA, et al. Inverse association of anti-inflammatory treatments and Alzheimer's disease: initial results of a co-twin control study. *Neurology* 1994;44:227–232.
111. Tang MX, Jacobs D, Stern Y, et al. Effect of oestrogen during menopause on risk and age at onset of Alzheimer's disease. *Lancet* 1996;348:429–432.
112. Yaffe K, Sawaya G, Lieberburg I, Grady D. Estrogen therapy in postmenopausal women: effects on cognitive function and dementia. *JAMA* 1998;279:688–695.
113. Farlow M, Gracon SI, Hershey LA, et al. for the Tacrine Study Group. A controlled trial of tacrine in Alzheimer's disease. *JAMA* 1992;268:2523–2529.
114. Knapp MJ, Knopman DS, Solomon PR, et al. SI for the Tacrine Study Group. A 30-week randomized controlled trial of high dose tacrine in patients with Alzheimer's disease. *JAMA* 1994;271:985–991.
115. Kompoliti K, Goetz CG, Boeve BF, et al. Clinical presentation and pharmacological therapy in corticobasal degeneration. *Arch Neurol* 1998;55:957–961.

Corticobasal Degeneration.
Advances in Neurology, Vol. 82,
edited by I. Litvan, C. G. Goetz, and A. E. Lang.
Lippincott Williams & Wilkins, Philadelphia © 2000.

5

Epidemiologic Aspects

Daniel M. Togasaki* and Caroline M. Tanner†

†*Department of Clinical Research,* *†*The Parkinson's Institute, Sunnyvale, California 94089-1605*

INTRODUCTION

Corticobasal degeneration (CBD) is a rare disorder that was first described by Rebeiz and colleagues (1,2). It did not become widely recognized until after 1985, when a clinicopathologic correlation case was published in the *New England Journal of Medicine* (3). Although awareness of the disease has increased, it is rarely diagnosed. The diagnostic criteria for CBD have not been completely defined, leading to difficulties for characterization of the disorder and epidemiologic study. This chapter will attempt to describe what little is known about the epidemiology of CBD and provide examples of some of the pitfalls of attempting further characterization in view of the extent of unknown information.

BASICS OF EPIDEMIOLOGY

Epidemiologic analysis is an important component of the study of disease. Parkinson's disease has been subjected to study, but other parkinsonian syndromes, such as CBD, have been more difficult to examine, generally because of the much smaller number of cases available in the population. Nevertheless, elucidation of the etiology and risk factors for the development of these syndromes will benefit from epidemiologic study.

Some basic terms used in epidemiology are defined in Table 1. Some of the calculations used for characterization of diagnostic tests are illustrated in Table 2.

DIAGNOSIS OF CBD

The definition of the clinical syndrome of CBD is still evolving. Ideally, the complete and accurate characterization of the clinical syndrome is contingent on diagnosing all subjects who have the disease and excluding subjects who do not. The apparent rareness of the disease makes it a formidable task to accumulate a sufficient number of cases to analyze and obtain meaningful results, as well as making it difficult for physicians to gain familiarity with and to recognize the syndrome.

The basic clinical descriptions and pathologic findings were initially published by Rebeiz (2), and were subsequently used to diagnose other patients. The classic presentation is as an akinetic-rigid syndrome that responds poorly to L-dopa coupled with focal, and usually asymmetric, cortical deficits (i.e., apraxia, alien limb, cortical sensory deficits). Later patient series often did not include pathologic confirmation for the vast majority of the cases (4,5). Other studies, which have included pathologic examination, have indicated that the classic symptomatology is associated with the classic pathologic features, including degenerating achromatic neurons and asymmetric frontoparietal cortical atrophy (6–8).

There is, however, a great deal of overlap between CBD and other clinical syndromes. This makes it problematic for even experienced movement disorder specialists to make an accurate diagnosis. One of the authors (DMT) has participated in a clinicopathologic conference with 10 other movement disorder specialists in which the consensus diagnosis was CBD, but the pathologic

TABLE 1. *Basic terminology used in epidemiology*

Term	Definition
Epidemiology	The study of the distribution of disease in populations
Incidence	The number of people in a population who newly develop the disease of interest within a given period of time (usually per year)
Incidence rate	The incidence per unit of population (usually per 100,000)
Prevalence	The number of people in a population who have the disease of interest at a given point in time
Prevalence rate	The prevalence per unit of population (usually per 100,000)
Odds ratio	The risk that a person with a specific risk factor will develop the disease of interest divided by the risk for a person without the factor
Bias	Any systematic flaw in an epidemiologic study that results in an erroneous estimation of an outcome parameter
Sensitivity	The ability of a test to identify persons who have the disease of interest
Specificity	The ability of a test to exclude persons who do not have the disease of interest
Positive predictive value	The ability of a positive result on a test to identify those who have the disease of interest (true positives)
Negative predictive value	The ability of a negative result on a test to identify those who do not have the disease of interest (true negatives)
Population-based study	An epidemiologic study that evaluates all members of a population using predefined methods. The population can be defined by geographic or political boundaries (a community), or by other parameters (such as patients at a medical clinic)
Case-control study	An epidemiologic study that compares persons with a disease to unaffected persons who are otherwise similar (usually a retrospective study)
Cohort study	An epidemiologic study that follows a group of persons over time and monitors them for the development of the disease and for the presence of putative risk factors (usually a prospective study)

diagnosis turned out to be Alzheimer's disease. In one study, among nine patients who fulfilled a set of diagnostic clinical criteria for CBD, to varying degrees (four were "clinically possible," three were "clinically probable," and two were "clinically definite," as defined by the authors), and later underwent postmortem examination, only one was diagnosed as having CBD at pathologic examination (9).

Litvan and colleagues (10) investigated the validity of the clinical diagnosis of CBD in determining the presence of the characteristic pathology. The case histories of 105 patients pathologically diagnosed with progressive supranuclear palsy (PSP), Lewy body disease, CBD, and other Parkinsonian disorders, were presented to a group of neurologists trained in movement disorders who then provided clinical diagnoses. Of the patients who had CBD, 35% were clinically diagnosed based on their history and physical examination findings early in the disease, and 48.3% were diagnosed when information was included from later in their course. For the patients who did not have CBD pathologically, 99.6% did not receive a diagnosis of CBD, both early and late in their course. This meant that most of the patients with pathologic diagnosis were not detected by clinical examination, but that almost all of the patients without CBD on pathologic examination were excluded from a diagnosis of CBD clinically.

These results suggest that even clinicians trained to recognize CBD have difficulty with diagnostic accuracy. The study by Litvan and colleagues (10) suggests that many, if not most, of CBD cases are missed by clinical diagnosis, which could bias the characterization of the disease by only including a subset of the patients.

TABLE 2. *Calculations used for characterization of diagnostic tests*

	Disease	No disease
Testing Positive	A	B
Testing Negative	C	D

Sensitivity = A ÷ (A + C); Specificity = D ÷ (D + B); Positive predictive value = A ÷ (A + B); Negative predictive value = D ÷ (C + D).

Other diseases have also been misdiagnosed as CBD, including Alzheimer's disease, progressive supranuclear palsy, Pick's disease, Parkinson's disease, multiple system atrophy, and Lewy body dementia (11,12). Any study trying to characterize CBD requires pathologic confirmation of all cases, so patients with other diagnoses are not included; that could invalidate any conclusions about demographics or risks.

It has been suggested that over half of the pathologically diagnosed cases of CBD would not even have been considered for clinical evaluation because they do not present with the "classic" symptomatology (which includes a movement disorder), but rather present primarily with dementia (13). It seems this has, in fact, occurred and that the clinical syndrome of CBD has been mischaracterized by the inclusion of only a subset of patients, having ignored all those who deviated from the initial description. The consensus clinical criteria for the diagnosis of CBD likely will need to be expanded.

To make matters even more complicated, the pathologic features of CBD have considerable overlap with other disorders, especially Pick's disease and PSP (14–16). This situation confuses things further, as pathologic diagnosis has been the "gold standard" for defining CBD. Recently, a series of commentaries was published discussing whether frontotemporal degeneration, Pick's disease, and CBD are one entity or three (17–19). Kertesz and colleagues (20) have suggested using the term Pick complex to lump these three diagnoses together, both clinically and pathologically. If this is the case, then the disease CBD does not have a definitive diagnostic feature. Making the diagnosis for CBD would be muddled, with uncertainty for both the clinical and pathologic criteria.

Despite this controversy, pathologic criteria might be diagnostically definitive. It has been reported that CBD is distinctive in its distribution of tau-immunoreactive inclusions in the distal processes of astrocytes, which would allow differentiation from the other syndromes mentioned in the preceding paragraph (14). Further confirmation will be needed, but if this holds up, there may be a need for additional staining of tissue to detect the distribution of tau for all cases in epidemiologic studies of CBD.

DESCRIPTIVE EPIDEMIOLOGY OF CBD

The descriptive epidemiology of CBD is derived entirely from case reports and case series from specialized movement disorders clinics. No community-based series have been published. Approximately 100 cases have been reported, although most do not have pathologic confirmation.

There are some problems with using such results to generalize to the characteristics of CBD in the population-at-large. There is a large bias in referrals to specialized clinics and tertiary care centers. More problematic cases of parkinsonism (usually meaning those that are more difficult to diagnose or treat), are referred more often than those that are straightforward (such as idiopathic Parkinson's disease). Because such clinics often require traveling to a distant location, the patients who are seen have to be able to afford and tolerate the trip. This often leads to a bias favoring patients who are less severely ill, are better off economically, or are living in urban areas where there is a greater likelihood that such centers are easily accessible. Having the knowledge to request referral for more specialized care also favors the more informed patient (which could reflect more education or greater access to medical information). In addition, as was described in more detail previously, the specialization of a clinic for movement disorders adds an additional bias in that a specific group of patients is examined, possibly excluding others whose disease is not clinically dominated by a movement disorder. The interaction of these biases does not lead to an easy assessment regarding whether the percentage of patients in these specialized settings leads to an overestimation or an underestimation of the number of CBD patients in the general population.

With these considerations in mind, we have summarized the available information in the following.

Age of Onset

The age of onset for the reported cases of CBD is late adulthood. One study reported onset at 63 ± 7.7 (mean ± SD) years of age (8). The youngest reported clinically diagnosed case is 40 (5), and 45 for a pathologically diagnosed case (8).

The symptoms progressively worsen as more areas of the brain become affected. Death usually occurs 5 to 10 years (7.9 ± 2.6) after onset (8).

Incidence and Prevalence

The incidence and prevalence of CBD is unknown, although it would undoubtedly qualify as an orphan disease, which is one having a prevalence in the United States of 200,000 or less. There have been no population-based studies investigating the extent of CBD in the community, as it is such a rare disorder. Most publications describe one or a few cases, or have been a series of cases from a movement disorders clinic collected over a number of years. One large movement disorders clinic has reported that CBD constitutes 0.9% of the patients with parkinsonism (18 of 2052) (21). For comparison, that same series reported 77.7% of the parkinsonian patients had Parkinson's disease (1595 of 2052).

Using the information summarized herein, we have attempted to estimate the incidence and prevalence of CBD in the general population. We stress that the accuracy of these calculations is dependent on the questionable validity of several assumptions that were necessary, as indicated in the following.

First, let us assume that CBD constitutes approximately 1% of the patients with parkinsonism seen at a movement disorders clinic. This number is probably an overestimation of the number for the general population of parkinsonian patients, since CBD is more likely to be referred to a specialized clinic. Second, assume that all patients with CBD manifest symptoms of either parkinsonism or (focal) cortical dysfunction or both, and that patients with parkinsonism constitute approximately one-half of the total. These are very crude estimates projected from a constrictingly limited amount of data, but are the best we can provide without additional studies.

Using those assumptions as a starting point, incorporating some of the information discussed previously regarding diagnosis, the following calculations can be performed. Of those patients at a movement disorders clinic who have parkinsonism, approximately 1% will have a clinical diagnosis of CBD. Clinically diagnosing CBD may miss one-half to two-thirds of the parkinsonian patients who would be diagnosed at postmortem examination (2% to 3%). Parkinsonian patients with CBD may underestimate the total number of CBD patients by one-half again (4% to 6%). This suggests that the number of people who will develop CBD in the population is about 4% to 6% of the number of those with parkinsonism. If the number of Parkinson's disease patients at the same movement disorders clinic is 78% of those with parkinsonism, then the number of patients who will develop CBD is 5.1% to 7.7% of the number of patients who will develop Parkinson's disease. This number would reflect the incidence rate of CBD in comparison with the incidence rate of Parkinson's disease. If the incidence rate of Parkinson's disease in the community is 12/100,000 each year (median value of studies reviewed in [22]), then the incidence rate of CBD would be 0.62/100,000 to 0.92/100,000 each year. Given that the duration of CBD is 7.9 years, the prevalence rate would be 4.9/100,000 to 7.3/100,000. If the prevalence rate for Parkinson's disease is 110/100,000 (median value of studies reviewed in [22]), then the prevalence rate of CBD would be 4.4% to 7.3% of that. Finally, if the population of the United States is 271,000,000 (23), then the number of persons with CBD would be 13,000 to 20,000.

The difficulties with the clinical diagnosis of CBD are highlighted by the study of Litvan and colleagues (10). If the clinical diagnosis is the screening test and the pathologic diagnosis is the definitive test, the reported sensitivity (35.0%) and specificity (99.6%) can be applied to calculate some practical numbers. Of 2000 patients with parkinsonism, if 2.5% of them have CBD by pathologic examination, there will be 50 with CBD. Clinical examination will identify 18 of these 50 (35%), but miss 32 (50 − 18 = 32). Of the 1950 remaining patients (without CBD pathologically), 1942 (99.6%) will be excluded from a diagnosis of CBD by clinical examination, but 8 (1950 − 1942 = 8) will be misidentified as having the disease. Thus, clinical diagnosis will correctly identify 18 cases, but will incorrectly identify eight cases that do not have the disease. In addition, 32 cases will be missed. Under these circumstances, the positive predictive value of a clinical diagnosis would be 69.2%, and the negative predictive value would be 98.4% (Table 3). The values for positive and negative predictive values will vary markedly from these numbers for populations that have a different overall prevalence of CBD.

In addition, because the diagnosis of CBD is based on the clinical syndrome, it is problematic to determine the accuracy of the numbers from any clinic because of the possibility of misdiagnosis, unless there has been confirmation at autopsy for each case, which is difficult to obtain. Death occurs a number of years after onset, necessitating long-term follow-up of the patients, who often have little incentive to return to a distant specialized clinic because there is no effective therapy. (They may have a minimal response to L-dopa, and are usually aggressively treated with antiparkinsonian medications despite poor alleviation of the symptoms.)

Risk Factors

Nothing is known about the etiology of the disease. There are no known risk factors for CBD, aside, possibly, from onset at older ages. It is possible that it may be harder to identify persons with CBD who are younger or older.

There is no clear gender preponderance and no clear ethnic preponderance. Essentially all of the published cases have been from North America, Europe, Australia, and Japan. This could reflect a true geographic or ethnic preponderance, or it could be due to physician awareness or a bias regarding publishing in the medical literature.

There is some suggestion that there may be a genetic factor in some of the cases, but the evidence is not strong. There is one family in which two brothers were diagnosed with CBD, but there is no pathologic confirmation (24). Two families with familial dementia were found to have pathologic changes consistent with CBD, but the clinical expression was not typical for CBD, and the syndrome was felt to be consistent with Pick's disease (25). The family of one other patient (from the original three cases) had several members that may have had degenerative neurologic disorders, but they were not examined, and their symptoms were poorly characterized (1). A pair of monozygotic twins, one of whom had clinical CBD, were discordant for the syndrome for at least seven years after diagnosis (26).

TABLE 3. *Positive and negative predictive values of clinical diagnosis of CBD*

	CBD by pathology	No CBD by pathology
Clinically CBD	18	8
Clinically No CBD	32	1942

Sensitivity = 18 ÷ (18 + 32) = 35%; Specificity = 1942 ÷ (1942 + 8) = 99.6%; Positive predictive value = 18 ÷ (18 + 8) = 69.2%; Negative predictive value = 1942 ÷ (32 + 1942) = 98.4%.

It is evident that not enough information is available yet to determine any risk factors for CBD. Determination of such risks will be a difficult and arduous task given the need for pathologic confirmation of the diagnosis, at which point the patient is unavailable for filling out questionnaires.

FUTURE EPIDEMIOLOGIC STUDY

As can be seen from this discussion, there is a great need for a specific and definitive diagnostic test for CBD. Clinical examination is not a useful diagnostic test, given its poor sensitivity, in conjunction with the rarity of the disease. Pathologic examination appears to be the definitive test, but it has limited utility for prospective studies, as one would need to include all potential subjects, and then eliminate those that do not meet criteria postmortem. A biomarker for CBD would be optimal, but such a test does not yet exist. This needs to be an area for further research. There has been little urgency motivating the development of a diagnostic test, as there is no useful therapy that can take advantage of antemortem diagnosis (27). The lack of useful therapies for CBD also precludes the ability to use a therapeutic trial as a diagnostic tool.

With a reliable diagnostic test, full characterization of the disease would be possible. The ability to accurately determine the clinical hallmarks of CBD requires the collection of a sufficiently large number of cases for analysis. It would also require that the cases be collected in an unbiased manner, meaning that they are representative of the population-at-large. The most unbiased method would be to screen all members of the population, or a randomly selected subset of the population. Given the low prevalence of CBD, the number of persons screened would pose a prohibitive obstacle (if the prevalence is 5 per 100,000, finding 50 persons with CBD requires screening 1,000,000). Using various criteria to preselect a subset of the population with a higher prevalence of CBD (a higher risk for developing CBD) would introduce bias that could affect the conclusions. For example, limiting the testing to persons older than 50 would have a higher yield, but would systematically exclude anyone who developed CBD at an earlier age, predetermining the conclusion that the disease only occurs in the elderly.

Assuming the diagnostic criteria can be settled, the next step would be investigation of the risk factors for the disease and attempts to determine its etiology. Such studies would use the tools of analytic epidemiology.

The most valid method for investigating risk factors is to use a population-based approach. In such a study, a group of persons is selected using unbiased methods, surveyed for a number of possible risk factors, and then monitored over time for the development of CBD. Information about additional risk factors can be included as monitoring progresses. For the same reason mentioned, however, this approach is logistically unfeasible for CBD, as well as for other rare diseases.

An investigation of risk factors for CBD would undoubtedly use a retrospective case-control design. A group of persons with the disease are compared with another group who do not have the disease, but have been matched in other ways (i.e., same age), and the presence or absence of possible risk factors is determined. This obviates the problem of having to examine and monitor a huge number of subjects, because no one is included unless he/she has been diagnosed previously with CBD (or he/she is a matched control). This approach faces the difficulty that a person's history with regard to a putative risk factor may not be available. Retrospective studies also are complicated by recall bias: Subjects with a disease are more likely to have searched their memory for potential risk factors, and are thus more likely to recall their presence than a normal subject.

CBD Registry

One approach to studying this disease would be the establishment of a registry for CBD, which would allow for the collection of cases from many different centers. This would likely be the only feasible way to accumulate sufficient cases for meaningful epidemiologic analyses. Before such a registry could be formed, however, diagnostic criteria would need to be finalized.

General features of such a registry would include enrollment by physician referral or by patient self-referral (i.e., over the Internet). Hopefully, the referral centers would include international representation, allowing for some degree of ethnic and geographic diversity. Information contained in such a registry for each enrollee would include clinical description, videotape recordings of the neurologic examination, names of persons available for future contact, and a form consenting to brain donation.

CONCLUDING REMARKS

The evolution of our understanding of CBD highlights the necessity of thorough examination of the clinical, pathologic, and diagnostic features of any disease. As our understanding has advanced, the number of disease entities diagnosed as, or related to, CBD has expanded. Current studies still are refining the diagnostic criteria for CBD. Learning the etiology of this disease will require identification of risk factors, an investigation that necessitates good epidemiologic study.

REFERENCES

1. Rebeiz JJ, Kolodny EH, Richardson EP. Corticodentatonigral degeneration with neuronal achromasia. *Arch Neurol* 1968;18:20–33.
2. Rebeiz JJ, Kolodny EH, Richardson EP. Corticodentatonigral degeneration with neuronal achromasia: a progressive disorder of late adult life. *Trans Am Neurol Assoc* 1967;92:23–26.
3. Case records of the Massachusetts General Hospital: Case 38-1985: case of corticonigral degeneration with neuronal achromasia. *N Engl J Med* 1985;313:739–748.

4. Riley DE, Lang AE, Lewis A, et al. Cortical-basal ganglionic degeneration. *Neurology* 1990;40:1203–1212.
5. Rinne JO, Lee MS, Thompson PD, Marsden CD. Corticobasal degeneration: a clinical study of 36 cases. *Brain* 1994;117:1183–1196.
6. Gibb WRG, Luthert PJ, Marsden CD. Clinical and pathological features of corticobasal degeneration. In: Streifler MD, Korczyn AD, Melamed E, Youdim MBH, eds. *Advances in neurology,* Vol. 53. New York: Raven Press, 1990: 51–54.
7. Lippa CF, Smith TW, Fontneau N. Corticonigral degeneration with neuronal achromasia: a clinicopathologic study of two cases. *J Neurol Sci* 1990;98:301–310.
8. Wenning GK, Litvan I, Jankovic J, Granata R, Maugome CA, McKee A, et al. Natural history and survival of 14 patients with corticobasal degeneration confirmed at postmortem examination. *J Neurol Neurosurg Psychiatry* 1998;64:184–189.
9. Boeve BF, Maraganore DM, Parisi JE, et al. Disorders mimicking the "classical" clinical syndrome of corticobasal ganglionic degeneration: report of nine cases. *Movement Disorders* 1996;11:351 (abst).
10. Litvan I, Agid Y, Goetz C, Jankovic J, Wenning GK, Brandel JP, et al. Accuracy of the clinical diagnosis of corticobasal degeneration: a clinicopathologic study. *Neurology* 1997;48:119–125.
11. Watts RL, Brewer RP, Schneider JA, Mirra SS. In: Watts RL, Koller WC, eds. *Movement disorders: neurologic principles and practice.* New York: McGraw-Hill; 1977: 611–621.
12. Kumar R, Bergeron C, Pollanen MS, Lang AE. In: Jankovic J, Tolosa E, eds. *Parkinson's disease and movement disorders, third edition.* Philadelphia: Williams & Wilkins, 1998:297–316.
13. Bergeron C, Pollanen MS, Weyer L, Black SE, Lang AE. Unusual clinical presentations of cortical-basal ganglionic degeneration. *Ann Neurol* 1996;40:893–900.
14. Feany MB, Mattiace LA, Dickson DW. Neuropathologic overlap of progressive supranuclear palsy, Pick's disease and corticobasal degeneration. *J Neuropathol Exp Neurol* 1996;55:53–67.
15. Jendroska K, Rossor MN, Mathias CJ, Daniel SE. Morphological overlap between corticobasal degeneration and Pick's disease: a clinicopathological report. *Mov Disord* 1995;10:111–114.
16. Schneider JA, Watts RL, Gearing M, Brewer RP, Mirra SS. Corticobasal degeneration: neuropathologic and clinical heterogeneity. *Neurology* 1997;48:959–969.
17. Nerary D. Frontotemporal dementia, Pick disease, and corticobasal degeneration: one entity or 3? 3. *Arch Neurol* 1997;54:1425–1427.
18. Kertesz A. Frontotemporal dementia, Pick disease, and corticobasal degeneration: one entity or 3? 1. *Arch Neurol* 1997;54:1427–1429.
19. Hachinski V. Frontotemporal dementia, Pick disease, and corticobasal degeneration: one entity or 3? *Arch Neurol* 1997;54–1429.
20. Kertesz A, Hudson L, Mackenzie IRA, Munoz DG. The pathology and nosology of primary progressive aphasia. Neurology 1994;44:2065–2072.
21. Stacy M, Jankovic J. Differential diagnosis of Parkinson's disease and the parkinsonism plus syndromes. *Neurol Clin* 1992;10:341–359.
22. Tanner CM, Hubble JP, Chan P. Epidemiology and genetics of Parkinson's disease. In: Watts RL, Koller WC, eds. *Movement disorders: neurologic principles and practice.* New York: McGraw-Hill, 1977:137–152.
23. United States Census Bureau, Population Division. Estimated as of November 1998.
24. Verin M, Rancurel G, De Marco O, Edan G. First familial cases of corticobasal degeneration. *Mov Disord* 1997;12(suppl 1):55 (abst).
25. Brown J, Lantos PL, Roques P, Fidani L, Rossor MN. Familial dementia with swollen achromatic neurons and corticobasal inclusion bodies: a clinical and pathological study. *J Neurol Sci* 1996;135:21–30.
26. Caselli RJ, Reiman EM, Timmann D, et al. Progressive apraxia in clinically discordant monozygotic twins. *Arch Neurol* 1995;52:1004–1010.
27. Kompoliti K, Goetz CG, Boeve BF, Maraganore DM, Ahlskog JE, Marsden CD, et al. Clinical presentation and pharmacogical therapy in corticobasal degeneration. *Arch Neurol* 1998;55:957–961.

Corticobasal Degeneration.
Advances in Neurology, Vol. 82,
edited by I. Litvan, C. G. Goetz, and A. E. Lang.
Lippincott Williams & Wilkins, Philadelphia © 2000.

6

Dystonia in Corticobasal Degeneration

Zeba Fatima Vanek* and Joseph Jankovic†

**Department of Neurology, University of California, Los Angeles, Los Angeles, California 90095-1769; and*
†Department of Neurology, Baylor College of Medicine, Houston, Texas 77030

INTRODUCTION

Although dystonia is commonly associated with corticobasal degeneration (CBD), the true frequency, nature, and extent of dystonic manifestations in CBD have not been well documented. Furthermore, some of the clinical observations on dystonic manifestations in CBD are either incomplete or not supported by postmortem confirmation of the diagnosis. In this chapter we present the available evidence for the nature, distribution, and frequency of dystonic features in CBD, based on the literature and our own database.

DIAGNOSTIC CRITERIA

The clinical diagnostic criteria for CBD, based on pathological confirmation, include: (a) chronic progressive course; (b) asymmetry at onset; (c) higher cortical dysfunction in the form of apraxia, cortical sensory dysfunction, or alien limb; and (d) movement disorders in the form of dystonia, myoclonus, with an akinetic-rigid syndrome resistant to L-dopa (1). Dystonia is defined as a syndrome of involuntary movements dominated by sustained muscle contractions causing twisting and repetitive movements or abnormal postures (2).

DEMOGRAPHICS

The small series of CBD cases reported in the literature describe the clinical characteristics in the patient population as a whole without distinguishing between the cases with or without dystonia. In our series of 66 patients with CBD evaluated over a 10-year period between 1988 and 1998, there were 44 (66.7%) women, with a female to male ratio of 2:1. Of the 39 patients with dystonia, there were 27 (69.2%) women, and of the 27 patients without dystonia, 17 (63%) were women. Similar to observations in the literature, the majority of our patients were Caucasians (92.4%) of Irish-Scottish-English descent (41%). The age at onset of CBD symptoms in our series ranged from 44 to 76 years (mean 64.7), which was similar to most reports in the literature (3,4). We did not find a statistically significant difference in the age at symptom onset between patients with and without dystonia (64.0 years vs. 65.4 years) or the duration of symptoms to the time of evaluation (4.2 years, range: 6 months to 12 years vs. 3 years, range: 1 to 6 years). It was not always possible to accurately differentiate historically the onset of dystonia from the onset of various other features of CBD.

EPIDEMIOLOGY

There have been no large epidemiological studies addressing the incidence or prevalence of CBD in general, or dystonia in CBD, in particular (5). Current data on clinical features of CBD is largely based on small autopsy series from movement disorder clinics rather than from population-based studies (6). In most such series, the occurrence or description of dystonia is either mentioned very briefly, or omitted altogether. In the earliest reports, dystonia was first mentioned in association with CBD in the initial description by Rebeiz (7). Since that time, the frequency of dystonia in CBD in most clinical series has been reported to range between 43% and 83% (3,7–16) (Table 1). Kompoliti et al. (17) reported the clinical presentation and treatment outcome of 147 patients from multiple centers diagnosed with CBD by movement disorders experts with no predetermined diagnostic criteria. In this retrospective meta-analysis, dystonia was found in 105 (71%) patients, seven of whom had autopsy confirmation of the diagnosis. In the largest series of pathologically established CBD cases, dystonia was found in seven of 14 (50%) of the patients (3).

We recently reviewed the clinical features in 66 patients with CBD evaluated at our center; four of the cases were pathologically proven (18). The presence and characteristics of dystonia were verified by a review of the medical records and videotapes. In this series of 66 CBD patients, 39 (59%) had at least one dystonic feature sometime during their illness.

CLINICAL FEATURES

The commonest initial symptom reported by patients with CBD is an asymmetric, progressive clumsiness and difficulty using one limb, usually an arm (3,6,16,17). In our series, 59 (89.4%) patients had onset of symptoms in one limb, with difficulty using one arm in 35 (53%). There is no information on the differences between the occurrence of associated features such as apraxia, higher cortical dysfunction, alien limb, and the various movement disorders in patients with and without dystonia. Although in our series alien limb phenomenon and dysphagia were more frequent in patients with dystonia, and tremor and depression were more common in patients without dystonia, no characteristic pattern predictive of associated dystonia emerged from the analysis of our database.

CHARACTERISTICS OF DYSTONIA IN CBD

Nearly all reports on CBD note the presence of dystonia, but detailed characterization of the dystonic features is lacking. In our series of 66 CBD patients we specifically focused on dystonia. Of the four cases of CBD whose diagnosis was confirmed by a postmortem examination, three had dystonia during the course of their illness. Accurate information on the onset of dystonia, in relation to the onset of the other manifestations of the disease was not always available in the literature nor in our series, but all patients had documentation about dystonia before the initiation of L-dopa or other dopaminergic therapy. There was no family history of a disorder resembling CBD, although six (15.4%) patients gave a history of a family member with a parkinsonian disorder. Six patients (15.3%) out of the 39 cases of

TABLE 1. *Frequency of dystonia in published series*

Authors	Number of patients in series, *N*	Patients with dystonia, *N* (%)	Distribution of dystonia
Rebeiz et al. (1968) (7), Watts et al. (1985) (8), Greene et al. (1990) (11), Lippa et al. (1990) (12), Paulus et al. (1990) (13), Riley et al. (1990) (14)	28	13 (46.4)	Limb
Obeso et al. (1985) (9), Gibb et al. (1989) (10), Sawle et al. (1991) (15), Rinne et al. (1994) (16),	36	30 (83.3)	Arm
Wenning et al. (1998) (3)	14	7 (50.0)	Limb: 6 (86%) Neck: 1 (14%)
Kompoliti et al. (1998) (17) (a multicenter study),	147	105 (71.4)	Not specified
Vanek and Jankovic (1999) (18)	66	39 (59.1)	Arm: 36 (92%) Leg: 11 (28%) Head, axial: 12 (31%)

CBD with dystonia gave a history of an antecedent event such as trauma or a transient ischemic attack, a few days to a year before the onset of their symptoms. The pathophysiological significance of these antecedent events, however, is not known.

Limb Dystonia

Most clinical and pathological series of CBD patients report limb dystonia to be the commonest dystonic manifestation. Rinne et al. (16) found early asymmetric limb dystonia in 12 of 30 (40%) patients, and subsequent fixed dystonic posturing of all limbs in 25 of 30 (83%) patients. Earlier cases reported by Rebeiz et al. (7) and later by Watts et al. (8), Greene et al. (11), Lippa et al. (12), and Riley et al. (14) reported the occurrence of limb dystonia in 43% to 83% of cases. In the 14 autopsy-confirmed cases of CBD reported by Wenning et al. (3), 43% of the patients had unilateral limb dystonia during their initial visit, with all evolving into an akinetic-rigid state before death (Table 1). None of the reported series, however, provide a detailed description of the dystonia.

One or more limb involvement was also the most common site for dystonia in our CBD population. Of the 39 patients with dystonia, 37 (95%) patients had dystonia affecting one or more limbs, with an arm affected in 36 (92%) patients. Although 11 (28%) patients developed leg dystonia, in only one patient, the leg was the predominant site of involvement. Three (8%) patients had dystonia in all four limbs.

The typical dystonic posture in our series consisted of the affected arm adducted at the shoulder, the elbows and wrists flexed and the arm extending in front or behind the body, with the dystonia becoming more pronounced while walking. The fingers were typically flexed at the metacarpophalangeal (MCP) joints, extended or flexed at the proximal interphalangeal (PIP) and distal interphalangeal (DIP) joints, exhibiting variable degrees of fixed postures, with or without associated contractures (Fig. 1). Overall, 17 (44%) cases exhibited adduction of the arm at the shoulder, 25 (64%) cases had flexion at the elbow, 20 (51%) flexion at the wrist, and 18 (46%) flexion at the MCP joint. Seven (18%) patients also had the thumb, index and middle fingers extended, and the fourth and fifth fingers flexed. In more advanced stages of the disease, some patients have developed more extended, rigid postures (Fig. 2).

Eleven (28%) patients in our series had foot or leg dystonia. Of these, seven (18%) had unilateral leg involvement, and four (10%) had dystonia in both legs. In only one patient, the leg was predominantly affected by the dystonia, and in all other patients the dystonia affected the arm

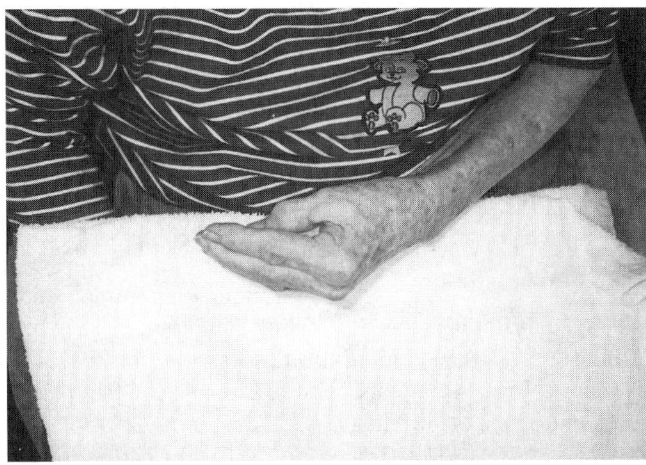

FIG. 1. Left-hand dystonic posture in a 77-year-old woman with moderately advanced CBD. The same hand also exhibited marked apraxia, involuntary grasp, and myoclonus.

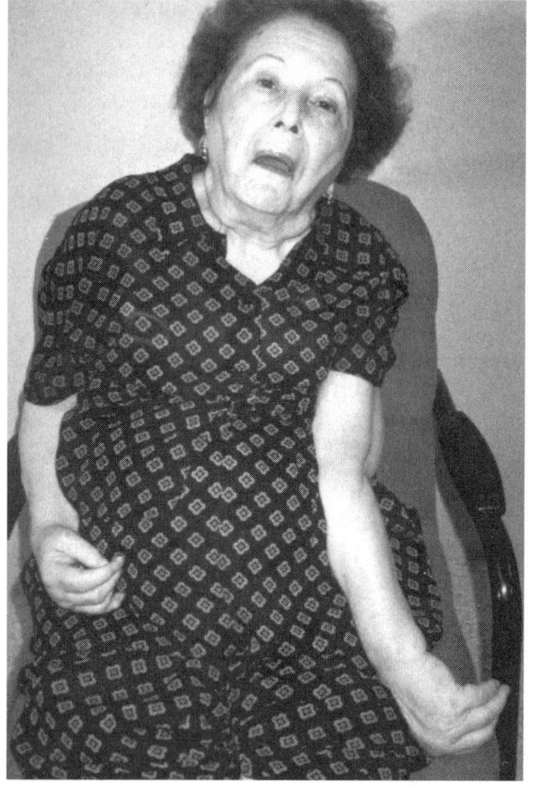

A

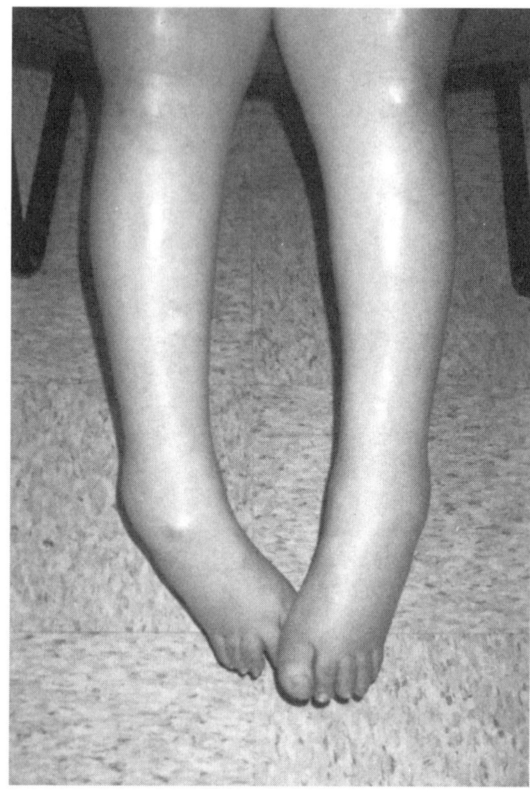

B

FIG. 2. A: This patient in advanced stages of CBD shows the typical dystonic posture of her left hand with adduction at the shoulder, hyperextension at the elbow, pronation of the forearm, and flexion of the hands. **B:** The same patient showing bilateral, right more than left inversion and flexion of the feet and extension of the toes.

more severely. We found the hips to be rotated in three, and flexed in two patients. The knees were dystonically flexed in four and extended in one advanced case. The dystonic posture in the feet resulted in foot inversion in 10 (26%) patients, but none had foot eversion. The foot was flexed in eight (21%), extended in one patient, the toes flexed in four and extended in four other patients.

Axial Dystonia

There were no cases of axial dystonia in the 30 patients described by Rinne et al. (16). Wenning et al. (3) found one patient in their 14 patients, and other authors do not mention the occurrence of axial dystonia. In our series, only 12 (31%) patients had early dystonia involving the head, neck, or trunk during the course of the disease, 10 of these patients had associated limb dystonia. This comprised of laterocollis in seven (18%), retrocollis in two, anterocollis in one, and torticollis in two patients. Only two patients had blepharospasm, none had oromandibular dystonia and nine (24%) patients had scoliosis, lordosis, or kyphosis.

Contractures and Pain

Although a common and often the most disabling symptom, there is little or no information in the literature on the occurrence of pain and contractures in CBD patients. In our patients with dystonia, 29 (74%) had fixed postures, and 24 (62%) had evidence of fixed contractures (Fig. 1). Contractures mainly affected the joints of the upper extremity in 22 (56%) patients, mostly the wrist and the fingers (19 patients, 49%). Some 11 (28%) patients also had contractures in the shoulder joints, and 6 (15%) had contractures affecting the ankles. Pain accompanying dystonia was seen in 16 (42%), and this mostly occurred in the dystonic hand. Variable degrees of rigidity, particularly affecting the dystonic limb, was seen in all patients.

Other Movement Disorders and Associated Features

Myoclonus has been reported to occur in 25% to 80.5% of patients with CBD (17,19,20). We found myoclonus in 39 (59.1%) of our CBD population. Of the 39 cases of CBD with dystonia, 24 (61.5%) patients had coexistent myoclonus, and in 23 (96%) of these patients, the myoclonus was present in the limb manifesting dystonia. There were 15 (55.5%) CBD patients with myoclonus, who did not have dystonia. Nine (23.1%) cases of CBD with dystonia in our series also had tremor in the dystonic limb, compared to 11 (40.74%) who had tremor in a limb without dystonia. Only two CBD patients with dystonia also exhibited choreic movements, which were also seen in two patients who did not have dystonia. All CBD patients with or without dystonia had rigidity and bradykinesia that was most pronounced in the dystonic limb.

Although the occurrence of apraxia in CBD is reported to be between 64.3% to 100%, it is difficult to distinguish this from the clumsiness caused by accompanying bradykinesia, rigidity, and dystonia (3,6,17,21–25). We found evidence of limb-kinetic apraxia in many patients with very mild dystonia or rigidity, but it was difficult to fully appreciate apraxia in the more advanced cases. The alien limb phenomenon has been described to range between 42.8% and 50.0% of all cases of CBD (9). In our series the alien limb phenomenon was seen in 23 (59.0%) cases who had dystonia, 18 had an alien hand, and five had an alien leg. This compared to 11 (40.7%) patients with alien limb found in the patients without dystonia. In nearly all cases, the alien limb phenomenon was seen in the dystonic limb. We found that 26 (66.7%) patients with dystonia had cortical sensory dysfunction compared to 13 (48.1%) patients who did not have dystonia. In all such cases, the sensory abnormality was also found in the dystonic limb.

IMAGING STUDIES

As with all other aspects of CBD, descriptions of the magnetic resonance imaging (MRI) findings in the literature, address the findings as a whole, and do not distinguish between patients with or without dystonia. Overall, an asymmetric pericentral cortical atrophy has been reported in about half of patients who have had conventional MRI (26–28). Although all patients in our series had an MRI of their brain, the results were available to us in 48. We found mild to moderately generalized atrophy in 23 out of 28 (82.1%) dystonia patients and 15 (75%) patients without dystonia. In nine (32.1%) patients with dystonia, the atrophy was asymmetric with a focal area more prominently affected by the atrophy on the contralateral side. Mild to moderately severe subcortical white matter changes were found in 12 (42.8%) patients with dystonia and in eight (40.0%) of the patients without dystonia.

NATURAL HISTORY AND PATHOLOGY

Relentless progression and ultimate death resulting from complications of immobility characterize the natural history of CBD.

Of the 39 patients with dystonia in our series, 15 had follow-up evaluations ranging from three months to nine years (mean: 3.1 years). Seven (18%) patients progressed to an advanced, akinetic-rigid-dystonic stage characterized by an expressionless face with open mouth and rigidly flexed or extended limbs (Fig. 2). Of the six cases of clinically diagnosed CBD who died, four had dystonia during the course of their illness. The pathological findings in four cases were similar to those reported by others, but they failed to identify any pathological marker for dystonia (7,11,13,15). The presence of pathology at many sites in the motor pathways makes it impossible to attribute the dystonia to a lesion at any particular site or draw pathophysiologic conclusions.

TREATMENT

Unfortunately, the symptoms and signs of CBD respond poorly to any form of therapy. This was found to be the observation in 40 cases reported by Goetz et al. (29), and more recently in the 147 case series reported by Kompoliti et al. (17). In the latter report, 128 (87%) patients received various forms of treatment. Overall, 32 patients received L-dopa, 12 were treated with a dopamine agonist, 12 clonazepam, 10 selegiline, and six received local botulinum toxin injections, during the course of their illness. Improvement in dystonia was allegedly seen in four patients given benzodiazepines, three cases given anticholinergics, and two cases given baclofen. Of the nine patients treated with botulinum toxin injections, six experienced improvement of their dystonia and the pain associated with it. Of the 39 cases of CBD with dystonia seen at our center, 17 had adequate follow-up data. Two patients had transient improvement of their myoclonus with clonazepam. Of the six patients in our series who were treated with local botulinum toxin injections into dystonic and painful areas, two had marked improvement of the dystonia and pain, and four had mild to moderate improvement. There were no complications attributed to botulinum toxin therapy. These combined data suggest that botulinum toxin may be used more widely in the future. Except for botulinum toxin injections, which may provide meaningful albeit transient benefit, very little if any benefit was noted with other therapies and the symptoms continued to progress relentlessly.

SUMMARY

Although a referral bias may have resulted in a higher proportion of atypical cases and consequently an overestimation of dystonia, asymmetric limb dystonia particularly affecting one arm initially was observed in 92% of all our CBD cases. Predominant leg dystonia is uncommon, and head, neck, or axial dystonia is rare. Dystonia is often associated with myoclonus, rigidity, apraxia, alien hand phenomenon, and sensory cortical signs in the affected limb, and there are no significant differences between the occurrence of these or other features, between patients with or without dystonia. There is no effective treatment for this relentless disorder except for temporary relief of dystonia and pain with local botulinum toxin injections. Further clinicopathologic studies are needed to elucidate the anatomical and physiologic substrates of dystonia in this disorder.

REFERENCES

1. Lang AE, Riley DE, Bergeron C. Cortical-basal ganglionic degeneration. In: Calne DB, ed. *Neurodegerative diseases.* Philadelphia: WB Saunders, 1994:877–894.
2. Jankovic J, Fahn S. Dystonic disorders. In Jankovic J, Tolosa E, ed. *Parkinson's disease and movement disorders,* 3rd ed. Baltimore: Williams & Wilkins, 1998: 513–551.
3. Wenning GK, Litvan I, Jankovic J, et al. Natural history and survival of 14 patients with CBGD confirmed at postmortem examination. *J Neurol Neurosurg Psychiatry* 1998;64:184–189.
4. Rivest J, Quinn N, Marsden CD. Dystonia in Parkinson's disease, multiple system atrophy, and progressive supranuclear palsy. *Neurology* 1990;40:1571–1578.
5. Tanner CM. Epidemiologic approaches to cortical-basal ganglionic degeneration. *Mov Disord* 1996;11:346–357.
6. Kumar R, Bergeron C, Pollanen MS, Lang AE. Cortical-basal ganglionic degeneration. In: Jankovic J, Tolosa E, eds. *Parkinson's disease and movement disorders,* 3rd ed. Baltimore: Williams & Wilkins, 1998:297–316.
7. Rebeiz JJ, Kolodny EH, Richardson EP Jr. Corticodentatonigral degeneration with neuronal. achromasia. *Arch Neurol* 1968;18:20–33.
8. Watts RL, Williams RS, Growdon JD, et al. Corticobasal ganglionic degeneration. *Neurology* 1985;35 Suppl 1: 178(abs).
9. Obeso JA, Rothwell JC, Marsden CD. The spectrum of cortical myoclonus. From focal reflex jerks to spontaneous motor epilepsy. *Brain* 1985;108:193–224.
10. Gibb WRG, Luthert PJ, Marsden CD. Corticobasal degeneration. *Brain* 1989;112:1171–1192.
11. Greene PE, Fahn S, Lang AE, et al. What is it? Case 1, 1990. Progressive unilateral rigidity, bradykinesia, tremulousness, and apraxia, leading to fixed postural deformity of the involved limb. *Mov Disord* 1990;5:341–351.
12. Lippa CF, Smith TW, Fontneau N. Corticonigral degeneration with neuronal achromasia. A clinicopathologic study of 2 cases. *J Neurol Sci* 1990;98:301–310.
13. Paulus W, Selim M. Corticonigral degeneration with neuronal achromasia and basal neurofibrillary tangles. *Acta Neuropathol* (Berl) 1990;81:89–94.
14. Riley DE, Lang AE, Lewis A, Resch L, Ashby P, Black S. Corticobasal ganglionic degeneration. *Neurology* 1990;40: 1203–1212.
15. Sawle GV, Brooks DJ, Marsden CD, Frackowiak RS. Corticobasal degeneration: a unique pattern of regional cortical oxygen hypometabolism and striatal fluorodopa uptake demonstrated by positron emission tomography. *Brain* 1991;114:541–556.

16. Rinne JO, Lee MS, Thompson PD, Marsden CD. Corticobasal degeneration: A clinical study of 36 cases. *Brain* 1994;117:1183–1196.
17. Kompoliti K, Goetz CG, Boeve BF, Maraganore DM, Ahlskog JE, Marsdeu CD, et al. Clinical presentation and pharmacological therapy in corticobasal degeneration. *Arch Neurol* 1998;55:957–961.
18. Vanek Z, Jankovic J. Dystonia in Corticobasal degeneration. Submitted, 1999.
19. Ashby P, Strafella A, Lang A. Cortical-basal ganglia degeneration-neurophysiology of stimulus-sensitive myoclonus. *Mov Disord* 1996;11:346–357.
20. Carella F, Ciano C, Panzica F, Scaioli V. Myoclonus in Cortical-basal ganglionic degeneration. *Mov Disord* 1997;12:598–603.
21. Heilman KM. The apraxia of cortical-basal ganglionic degeneration. *Mov Disord* 1996;11:3:346–357.
22. Doody RS, Jankovic J. The alien hand and related signs. *J Neurol Neurosurg Psychiatry* 1992;55:806–810.
23. Watts RL, Brewer RP. Cortical-basal ganglionic degeneration: classical clinical features and natural history. *Mov Disord* 1996;11:3:346–357.
24. Lindholm KM, Shannon KM, Stebbins GT. A comparison of apraxia in progressive supranuclear palsy and corticobasal ganglionic degeneration. *Mov Disord* 1996; 11:3:346–357.
25. Okuda B, Tachibana H. Cortical-basal ganglionic degeneration. *Neurology* 1995;45:1033–1034.
26. Gimenez-Roldan S, Mateo D, Benito C, Grandas F, Perez-Gilbert. Progressive supranuclear palsy and corticobasal ganglionic degeneration: differentiation by clinical features and neuroimaging techniques. *J Neural Transm* 1994;42:79–90.
27. Caselli RJ. Asymmetric cortical degeneration syndromes: clinico-pathologic considerations. *Mov Disord* 1996;11:3:346–357.
28. Caselli R J, Jack CR, Petersen RC, Wahnes HW, Yauagihara T. Asymmetric cortical degeneration syndromes: clinical and radiologic correlations. *Neurology* 1992;42: 1462–1468.
29. Goetz CG, Kompoliti A, Greene PE, et al. Pharmacological therapy in cortical-basal ganglionic degeneration. *Mov Disord* 1996;11:3:346–357.

Corticobasal Degeneration.
Advances in Neurology, Vol. 82,
edited by I. Litvan, C. G. Goetz, and A. E. Lang.
Lippincott Williams & Wilkins, Philadelphia © 2000.

7

Myoclonus in Corticobasal Degeneration and Other Neurodegenerations

Philip D. Thompson* and Hiroshi Shibasaki†

**University Department of Medicine, University of Adelaide, Adelaide, South Australia 5000, Australia; and †Department of Brain Pathophysiology, Kyoto University Graduate School of Medicine, Shogoin, Sakyo-Ku, Kyoto 606-8507 Japan*

INTRODUCTION

Myoclonus refers to a brief shock-like movement or a brisk muscle jerk. Myoclonus occurs in a considerable number of neurodegenerative diseases as one element of a complex and progressive motor decline. In some of these conditions, myoclonus may be a prominent clinical feature and of diagnostic significance (Table 1). For practical clinical purposes, these conditions may be grouped as myoclonic syndromes with accompanying cognitive deficits, suggesting the diagnosis of Alzheimer's disease or Creutzfeldt-Jakob disease in the elderly, or progressive metabolic neurodegeneration in younger age groups and myoclonic syndromes with other motor impairment such as an akinetic rigid or ataxic syndrome, suggesting corticobasal degeneration (CBD), multiple system atrophy, cerebellar degenerations, and other inherited neurodegenerations such as dentato-rubro-pallido-luysian atrophy or even Huntington's disease. Finally, it is always important to consider the possibility of a metabolic encephalopathy or drug toxicity (Table 2), since these are probably the commonest causes of myoclonus in the elderly.

This chapter reviews the clinical and physiological characteristics of myoclonus in these various conditions. However, even when equipped with a detailed clinical and physiological analysis of myoclonus, it may not be possible to diagnose the underlying pathology with accuracy.

MYOCLONUS IN CBD

Clinical Features

CBD typically presents as a unilateral motor disorder affecting the hand and arm more frequently than the lower limb (1). Myoclonus of one limb is evident in one-third of cases at the time of presentation and evolves in a further 20% over the following 2 years as the disease progresses. Approximately 50% of patients with corticobasal degeneration develop myoclonus during the course of the illness (2). A jerky tremor may precede the appearance of myoclonus in the same limb early in the condition (3,4).

Myoclonus is most conspicuous in distal muscles and is often superimposed on dystonic posturing of the affected limb, obscuring any underlying associated apraxic motor deficit. Action and reflex myoclonus are characteristic. Attempts to move the limb voluntarily are interrupted by trains of repetitive action myoclonus. Repetitive bursts of stimulus sensitive reflex myoclonus are elicited by cutaneous stimulation and tendon taps. The presence of spontaneous myoclonus in CBD is difficult to judge because of the action myoclonus in the setting of rigidity and alien limb movements that interfere with attempts to achieve complete relaxation.

TABLE 1. *Myoclonus in neurodegenerative conditions*

Myoclonus with cognitive decline
Alzheimer's disease
Creutzfeldt-Jakob disease
Paraneoplastic encephalopathy
Myoclonus with akinetic-rigid or ataxic syndromes
Corticobasal degeneration
Multiple system atrophy
Cerebellar degenerations
Huntington's disease
Dentato-rubro-pallido-luysian atrophy
Progressive myoclonus with epilepsy or ataxia
Mitochondrial encephalopathy with ragged red fibres (MERRF)
Lafora body disease
Unverricht-Lundborg disease (Baltic myoclonus)
Spinocerebellar degenerations
Sialidosis
Kuf's disease
Celiac disease

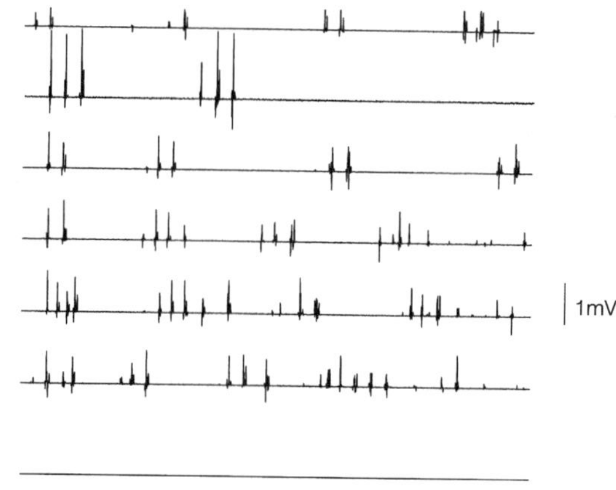

FIG. 1. Surface EMG recordings from abductor pollicis brevis during action myoclonus in a patient with CBD. The muscle bursts are of short duration and repetitive, occurring in clusters of two to five bursts. The interval between individual bursts tends to be stereotyped and of the order of 70 ms. (From ref. 5, with permission.)

Physiology

Electromyographic (EMG) Studies of Myoclonus

Studies of EMG activity in CBD confirm that myoclonus is predominantly action- or reflex-induced and that spontaneous myoclonus is uncommon. Action and reflex myoclonus is produced by short duration (25 to 50 ms) muscle discharges, simultaneously activating antagonist muscle pairs, in bursts of two to four discharges with interburst intervals of 60 to 80 ms (Fig. 1). These brief trains of high-frequency myoclonic discharges occur in clusters of two to three per second. In the case of action myoclonus, this activity continues throughout the period of voluntary muscle activation. The pattern of muscle activation throughout a limb is comparable during both action and stimulus sensitive reflex myoclonus, and is consistent with corticospinal activation (5).

TABLE 2. *Myoclonus associated with systemic illness, encephalopathy, and drug toxicity*

Myoclonus and metabolic encephalopathy
Hepatic failure
Renal failure
Respiratory failure
Electrolyte imbalance
Non–ketotic hyperglycemia
Myoclonus and drugs
L-dopa
Serotonin reuptake inhibitors
Monoamine oxidase inhibitors
Tricyclic antidepressants
Neuroleptics
Lithium
Opiates
Sympathomimetics
Bismuth

Electroencephalographic (EEG) Activity in CBD

Nonspecific slowing of EEG rhythms may be seen, but spike discharges are not present. There are no time-locked cortical spike or sharp wave discharges on backaveraged EEG in relation to the myoclonus in most cases.

In a recent report, Mima et al. (6) observed that clear cortical activity preceding myoclonus could be detected on backaveraged magnetoencephalography, but was not evident on EEG.

Cortical Somatosensory Evoked Potentials (SEP)

The parietal N20-P25-N35 components of the SEP may be poorly formed with a broad notched positive wave rather than the normal "W" shape waveform. In contrast, the prefrontal P22-N30 components are relatively preserved (Fig. 2). Borderline enlargement of the P25-N33 component of the cortical SEP was observed in only one of 14 cases (case 7) (5).

Reflex Myoclonus

Reflex myoclonus elicited by cutaneous stimuli such as pinprick, light touch, and tendon taps, and electrical digital sensory nerve stimulation may appear at intensities near or even below sensory perceptual threshold, and in some patients with cortical sensory loss (Fig. 3) (5,7). A C reflex corresponding to the stimulus sensitive reflex myoclonus may be elicited by mixed nerve stimulation at intensities below the motor threshold for a direct M response, indicating activation of large diameter sensory afferents (Fig. 3).

A striking and reproducible finding in CBD is the latency of C reflexes and reflex myoclonus. Following mixed ulnar and median nerve stimulation at the wrist C reflex latencies in hand muscles were of the order of 40 ms, and approximately 50 ms following stimulation of digital sensory nerves (4–9).

Origin of Myoclonus in CBD

Differences between Myoclonus in CBD and Typical Cortical Myoclonus

The major differences between myoclonus in CBD and "typical" cortical reflex myoclonus are summarized in Table 3. In both conditions, myoclonus may appear as focal, distally predominant, stimulus-sensitive reflex and action myoclonus. Hypersynchronous short duration bursts of muscle activity are common to both. Since the cortex is one of the major sites of pathological change in CBD, it is appropriate to consider the cortex a likely site of origin for the myoclonus. However, there are several differences between myoclonus in CBD and "typical" cortical reflex myoclonus. In contrast to "typical" cortical reflex myoclonus, myoclonus in CBD is not generally associated with enlarged or "giant" cortical somatosensory evoked potentials, cortical potentials do not precede each myoclonic jerk on back-averaged EEG, and the latency of reflex myoclonic jerks is shorter. The latency of reflex myoclonus in hand muscles after stimulation of the median nerve at the wrist is about 40 ms in CBD, in contrast to 50 to 60 ms in classical cortical reflex myoclonus. These differences are illustrated by comparing Figs. 2 and 4.

Pathophysiology of Myoclonus

Reflex cortical myoclonus involves a pathway beginning with activation of peripheral sensory receptors, traversing peripheral sensory afferents, ascending central sensory tracts before reaching the sensory cortex, and an efferent limb via the corticospinal tract. In addition to the conduction times in the major sensory afferent and motor efferent pathways (which can be estimated from measurement of SEP component latencies and the latency of muscle responses to magnetic brain stimulation), this reflex pathway includes a small interval for recruitment of cortical motoneurons and intracortical relay from the sensory input to activate the motor efferent pathway. Estimates of the cortical delay for generation of myoclonic activity in "typical" cortical reflex myoclonus associated with "giant" SEPs (6.9 ± 3.7ms) are significantly longer than for CBD (1.4 ± 0.8ms) (5).

Cortical Excitability

It is likely that enhanced cortical excitability contributes to the generation of repetitive myoclonus following motor cortical activation by voluntary movement (action myoclonus), in response to sensory afferent input (reflex myoclonus) or by magnetic stimulation. Magnetic brain stimulation, which is more sensitive to changes in cortical excitability than anodal electrical brain stimulation (10), induced repetitive muscle responses with interburst intervals of 70 ms in some patients with CBD and myoclonus. Such responses were not seen with electrical stimulation of the brain, in the same patient. The short latency EMG responses, and therefore the afferent discharges following muscle contraction, were comparable in size for both modes of brain stimulation. Thus, it is unlikely that reflex myoclonus alone could give rise to the repetitive activity occurring in response to

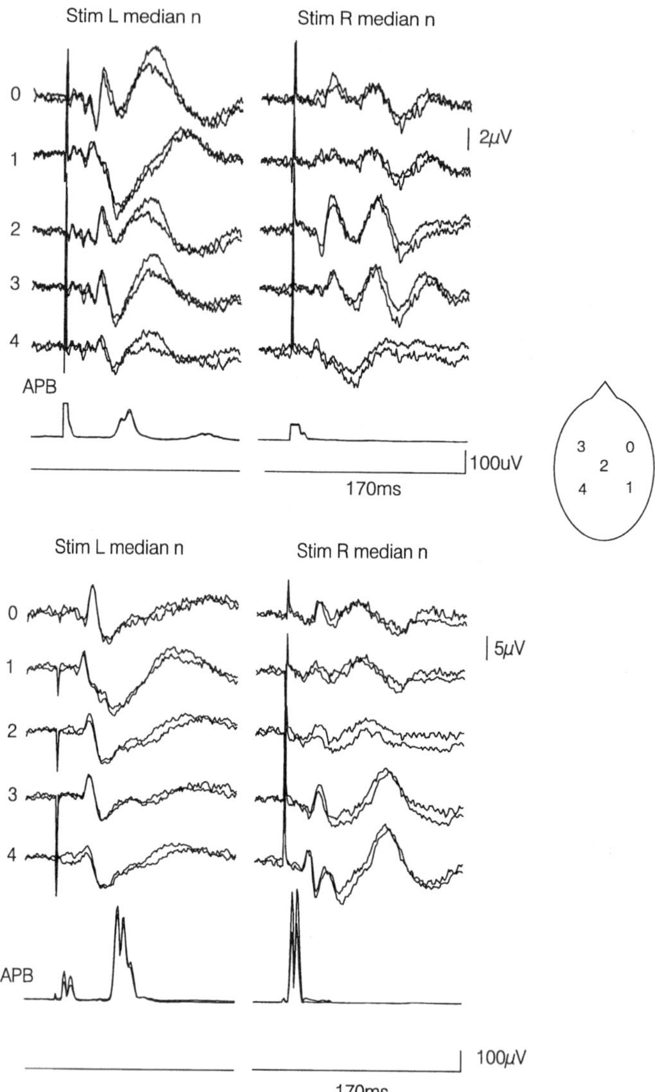

FIG. 2. Cortical somatosensory evoked potentials following median nerve stimulation at the wrist in two patients with CBD. Reflex myoclonus is evident in abductor pollicis brevis (APB) in both. In the upper panels there is loss of the normal P1-N2 component in the parietal leads, whereas the precentral waveforms are relatively preserved. This is evident over both hemispheres following stimulation of the right and left median nerves even though reflex myoclonus was present only on stimulation of the left median nerve. Note that the stimulus threshold for eliciting reflex myoclonus was less than that required to elicit an M wave in APB. In the lower panels, left median nerve stimulation elicited reflex myoclonus, a prominent right parietal N1 (N20) followed by an abnormal P1-N2 component. Stimulation of the right median nerve in this case produced a normal parietal SEP configuration. (From ref. 5, with permission.)

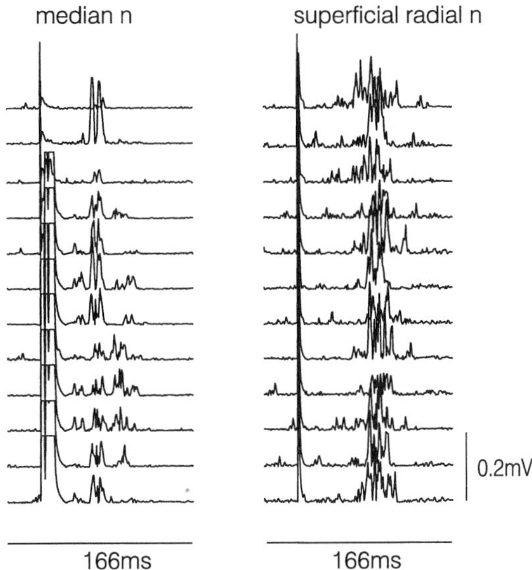

FIG. 3. Reflex myoclonus in a patient with CBD. Surface EMG recordings of reflex myoclonus in abductor pollicis brevis following stimulation of the median nerve at the wrist (*left traces*) at increasing stimulus intensities elicited reflex myoclonus at intensities below the threshold for an M response. Stimulation of the superficial radial nerve (*right traces*) also evoked reflex myoclonus in APB in this case. Stimuli were delivered 25 ms after start of sweep. (From ref. 5, with permission.)

magnetic but not electrical stimulation. The simplest explanation is that magnetic stimulation revealed enhanced cortical excitability in CBD. Cortical hyperexcitabilty in CBD was also demonstrated by Lu et al. in two cases, where the silent period to magnetic brain stimulation was shorter on the affected side, consistent with impaired cortical inhibitory systems (11).

Transcortical Reflexes and Cortical Myoclonus

Cortical reflex myoclonus is thought to be mediated by long latency reflexes traversing the sensorimotor cortex. The intracortical component of the long latency reflexes generating reflex myoclonus in CBD is significantly shorter than the intracortical processing of sensory input in "typical" cortical reflex myoclonus. This may reflect changes in cortical excitability as described herein. The timing of reflex activity may also reflect enhancement of different components of the long latency reflexes. Long latency transcortical reflexes elicited by peripheral sensory stimulation (e.g., peripheral nerve stimulation or muscle stretch) generate at least three periods of enhanced motor cortex excitability each with a preferred timing of onset (5). On latency considerations, reflex myoclonus in CBD appears to utilize the first period of transcortical excitability occurring 40 ms after stimulation. This period may reflect direct sensory relay from ventrolateral thalamic nuclei to motor cortex. In contrast, cortical reflex myoclonus appears based on the second period of transcortical excitability, 50 to 60 ms after stimulation, conveyed by lemniscal input to the principal sensory relay nuclei of the thalamus, either directly or via the cerebellum, then through thalamocortical relays to sensory

TABLE 3. *Comparison of the major clinical and electrophysiological characteristics of "typical" cortical myoclonus and myoclonus in corticobasal degeneration*

	Cortical reflex myoclonus	Corticobasal degeneration
Clinical characteristics	Focal, multifocal action stimulus sensitive (reflex)	Focal action stimulus sensitive (reflex)
EMG	Hypersynchronous short-duration bursts	Hypersynchronous short-duration bursts
SEP	"Giant" P25-N33 > 10uV	Small, disorganized
Backaveraged EEG	Time-locked positive spike	No potential
Latency of reflex myoclonus	~50–60 ms (hand)	~40 ms (hand)

EEG, electroencephalographic activity; EMG, electromyographic activity; SEP, somatosensory evoked potential

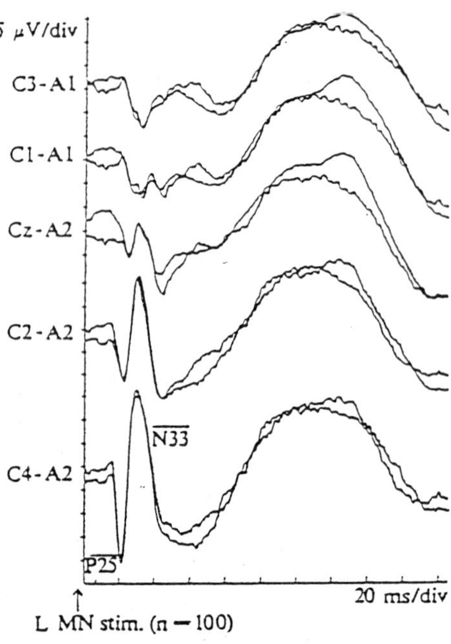

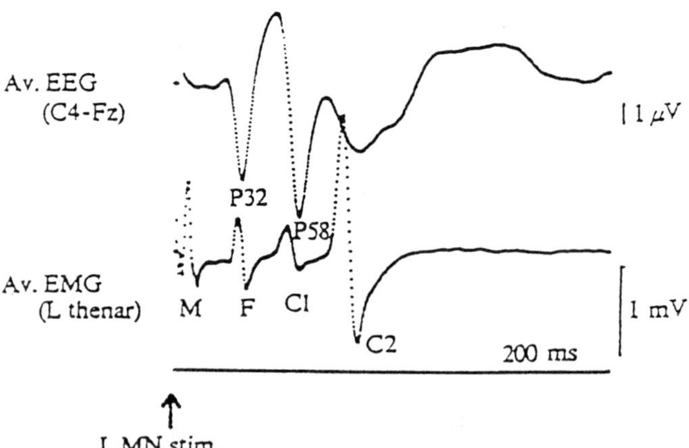

FIG. 4. Cortical somatosensory evoked potentials (*upper panel*) and cortical reflex myoclonus (*lower panel*) in two patients with progressive myoclonic epilepsy and typical physiological features of cortical reflex myoclonus. Following left median nerve (LMN) stimulation, high amplitude P25-N33 components of the SEP are recorded, maximal over the right central electrodes (C2 and C4), and 10 ms later, similar potentials of smaller amplitude are seen over the left central (C3 and C1) electrodes. In the lower panel, median nerve stimulation elicits double positive peaks of "giant" cortical SEP and the direct M wave in the thenar muscles is followed by an F wave (latency 26 ms), and two C reflexes (C1 at 48 ms, and C2 at 73 ms). The latency difference between the two positive peaks of the SEP P32-P58 is comparable to the interval between the double C reflexes (25 ms). Traces are the average of 64 responses. (From ref. 13, with permission.)

cortex. Corticocortical relays then transfer the sensory information to sensory areas 3, 1, and 2 of the cortex before a final relay to the motor cortex (area 4). These pathways may be important in the generation of "giant" cortical SEPs in "typical" cortical reflex myoclonus (12,13).

The cortical pathology in CBD may lead to alterations in the balance of inhibitory and excitatory inputs to cortical neurons resulting in enhanced cortical excitability. Accordingly, reflex myoclonus in CBD may be based on pathological enhancement of responses of motor cortical areas to direct sensory input or exaggeration of inputs relayed through thalamocortical loops. The observation that stimulus sensitive reflex myoclonus was present in some patients with sensory loss affecting cutaneous sensation (pinprick, light touch) and joint position sense in the affected hand is consistent with a direct relay of sensory input to motor cortex (5). Chen et al. (7) also concluded that exaggeration of short latency cutaneous cortical reflexes contributed to myoclonus in CBD. Abnormal thalamic metabolism contralateral to myoclonus in CBD on functional imaging studies also points to a role of thalamocortical connections in the development of myoclonus in this condition (14–16). However, thalamotomy has not been effective in improving motor function (7,8), although myoclonus was reported to improve transiently in one case (4).

MYOCLONUS IN ALZHEIMER'S DISEASE

Multifocal stimulus sensitive myoclonus and generalized myoclonus are common in the later stages of sporadic Alzheimer's disease, and myoclonus is increasingly recognized as a major clinical feature in inherited forms of the disease. Myoclonus may be prominent in familial Alzheimer's disease and accompanied by seizures, particularly in chromosome 14 linked pedigrees with mutations in the presenilin 1 gene.

In a study of apparently sporadic Alzheimer's disease and myoclonus, Wilkins et al. found EMG bursts of 20 to 80 ms duration, variable stimulus sensitivity and variable C reflex latencies ranging from 36 to 75 ms (17). Cortical SEPs were enlarged in one patient and a negative cortical potential preceding the myoclonus over the contralateral central head area was identified in four (latencies from negative potential to myoclonus ranged from 25 to 40 ms). In the same study, three patients with myoclonus and Alzheimer's disease associated with trisomy 21 (Down syndrome) were also studied (17). In one, a giant SEP was recorded and in two a contralateral negative potential was present in the EEG 37 and 45 ms before the myoclonus. Intracortical spread, typical of cortical myoclonus, also was present in one. In two patients, one with sporadic Alzheimer's disease and one associated with Down syndrome, long duration bifrontal negative waves beginning 50 to 100 ms and 180 ms before the jerk were recorded.

These results suggest that myoclonus may be of either cortical or subcortical origin in Alzheimer's disease, a notion supported by Ugawa et al. in a study of seven patients with dementia and myoclonus (18). A cortical origin was confirmed in three cases (with cortical spike discharges preceding myoclonus on jerk-locked averaging). Two of these cases had enlarged cortical SEPs and long latency (cortical) reflex myoclonus. In three cases, backaveraged EEG revealed a contralateral broad negative wave preceding the onset of myoclonus by 60 to 100 ms. Cortical SEPs were normal and reflex myoclonus was not present in these cases, consistent with a subcortical origin of the myoclonus. In two patients with this pattern, periodic discharges were evident on EEG (Fig. 5), similar to the findings in Creutzfeldt-Jakob disease (to be discussed).

MYOCLONUS IN CREUTZFELDT-JAKOB DISEASE

Multifocal distal or generalized stimulus sensitive myoclonus, typically in response to a loud noise, and occasionally rhythmic myoclonus, may all appear in the course of Creutzfeldt-Jakob disease. Electroencephalography shows a loss of normal background rhythms with slow waves of variable amplitude, distribution, and morphology. Most characteristic are periodic discharges consisting of bilaterally synchronous sharp waves (duration 200 to 400 ms) repeating at a frequency of 0.5 to 1 Hz. The combination

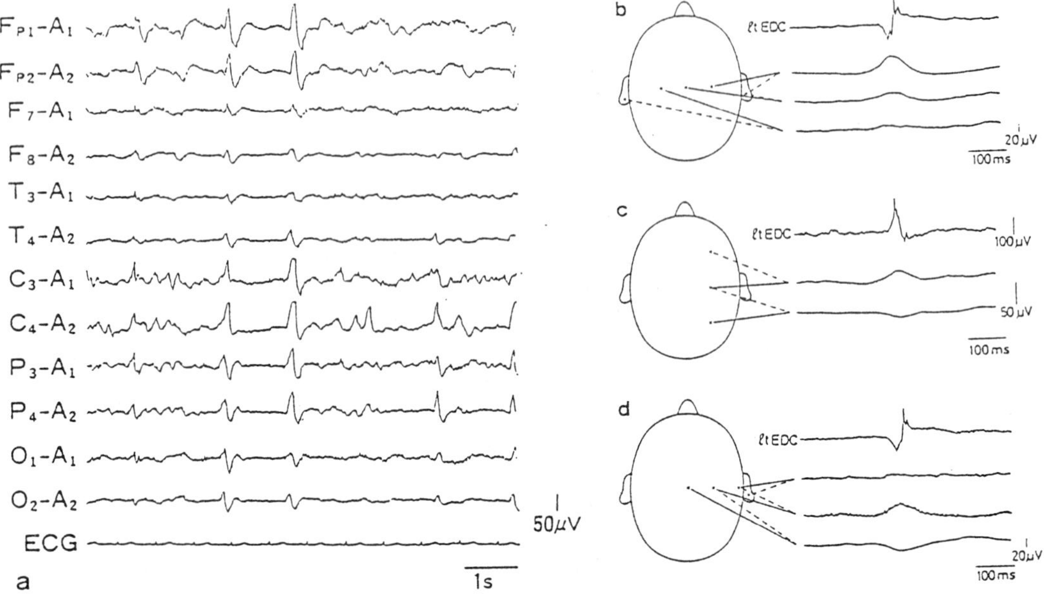

FIG. 5. A: Conventional EEG recording in a patient with Alzheimer's disease showing quasiperiodic discharges (*left panel*). **B,C,D:** In the right-hand panel, the topography of a negative EEG wave recorded by jerk-locked averaging in relation to myoclonus in the left extensor digitorum communis (lt EDC) is shown. The onset of the cortical potential preceded the myoclonic jerk by 60 to 80 ms. SEPs were not enlarged and no reflex myoclonus was present. These features and the distribution of the potential suggest a subcortical origin for the myoclonus. (From ref. 18, with permission.)

of dementia, myoclonus, and periodic EEG discharges was encountered in 53% of 209 consecutive cases of experimentally transmitted Creutzfeldt-Jakob disease (19).

There is an inconsistent relationship between the periodic sharp activity and myoclonus in Creutzfeldt-Jakob disease. Shibasaki et al. reported the results of jerk-locked averaging in two patients with Creutzfeldt-Jakob disease and spontaneous myoclonus (20). In one patient with multifocal EEG spikes, without a clear relationship to the myoclonus in the raw record, jerk-locked averaging revealed a sharp wave (duration 100 to 130 ms) over the contralateral central region, starting 50 to 85 ms before the onset of myoclonus. The other patient displayed typical periodic discharges in the EEG (at a frequency of 1 Hz), which appeared to be related to the myoclonus in raw records. Jerk-locked averaging of the EEG showed a widely distributed, predominantly contralateral, negative potential preceded the myoclonic jerks with a peak latency 60 ms before the onset of myoclonus (Fig. 6). The wave continued to spread to both frontal areas. The distribution of the cortical discharge and the long interval to the onset of myoclonus suggest a subcortical origin for the myoclonus.

Cortical reflex myoclonus may also be seen in Creutzfeldt-Jakob disease. Photic reflex myoclonus of cortical origin was demonstrated in two further patients by Shibasaki and Neshige (21). The EEG of both patients exhibited typical periodic discharges as described, and in one somaesthetic reflex myoclonus was also present. Cortical responses to flash were enhanced, and SEPs were enlarged in one (Fig. 7).

MYOCLONUS IN MULTIPLE SYSTEM ATROPHY

Myoclonus is estimated to occur in approximately 30% of patients with multiple system atrophy (22), possibly more frequently in the striatonigral than the olivopontocerebellar form.

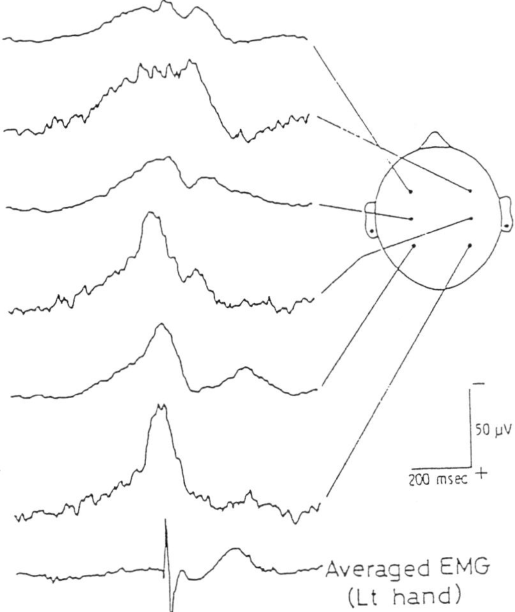

FIG. 6. Averaged EEGs and EMG obtained by jerk-locked averaging with respect to the myoclonic EMG (average of 32 samples) from a patient with Creutzfeldt-Jakob disease who exhibited bilaterally synchronous periodic sharp EEG complexes (at a frequency of 1 Hz), which appeared to be related to myoclonic activity of the left hand. Each scalp electrode is referred to the ipsilateral earlobe. The myoclonic EMG discharge from the left hand is preceded by a sharp negative potential that is maximal at the right centroparietal region and widely distributed. The distribution of this potential suggests a subcortical origin. (From ref. 20, with permission.)

Typical cortical reflex myoclonus is well recognized in patients with a predominantly cerebellar presentation of multiple system atrophy (23). In a study of 24 patients with multiple system atrophy, radiological evidence of olivopontocerebellar degeneration, parkinsonism, ataxia, and stimulus sensitive reflex myoclonus, 23 were found to have reflex myoclonus to sensory stimuli (cutaneous stimulation and muscle stretch) (24). The myoclonus was shown to have the characteristics of cortical reflex myoclonus with enlargement of the P25-N33 component of the cortical SEP (mean amplitude 10.3 μV, range 1.2 to 31.2 μV) and in 16 patients, reflex responses were recorded in forearm muscles after stimulation of the median nerve at the wrist at latencies ranging from 30 to 50 ms (mean 39.9 ms) (24). Only three of the 24 had action or spontaneous myoclonus. In another report of three patients with multiple system atrophy, SEPs were not enlarged in the two examined and reflex facilitation of muscle activity in forearm flexors occurred at longer latencies (51 to 63 ms) (7).

Artieda and Obeso, in a further report (25) identified a striking pattern of photic cortical reflex myoclonus with generalized muscle jerks following flash stimulation (at frequencies between 1 and 15 Hz) in five patients with multiple system atrophy (four with radiological evidence of olivopontocerebellar atrophy and postmortem changes of striatonigral degeneration in one). All had reflex myoclonus induced by sensory stimulation. Flash stimulation induced a positive occipital potential and was followed 8 to 12 ms later by a frontal wave with an anterior pre-Rolandic distribution. In contrast, sensory stimulation (peripheral nerve) was followed by an enlarged cortical SEP distributed over the parieto-Rolandic areas. The authors postulated activation of the occipital cortex by the flash followed by intracortical conduction to premotor areas and subsequently, activation of the motor cortex and the generation of a myoclonic jerk. Muscle responses were recorded in limb muscle with intermuscle intervals consistent with corticospinal conduction.

It is common for patients with an akinetic rigid or striatonigral form of multiple system atrophy to exhibit myoclonus at some stage during the illness. The origin of this form of myoclonus is unclear, and has received little attention to date. On the basis of personal observations, the majority do not appear to have a cortical origin. In a detailed study of one case of preserved striatonigral degeneration, myoclonus was shown to originate in the brainstem (26).

MYOCLONUS IN HUNTINGTON'S DISEASE

Myoclonus is a rare finding in Huntington's disease. In a study of three patients from two families in whom the diagnosis of Huntington's disease was confirmed by DNA analysis, myoclonus was a striking feature and exhibited many of the features of cortical myoclonus (27).

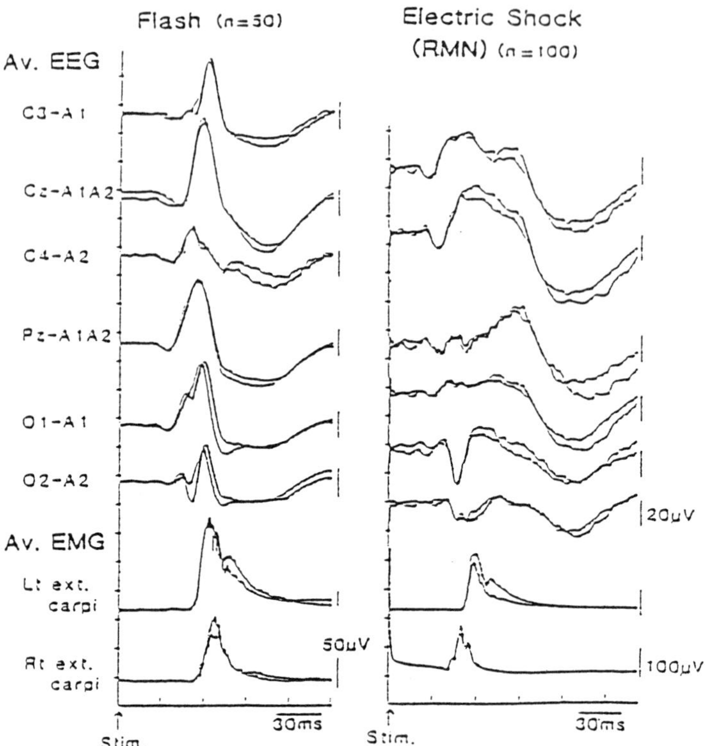

FIG. 7. Averaged EEG and EMG from patient with Creutzfeldt-Jakob disease and myoclonus. Reflex myoclonus to flash (*left panel*) and peripheral nerve stimulation (*right panel*) is present. On peripheral nerve stimulation, the cortical SEPs are enlarged. Following right median nerve (RMN) stimulation, a giant SEP was first seen over the left central electrode (C3), then over the right central electrode (C4). The C reflex was first elicited in the right wrist extensor, and then the left. These findings are consistent with typical somatosensory cortical myoclonus. (From ref. 21, with permission.)

Action and stimulus sensitive myoclonus were prominent. Backaveraged EEG revealed spike discharges preceding myoclonus. Intracortical spread of spike waves accompanied reflex and action myoclonus leading to generalized multifocal myoclonus. Striking photic reflex myoclonus was also demonstrated (Fig. 8).

The latency of reflex myoclonus (C reflexes) in hand muscles induced by peripheral nerve stimulation (approximately 40 ms) was similar to that in CBD and unlike typical cortical myoclonus. Reflex myoclonus was repetitive with bursts of muscle activity and cortical waves separated by intervals of approximately 20 ms. Cortical SEPs were disorganized and small, consistent with previous studies of the cortical SEP in Huntington's disease (without myoclonus). Preservation of the cortical SEP with borderline enlargement of the P1-N2 component was described by Carella et al. (28) in a patient with Huntington's disease, action myoclonus and reflex myoclonus in hand muscles 40 ms after stimulation of the median nerve at the wrist.

Myoclonus in Huntington's disease, therefore, may display the features of (a) myoclonus preceded by time-locked cortical discharges; (b) short latency reflex myoclonus (of the type seen in corticobasal degeneration) with disorganized SEPs; and (c) photic reflex myoclonus.

MYOCLONUS IN DENTATO-RUBRO-PALLIDO-LUYSIAN ATROPHY

Myoclonus is recognized as a prominent feature of some families with this rare condition. Most of the myoclonus-epilepsy phenotypes appear to originate in Japan. Physiological studies of myoclonus have not been reported to our

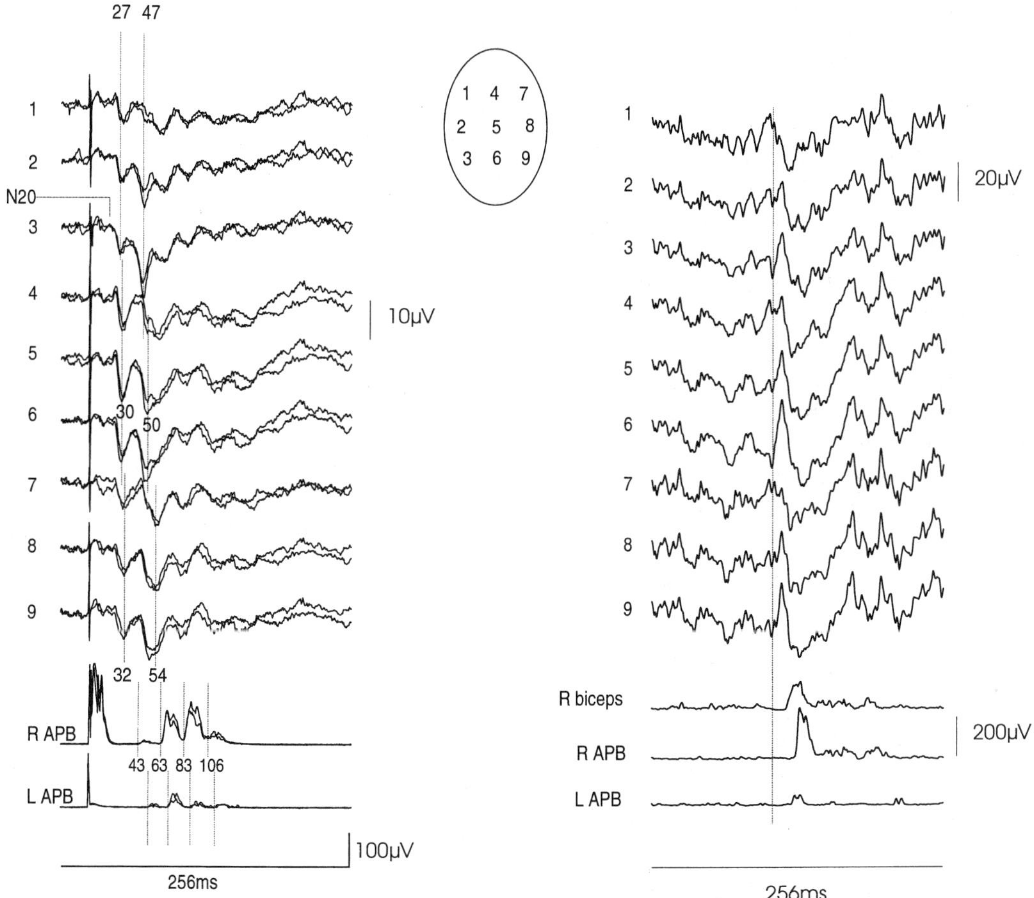

FIG. 8. Cortical somatosensory evoked potentials following stimulation of the right median nerve at the wrist (*left panel*) and back-averaged EEG preceding myoclonic jerks in the right abductor pollicis brevis (APB) (*right panel*) in a 31-year-old woman with myoclonus and Huntington's disease. The somatosensory evoked potential from electrode 3 shows a small N20 response followed by positive waves that spread at short intervals to the paramedian and right-sided scalp electrodes. The left parietal electrode shows a positivity in frontal and parietal electrodes at 27 ms followed by another positive wave, 20 ms later. This second positivity is largest over central and postcentral leads and also spreads across to the contralateral side. Following stimulation of the median nerve, reflex responses were recorded in APB at 43, 63, 83 and 106 ms with later smaller responses occurring in left APB about 10 ms after those on the right. Backaveraged EEG triggering from the right APB revealed a positive cortical discharge over the left parietal region (best seen in electrodes 3 and 6) preceding myoclonus by 20 ms. (From ref. 27, with permission.)

knowledge, and the nature of myoclonus in this condition remains to be elucidated.

MYOCLONUS IN CEREBELLAR DEGENERATIONS

In some cerebellar degenerations striking, and typical, cortical reflex myoclonus is found. In addition to primary CBD, the differential diagnosis of a progressive ataxic syndrome with myoclonus will overlap with the inherited metabolic encephalopathies. Approximately 40% of cases with a progressive ataxic syndrome and myoclonus remain with a diagnosis of "spinocerebellar degeneration" despite extensive investigation (see Table 1) (29).

MYOCLONUS IN INHERITED METABOLIC ENCEPHALOPATHIES

Seizures, dementia, and ataxia usually accompany myoclonus caused by these conditions. Most begin in childhood or adolescence but many well-documented examples of late presentations of metabolic encephalopathies with myoclonus are to be found in the literature. The commoner examples are listed in Table 1. Mitochondrial encephalopathies are perhaps the commonest identified cause within this group. Physiological findings from a patient with a mitochondrial encephalomyopathy with ragged red fibers are shown in Fig. 9. In the great majority of these cases, myoclonus conforms to a stereotyped pattern of "typical" cortical reflex myoclonus. This includes distally predominant action, reflex, and stimulus sensitive myoclonus on clinical examination and physiological evidence of enlarged cortical SEPs, C reflexes (latency 50 to 60 ms) following mixed or cutaneous peripheral nerve stimulation, contralateral cortical EEG spike discharges preceding myoclonus on backaveraged EEG, and intracortical spread of spike discharges during action and reflex myoclonus (30).

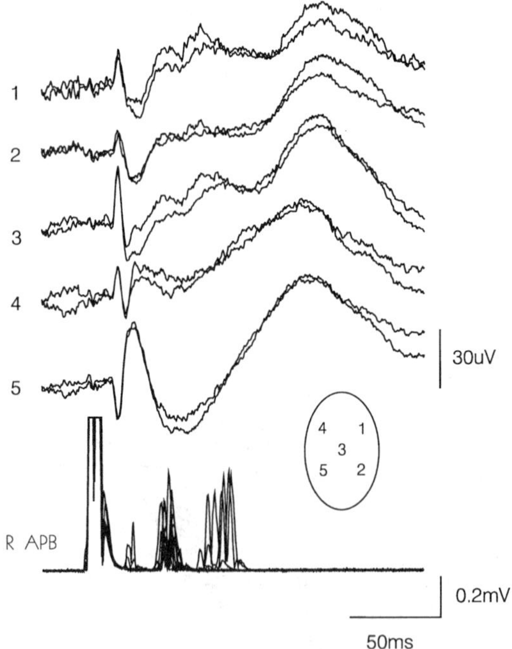

FIG. 9. Enlarged P1-N2 component of the cortical SEP in a 22-year-old woman with cortical reflex myoclonus and a clinical picture of myoclonic epilepsy and ragged red fibers with a mitochondrial DNA mutation. Reflex myoclonus is evident in the right abductor pollicis brevis after stimulation of the right median nerve. Following an M wave, an F response (latency 27 ms) is followed by two C reflexes, the first at 48 ms and the second at variable timings around 80 ms. (From ref. 30, with permission.)

CONCLUSION

The mechanisms responsible for myoclonus in these various degenerative diseases remain the subject of investigation. Future research will explore the role of the cortex in myoclonus in more detail using new measurements of the excitability of primary sensorimotor cortex using magnetic brain stimulation and detailed mapping of cortical function using magnetoencephalography.

REFERENCES

1. Thompson PD, Marsden CD. Corticobasal degeneration. In: Rossor M, ed. *Unusual dementias.* London: Bailliere Tindall, 1992:677–686.
2. Rinne JO, Lee MS, Thompson PD, Marsden CD. Corticobasal degeneration. A clinical study of 36 cases. *Brain* 1994;117:1183–1196.
3. Lang AE, Riley DE, Bergeron C. Cortical-basal ganglionic degeneration. In: Calne DB, ed. *Neurodegenerative diseases.* Philadelphia: WB Saunders, 1994:877–894.
4. Brunt ERP, van Weerden TW, Pruim J, Lakke JWPF. Unique myoclonic pattern in corticobasal degeneration. *Mov Disord* 1995;10:132–142.
5. Thompson PD, Day BL, Rothwell JC, Brown P, Britton TC, Marsden CD. The myoclonus in corticobasal degeneration. Evidence for two forms of cortical reflex myoclonus. *Brain* 1994;117:1197–1207.
6. Mima T, Nagamini T, Ikeda A, Yazawa S, Kimura J, Shibasaki H. Pathogenesis of cortical myoclonus studied by magnetoencephalography. *Ann Neurol* 1998; 43: 598–607.
7. Chen R, Ashby P, Lang AE. Stimulus sensitive myoclonus in akinetic rigid syndromes. *Brain* 1992;115: 1875–1888.
8. Riley DE, Lang AE, Lewis A, Resch L, Ashby P, Blank S, Hornykiewicz O. Cortical-basal ganglionic degeneration. *Neurology* 1990;40:1203–1212.
9. Carella F, Scaioli V, Franceschetti S, Girotti F, Giovannini P, Ciano C., Caraceni T. Focal reflex myoclonus in corticobasal degeneration. *Funct Neurol* 1991;6:165–170.
10. Day BL, Dressler D, Maertens de Noordhout A, Marsden CD, Rothwell JC, Thompson PD. Electrical and magnetic stimulation of human motor cortex: surface EMG and single unit responses in arm muscles. *J Physiol* 1989;412:449–473.

11. Lu CS, Ikeda A, Terada K, et al. Electrophysiological studies of early stage corticobasal degeneration. *Mov Disord* 1998;13: 140–146.
12. Hallett M, Chadwick D, Marsden CD. Cortical reflex myoclonus. *Neurology* 1979;29:1107–1125.
13. Shibasaki H, Yamashita Y, Neshigi R, Tobimatsu S, Fukui R. Pathogenesis of giant somatosensory evoked potentials in progressive myoclonic epilepsy. *Brain* 1985;108:225–240.
14. Sawle GV, Brooks DJ, Marsden CD, Frackowiak RSJ. Corticobasal degeneration. *Brain* 1991;114:541–556.
15. Eidelberg D, Dhawan V, Moeller JJ, Sidtis JJ, Ginos JZ, Powells JM. The metabolic landscape of cortico-basal ganglionic degeneration: regional asymmetries studied with positron emission tomography. *J Neurol Neurosurg Psychiatry* 1991;54:856–862.
16. Blin J, Vidailhet M, Pillon B, Dubois B, Feve JR, Agid Y. Corticobasal degeneration: decreased and asymmetrical glucose consumption as studied with PET. *Mov Disord* 1991;7:348–354.
17. Wilkins DE, Hallett M, Berardelli A, Walshe T, Alvarez N. Physiologic analysis of the myoclonus of Alzheimer's disease. *Neurology* 1984;34:898–903.
18. Ugawa Y, Kohara N, Hirasawa H, Kuzuhara S, Iwata M, Mannen T. Myoclonus in Alzheimer's disease. *J Neurol* 1987;235:90–94.
19. Brown P. Transmissible human spongiform encephalopathy (infectious cerebral amyloidosis): Creutzfeldt-Jakob disease, Gerstmann-Straussler-Schinker syndrome, and Kuru. In: Calne D, ed. *Neurodegeneration.* Philadelphia: WB Saunders, 1994:839–876.
20. Shibasaki H, Motomura M, Yamashita Y, Shii H, Kuroiwa Y. Periodic synchronous discharge and myoclonus in Creutzfeldt-Jakob disease: diagnostic application of jerk-locked averaging method. *Ann Neurol* 1981;9:150–156.
21. Shibasaki H, Neshige R. Photic cortical reflex myoclonus. *Ann Neurol* 1987;22:252–287.
22. Wenning GK, Quinn NP. In: Quinn, NP ed. *Multiple system atrophy in* parkinsonism. London: Bailliere Tindall, 1997: 187–204.
23. Obeso JA, Rothwell JC, Marsden CD. The spectrum of cortical myoclonus. *Brain* 1985;108:193–224.
24. Rodriguez ME, Artieda J, Zubieta JL, Obeso JA. Reflex myoclonus in olivopontocerebellar atrophy. *J Neurol Neurosurg Psychiatry* 1994;57:316–319.
25. Artieda J, Obeso JA. The pathophysiology and pharmacology of photic cortical reflex myoclonus. *Ann Neurol* 1993;34:175–184.
26. Houston PD, Lim CL, Fung V, Yiannikas C, Morris JGL. Brainstem myoclonus in a patient with non Dopa responsive parkinsonism. *Move Disord* 1996;11:404–410.
27. Thompson PD, Bhatia KP, Brown P, Davis MB, Pires M, Quinn NP, et al. Cortical myoclonus in Huntington's disease. *Mov Disord* 1994;9:633–641.
28. Carella F, Scaioli V, Ciano C, Birelli S, Oliva D, Girotti F. Adult onset myoclonic Huntington's disease. *Move Dis* 1993;8:201–205.
29. Marsden CD, Harding AE, Obeso JA, Lu CS. Progressive myoclonic ataxia (The Ramsay Hunt syndrome). *Arch Neurol* 1990;47:1121–1125.
30. Thompson PD, Hammans SR, Harding AE. Cortical reflex myoclonus in patients with the mitochondrial DNA transfer RNA Lys (8344) (MERRF) mutation. *J Neurol* 1994;241:335–340.

Corticobasal Degeneration.
Advances in Neurology, Vol. 82,
edited by I. Litvan, C. G. Goetz, and A. E. Lang.
Lippincott Williams & Wilkins, Philadelphia © 2000.

8

Parkinsonism in Corticobasal Degeneration

Anthony E. Lang

Division of Neurology, Toronto Western Hospital, Toronto, Ontario, M5T 2S8, Canada

INTRODUCTION

This chapter will discuss the occurrence, nature, and possible pathogenesis of Parkinsonian features seen in patients with corticobasal (cortical-basal ganglionic) degeneration (CBD). Parkinsonism is a syndrome typically defined as consisting of the combination of at least two of the four cardinal features—akinesia, rigidity, tremor, and postural disturbance. It has been recognized since the first descriptions of CBD that these features are extremely common early manifestations and most clinical series have found that an akinetic-rigid syndrome eventually develops in all patients with this disorder. For example, in a recent case series of 147 patients from eight movement disorders centers (1) at least one Parkinsonian feature developed in all; 95% had at least two Parkinson signs and eight had one each (four gait only, two rigidity only, one bradykinesia only, and one tremor only). However, accepted diagnostic criteria for CBD (2,3) universally demand the presence of an akinetic-rigid syndrome and most large published series originate from movement disorders centers, raising the strong possibility of referral bias.

In dealing with the topic of Parkinsonism in CBD, a number of questions need to be considered: (a) What are the proportions of patients who: present with Parkinsonism, present with other symptoms and signs but also demonstrate Parkinsonian features either early or later in the course of the illness, and do not develop the features of Parkinsonism at all during the course of the disease? (b) What are the sources of potential confusion in establishing the signs and symptoms as those of Parkinsonism? (c) What are the pathological substrates that account for the Parkinsonism in CBD? (d) What is the response of the Parkinsonian features to therapeutic interventions? In attempting to address these questions, the issue of diagnostic accuracy becomes critical. As stated, clinical diagnostic criteria for the syndrome of CBD uniformly include akinesia and rigidity. However, there have also been many cases in which the typical pathology of CBD was associated with "atypical" clinical presentations; usually the diagnosis of CBD in these cases was not possible in life. Furthermore, in recent years there have been several cases reported that presented with the "classical" syndrome (i.e., fulfilling all established clinical diagnostic criteria) where postmortem revealed an alternative pathology (4). Thus, in the absence of pathological confirmation, there is an unavoidable degree of diagnostic uncertainty that will impact on the accuracy of the responses to the questions listed. Because most studies of "CBD patients" to date have lacked pathological confirmation for the majority of the cases reported, it must be acknowledged that the presence of the classical clinical features that encouraged or permitted the diagnosis in life may have had an important influence on the reported results. This especially applies to studies claiming to establish characteristic "patterns" of dysfunction that could be used to distinguish this disorder from other forms of Parkinsonism. Examples of this problem are attempts to distinguish CBD from other disorders using neuropsychological, eye movement, or positron emission tomography (PET) criteria.

In attempting to address the question of Parkinsonism in CBD we will emphasize reports of cases with pathologically proven disease in which sufficient clinical information was provided. For the purposes of this review, 68 patients with CBD were included (5–36). Two large series were not included because of insufficient information on individual patients (21,37). The clinical features described in these two series were distinctly different and may have related to the sources of referral of the brains. In the study of Wenning et al. (37) in which most of the 14 patients came from movement disorders clinics, early Parkinsonian features were the rule. The 12 patients studied by Feaney et al. (21) came predominantly from dementia clinics (D. Dickson, personal communication) and most presented with cognitive and behavioral disorders. Despite the major advantages of restricting our review to pathologically proven cases with sufficient clinical information, it must be acknowledged that there may be similar obvious or covert sources of bias in any of these reports (e.g., referral bias, the tendency to report unusual cases, etc.).

PRESENTING SYMPTOMS

Twenty-four of the 68 cases reviewed presented with isolated signs and symptoms of Parkinsonism and 44 patients presented with symptoms incompatible with typical Parkinson's disease. In Table 1, I have attempted to subdivide this latter group into four categories, depending on the occurrence and timing of the development of Parkinsonian features:

1. Those who presented with or had the very early development of additional Parkinsonism;
2. Those who developed these features midway through the course of their disease;
3. Those who developed features only late in their illness;
4. Those where no features of Parkinsonism were described at all.

In the majority, Parkinsonism developed in the early (32/68) or middle stages (18/68) of the disease. Twelve patients developed some features of Parkinsonism only late in the course, whereas six patients were classified as not demonstrating any of these features in life (28,32,34,35). As will be discussed, there may have been other explanations for features interpreted as Parkinsonism, and so this latter figure may be an underestimate.

As mentioned, Wenning et al. (37) found that a high proportion of patients presented with Parkinsonian features. At the first neurological visit, on average 3 years after symptom onset, the most commonly encountered "extrapyramidal" fea-

TABLE 1. *Features and timing of the occurrence of parkinsonism in sixty-eight pathologically proven cases of CBD*

	Parkinsonism				
Presenting features	Early	Mid	Late	None	Total
Isolated Parkinsonism	24	—	—	—	24 (35%)
Cognitive/behavioral	3	10	5	5	23 (34%)
Primary progressive aphasia/word finding difficulties	—	3	6	—	9 (13%)
Apraxia/cortical motor limb features	1	4	1	1	7 (10%)
Sensory disturbances	3	—	—	—	3 (4%)
Other	1	1	—	—	2 (3%)
Total	32 (47%)	18 (26%)	12 (18%)	6 (9%)	68

CBD, Corticobasal Degeneration.
Table 1 is a presentation of features and timing of the occurrence of Parkinsonism in sixty-eight pathologically proven cases of CBD. The far left column lists the presenting feature and the far right column gives the total number (and percent of the entire 68 cases) of patients presenting in this fashion. The middle columns under "Parkinsonism" give the numbers of patients who presented with a specific feature who developed Parkinsonian features in the early, mid, or late stages of their illness or who failed to demonstrate Parkinsonism in life (i.e., "None"). The bottom row gives the total numbers of patients who demonstrated Parkinsonism beginning in the early, mid, or late disease stages or who were not described as developing Parkinsonism at any time over the entire course of their illness (none).

tures included limb rigidity in 79%, bradykinesia in 71%, and postural imbalance in 45%, followed by limb dystonia in 43%. However, the majority of their 14 patients had come from movement disorders clinics. Recently, we (35) reviewed the experience of the Canadian Brain Tissue Bank, which receives referrals from a number of sources including dementia and movement disorders clinics. Prior to death only four of the 13 cases reviewed had a clinical diagnosis of CBD (in contrast to 50% of those reviewed by Wenning et al.). Nine had early cognitive disturbances; six had a diagnosis of Alzheimer's disease prior to death (in contrast to 21% of the cases presenting with cognitive problems [Wenning et al.]). Five patients had early language dysfunction including reduced speech output. Five patients had the relatively early onset of Parkinsonian features that accompanied prominent cognitive disturbances in three. In two of the 13 patients, no features of Parkinsonism were noted over the course of their illness. This series may be more representative of the true picture of CBD than other series since it draws from both dementia and movement disorders referrals. It might even be more representative than the collection of cases summarized in Table 1, since this series of 68 cases is comprised of reports of single or very small numbers of cases that could be influenced by reporting biases mentioned earlier.

CLINICAL FEATURES AND SOURCES OF DIAGNOSTIC CONFUSION

The clinical features of Parkinsonism described in patients with CBD include tremor, rigidity, bradykinesia or clumsiness of a limb, and gait and postural disturbances. Tremor is typically a postural and action (or "intention") tremor. It is often described as irregular and "jerky" and may evolve into the characteristic stimulus sensitive myoclonus. It is likely that this component accounts for the rare mention of tremor at rest (6,19,37) and it is unclear whether a classical pill-rolling tremor of Parkinson's disease ever occurs in this disorder. Rigidity is possibly the commonest Parkinsonian feature documented in CBD. Most often this is asymmetrically present in the limbs, the arm typically affected more than the leg. Occasionally, the leg is more severely affected than the arm and less often axial tone is increased more than limb tone. The rigidity of CBD can reach extreme proportions. In milder forms, rigidity is indistinguishable from that found in Parkinson's disease (PD), including the presence of cogwheeling. However, in the case of extreme rigidity the distinction is readily apparent. There may be important contributions from the dystonic posturing ("dystonic rigidity"), from additional spasticity, and particularly from paratonia. It is likely that a number of the patients classified as having early Parkinsonism on the basis of "rigidity" in a limb actually had paratonia owing to the early pathological involvement of frontal cortex and subcortical white matter.

Many of the cases reviewed were described as having clumsiness of a limb (most often the hand) interfering with the accurate performance of a variety of tasks. This was often interpreted as akinesia or bradykinesia, especially if accompanied by increased tone in the same limb. Obviously, there are a number of motor deficits found in patients with CBD aside from bradykinesia that could result in "clumsiness," including tremor, myoclonus, dystonia, ideomotor apraxia, pyramidal deficits, cortical sensory dysfunction, and alien limb phenomenon. However, all of these should have been evident on examination and they were taken into account whenever mentioned in formulating Table 1. An important potential source of confusion (and controversy) with bradykinesia that will remain a persistent problem after all of these other disturbances are excluded is "limb kinetic apraxia" (LKA). Okudo and Tachibana (38) have argued that LKA, defined as a breakdown of previously skilled movements manifested by difficulty in making fine finger movements, is the commonest form of apraxia seen in CBD. Leiguarda et al. (39) briefly reviewed the longstanding debate surrounding the validity of this concept. In general they agreed with Okuda and Tachibana inasmuch as "the disruption of movement seen in lesions of the corticospinal pathway, or *as seen in Parkinson's disease* (my emphasis), can seldom be fully explained by weakness, akinesia, abnormal posture or tone" indicating an "additional breakdown of the movement pattern or formula—Liepmann's innervatory engram—that suggests a higher motor disorder or apraxia." Very few of the reports on CBD acknowledge or consider the possible contribution of this motor disorder to the patient's symptomatology. Interestingly, when it is specifically sought, LKA is extremely common and may account for most of the early symptoms of "clumsiness" (32). In such cases, bradykinesia is often not considered as an initial feature unless it occurred in the context of another Parkinsonian sign such as rigidity. This issue requires careful future evaluation, applying strict definitions of the motor disturbances constituting bradykinesia and LKA. Recently, Denes et al. (40) proposed the following five criteria to classify movement error as limb kinetic apraxia:

1. Awkwardness and clumsiness of the movement in the absence of elementary motor and sensory deficit, or ataxia, and in the presence of normal muscle tone;
2. Absence of voluntary-automatic dissociation (i.e., the motor impairment should equally affect both movements performed in daily living activities and those performed in the testing sessions);
3. The motor impairment should affect equally the execution of both symbolic and meaningless gestures;
4. Constancy of the impairment throughout the various observations;
5. Normal conceptual knowledge of the movements.

Distinguishing these deficits from motor dysfunction that many investigators might accept within the realm of bradykinesia (especially severe forms of this) may be quite difficult. As will be discussed, this clinical conundrum is typical of the problems faced when attempting to delineate clinical-pathological correlations in CBD. In the face of widespread pathology, does one explain the initial clumsiness and increase in tone (? Parkinsonism) on the basis of disease involvement of the basal ganglia, the premotor cortex, or a disruption between the two?

Finally, gait disturbances and postural instability resulting in falls are common features in CBD especially later in the course of the illness. At least seven of the 68 cases reviewed developed early leg symptoms (3,6,11,16,29,31) and in the study of 14 patients by Wenning et al. (37) (most from movement disorders clinics) at first visit, after 35.5 months of symptoms, a gait disorder, postural instability, and falls were recorded in 43%, 45%, and 43% respectively, whereas at the last visit, 37.4 months later, these features were present in 100%, 92%, and 69%. Often the gait is described as short-strided and shuffling, similar to that of Parkinson's disease. However, several reports indicate a wide base that would be atypical of PD and other features such as apraxia, and cortical sensory loss in the leg must be considered, especially in accounting for unsteadiness and falls.

The presence and severity of Parkinsonian features may influence the survival of patients with CBD. Wenning et al. (37) found that patients with bilateral bradykinesia (or a frontal syndrome or both) or those that exhibited two of three extrapyramidal features (tremor, rigidity, bradykinesia) at their first examination had a shorter survival than those who did not. In our series (35), the five patients with an earlier onset of Parkinsonism (within less than 3 years of symptom onset) had a 4.8 year survival (range 3 to 7 years), whereas the eight who developed Parkinsonism later or not at all survived for 6.9 years (range 5 to 10 years).

CLINICAL-PATHOLOGICAL CORRELATIONS

CBD is a progressive neurodegenerative disorder that involves a number of cortical and subcortical regions. These changing and widespread characteristics make it exceedingly difficult to establish the exact pathological substrate(s) for the Parkinsonian features. In addition, as previously outlined, there are a number of potential sources of confusion with respect to the clinical nature of the Parkinsonian features that further confounds this exercise. The dopaminergic cells of the substantia nigra compacta (SNc) are almost uniformly affected by the pathology of CBD. [18F]fluoro-L-dopa (F-dopa) PET scans demonstrate asymmetrical reduction in striatal uptake that correlates with the clinically most affected side (41). In contrast to the pattern of striatal F-dopa uptake in Parkinson's disease, where activity in the putamen is reduced much more than in the caudate, in cases of CBD (mostly clinically diagnosed) reduction in F-dopa uptake in the caudate and the putamen has been equivalent. This suggests that the lateromedial gradient of involvement of the SNc typical of PD should not be evident in the pathology of CBD. Indeed, where it is mentioned, most but not all pathological studies have reported a relatively uniform distribution of degeneration within the nigra (as well as involvement of other dopaminergic cell groups in the midbrain). Rare cases have demonstrated little or no involvement of this region (9,34). Interestingly, these cases manifested predominant language and cognitive dysfunction with little or no unequivocal Parkinsonian features evident in life. This experience might suggest that the primary substrate for the Parkinsonism in CBD is the degeneration of the SNc. However, there are major problems with this simple explanation. The pathology of CBD also affects several other components of the cortico-striato-pallido-thalomo-cortical motor loop (42), including the putamen, lateral and medial segments of the globus pallidus, the lateral thalamus, and premotor cortices. The cases lacking SNc involvement and Parkinsonism also lacked involvement in these other motor control regions (9,34). In addition, occasional cases have been described where severe SNc involvement occurred in the absence of other basal ganglia pathology and the patient demonstrated very little true Parkinsonism (27). Where Parkinsonism was evident in life, the extent of the pathological involvement of these other areas, especially the basal ganglia, has varied considerably from case to case, ranging from no changes or only the presence of rare chromatolytic neurons to severe gliosis and neuronal loss. Generally it is not possible to establish a clear correlation between the presence or degree of Parkinsonism and the relative involvement of these potentially relevant structures. The fact that the pathology is available only at the end stages of the disease in most cases further hampers these attempts.

As will be discussed briefly in the following section, the response of the Parkinsonian features in CBD to dopaminergic therapy is usually quite poor. This is probably owing to the additional involvement of areas "downstream" from the nigrostriatal dopamine neurons. Interestingly, two patients who were said to have obtained benefit from L-dopa (8,28) demonstrated no involvement of basal ganglia aside form the severe depletion of neurons in the SNc. Future research studies combining various functional imaging techniques such as PET, magnetic resonance spectroscopy (MRS) (43), and fMRI with subsequent pathological confirmation of the diagnosis will be necessary to further our understanding of these clinicopathological correlations.

TREATMENT OF PARKINSONISM

Unfortunately, little can be said about the effective treatment of Parkinsonian features found in patients with CBD. At one time or another, most of these patients are given trials of a variety of anti-Parkinson medications, including L-dopa, dopamine agonists, amantadine, and anticholinergics. Generally, these have been completely ineffective, although as mentioned previously, rare examples of benefit are described and this may indicate a relative preservation of both the dopamine receptors in the striatum and the striato-pallido-thalamo-cortical connections. Drug trials were mentioned for 18 of the 68 patients reviewed. In addition to the responses already mentioned, two others were said to have had transient or mild improvement and the remainder failed to benefit. In the study by Wenning et al., four of the 14 patients received L-dopa, three had no benefit, and one was said to have had "a moderate (30% to 50%) response of unknown duration" (37). Ninety-two percent of 147 clinically diagnosed cases reviewed by Kompoliti et al. (1) had received dopaminergic drugs; 24% obtained some benefit, 71% did not improve, and 5% experienced worsening of Parkinsonian features, dystonia, myoclonus, or gait dysfunction. L-dopa accounted for most of these trials and most of the positive drug responses; 25 of the 33 showing some improvement had benefit in Parkinsonian features.

Very few patients with CBD have undergone functional neurosurgery for their Parkinsonism. We performed a Vim thalamotomy in one patient for severe arm dystonia before she had developed other features that permitted the correct diagnosis. The procedure had no effect whatsoever on the dystonia or the subsequent development of stimulus-sensitive myoclonus, and rigidity. Fazzini et al. (44) reported that medial pallidotomy was ineffective in improving one patient with CBD and the author is aware of one or two other patients similarly treated at other institutions who also failed to benefit from this procedure. Our group has been asked to consider this therapy or deep brain stimulation in a number of patients; however, knowing the widespread nature of the pathology and the complex basis of the clinical disability, we have advised against such surgery in all cases.

CONCLUSIONS

Parkinsonian features are extremely common in patients suffering from CBD. They contribute greatly to the extent of disability and probably shorten survival. Other clinical features present in these patients, such as paratonia and limb kinetic apraxia owing to involvement of premotor cortical areas, could be mistaken for Parkinsonism and may account for some of the descriptions of "rigidity" and "bradykinesia" in the literature. Attempts at establishing clinicopathological correlations for the Parkinsonism are further confounded by the widespread and progressive nature of the pathology. Involvement of the SNc almost certainly contributes but pathological changes in other components of the basal ganglia-cortical motor loop are also important. To date, treatment has been unsatisfactory. It is likely that symptomatic or "palliative" therapy, for example, attempting to alter neurotransmitter function as used in Parkinson's disease, will remain ineffective and advances in this field will require a greater understanding of the cause of the disorder or the pathogenetic mechanisms underlying the progressive neuronal and glial pathology.

ACKNOWLEDGMENT

This work was partially supported by a Centre of Excellence grant from the National Parkinson Foundation (Miami).

REFERENCES

1. Kompoliti K, Goetz CG, Boeve BF, et al. Clinical presentation and pharmacological therapy in corticobasal degeneration. *Arch Neurol* 1998;55:957–961.
2. Lang AE, Riley DE, Bergeron C. Cortical-basal ganglionic degeneration. In: Calne DB, ed. *Neurodegenerative diseases.* Philadelphia: WB Saunders, 1994:877–894.
3. Watts RL, Mirra SS, Richardson EP. Cortical-basal ganglionic degeneration. In: Marsden CD, Fahn S, eds. *Movement disorders III.* Oxford: Butterworth Heinemann, 1994:282–299.
4. Kumar R, Bergeron C, Pollanen M, Lang AE. Cortical-basal ganglionic degeneration. In: Jankovic J, Tolosa E, eds. *Parkinson's disease and movement disorders.* Baltimore: Williams & Wilkins, 1998:297–316.
5. Rebeiz JJ, Kolodny EH, Richardson EP. Corticodentatonigral degeneration with neuronal achromasia. *Arch Neurol* 1968;18:20–33.
6. Gibb WRG, Luthert PJ, Marsden CD. Corticobasal degeneration. *Brain* 1989;112:1171–1192.
7. Riley DE, Lang AE, Lewis A, et al. Cortical-basal ganglionic degeneration. *Neurology* 1990;40:1203–1212.
8. Lippa CF, Smith TW, Fontneau N. Corticonigral degeneration with neuronal achromasia. *J Neurol Sci* 1990; 98:301–310.
9. Lippa CF, Cohen R, Smith TW, Drachman DA. Primary progressive aphasia with focal neuronal achromasia. *Neurology* 1991;41:882–886.
10. Sakurai Y, Hashida H, Uesugi H, et al. A clinical profile of corticobasal degeneration presenting as primary progressive aphasia. *Eur Neurol* 1996;36:134–137.
11. Eberhard DA, Lopes MBS, Trugman JM, Brashear HR. Alzheimer's disease in a case of cortical basal ganglionic degeneration with severe dementia. *J Neurol Neurosurg Psychiatry* 1996;60:109–110.
12. Rey GJ, Tomer R, Levin BE, Sanchez-Ramos J, Bowen B, Bruce JH. Psychiatric symptoms, atypical dementia, and left visual field inattention in corticobasal ganglionic degeneration. *Mov Disord* 1995;10:106–110.
13. Greene PE, Fahn S, Lang AE, Watts RL, Eidelberg D, Powers JM. What is it? Case 1 1990: progressive unilateral rigidity, bradykinesia, tremulousness, and apraxia, leading to fixed postural deformity of the involved limb. *Mov Disord* 1990;5:341–351.
14. Brown J, Lantos PL, Roques P, Fidani L, Rossor MN. Familial dementia with swollen achromatic neurons and corticobasal inclusion bodies: a clinical and pathological study. *J Neurol Sci* 1996;135:21–30.
15. Bergeron C, Pollanen MS, Weyer L, Black SE, Lang AE. Unusual clinical presentations of cortical-basal ganglionic degeneration. *Ann Neurol* 1996;40:72–79.
16. Rinne JO, Lee MS, Thompson PD, Marsden CD. Corticobasal degeneration. A clinical study of 36 cases. *Brain* 1994;117:1183–1196.
17. Paulus W, Selim M. Corticonigral degeneration with neuronal achromasia and basal neurofibrillary tangles. *Acta Neuropathol* 1990;81:89–94.
18. Case 38-1985. Case records of the Massachusetts General Hospital. *N Engl J Med* 1985;313:739–748.
19. Case 16-1986. Case records of the Massachusetts General Hospital. *N Engl J Med* 1986;314:1101–1111.
20. Ikeda K, Akiyama H, Iritani S, et al. Corticobasal degeneration with primary progressive aphasia and accentuated cortical lesion in superior temporal gyrus:

Case report and review. *Acta Neuropathol (Berl)* 1996;92:534–539.

21. Feany MB, Ksiezak-Reding H, Liu W-K, Vincent I, Yen S-HC, Dickson DW. Epitope expression and hyperphosphorylation of tau protein in corticobasal degeneration: differentiation from progressive supranuclear palsy. *Acta Neuropathol (Berl)* 1995;90:37–43.
22. Mitsuyama Y, Masuda K, Inoue T, Koono M, Koga S, Nakamura J. Primary progressive dementia with swollen chromatolytic neurons. *Dementia* 1992;3:223–231.
23. Buée-Scherrer V, Hof PR, Buée L, et al. Hyperphosphorylated tau proteins differentiate corticobasal degeneration and Pick's disease. *Acta Neuropathol (Berl)* 1996;91:351–359.
24. Mori H, Nishimura M, Namba Y, Oda M. Corticobasal degeneration: a disease with widespread appearance of abnormal tau and neurofibrillary tangles, and its relation to progressive supranuclear palsy. *Acta Neuropathol (Berl)* 1994;88:113–121.
25. Horoupian DS, Chu PL. Unusual case of corticobasal degeneration with tau/Gallyas-positive neuronal and glial tangles. *Acta Neuropathol (Berl)* 1994;88:592–598.
26. Uchihara T, Mitani K, Mori H, Kondo H, Yamada M, Ikeda K. Abnormal cytoskeletal pathology peculiar to corticobasal degeneration is different from that of Alzheimer's disease or progressive supranuclear palsy. *Acta Neuropathol (Berl)* 1994;88:379–383.
27. Halliday GM, Davies L, McRitchie DA, Cartwright H, Pamphlett R, Morris JGL. Ubiquitin-positive achromatic neurons in corticobasal degeneration. *Acta Neuropathol (Berl)* 1995;90:68–75.
28. Jendroska K, Rossor MN, Mathias CJ, Daniel SE. Morphological overlap between corticobasal degeneration and Pick's disease: a clinicopathological report. *Mov Disord* 1995;10:111–114.
29. Schneider JA, Watts RL, Gearing M, Brewer RP, Mirra SS. Corticobasal degeneration: neuropathologic and clinical heterogeneity. *Neurology* 1997;48:959–969.
30. Kawasaki K, Iwanaga K, Wakabayashi K, et al. Corticobasal degeneration with neither argyrophilic inclusions nor tau abnormalities: a new subgroup? *Acta Neuropathol (Berl)* 1996;91: 140–144.
31. Takahashi T, Amano N, Hanihara T, et al. Corticobasal Degeneration: widespread argentophilic threads and glia in addition to neurofibrillary tangles. Similarities of cytoskeletal abnormalities in corticobasal degeneration and progressive supranuclear palsy. *J Neuro Sci* 1996;138; 66–77.
32. Tsuchiya K, Ikeda K, Uchihara T, Oda T, Shimada H. Distribution of cerebral cortical lesions in corticobasal degeneration: a clinicopathological study of five autopsy cases in Japan. *Acta Neuropathol (Berl)* 1997;94: 416–424.
33. Wakabayashi K, Oyanagi K, Makifuchi T, Ikutu F, Homma A, Homma Y. et al. Corticobasal degeneration: etiopathological significance of the cytoskeletal alterations. *Acta Neuropathol (Berl)* 1994;87:545–553.
34. Clark AW, Manz HJ, White CL, Lehmann J, Miller D, Coyle JT. Cortical degeneration with swollen chromatolytic neurons: its relationship to Pick's disease. *J Neuropathol Exp Neurol* 1986;45:268–284.
35. Grimes DA, Lang AE, Bergeron C. Dementia is the most common presentation of cortical-basal ganglionic degeneration. *Neurology* 1998;50(suppl 4):A96.
36. Hauser, RA 1998. Personal communication
37. Wenning GK, Litvan I, Jankovic J, et al. Natural history and survival of 14 patients with corticobasal degeneration confirmed at postmortem examination. *J Neurol Neurosurg Psychiatry* 1998;64:184–189.
38. Okuda B, Tachibana H. The nature of apraxia in corticobasal degeneration. *J Neurol Neurosurg Psychiatry* 1994; 57:1548–1549.
39. Leiguarda R, Lees AJ, Merello M, Starkstein S, Marsden CD. The nature of apraxia in corticobasal degeneration. *J Neurol Neurosurg Psychiatry* 1994;57:455–459.
40. Denes G, Mantovan MC, Gallana A, Cappelletti JY. Limb-kinetic apraxia. *Mov Disord* 1998;13:468–476.
41. Sawle GV, Brooks DJ, Marsden CD, Frackowiak RS. Corticobasal degeneration. A unique pattern of regional cortical oxygen hypometabolism and striatal fluorodopa uptake demonstrated by positron emission tomography. *Brain* 1991;114:541–556.
42. Alexander GE, DeLong MR, Strick PL. Parallel organization of functionally segregated circuits linking basal ganglia and cortex. *Ann Rev Neurosci* 1986;9: 357–381.
43. Tedeschi G, Litvan I, Bonavita S, et al. Proton magnetic resonance spectroscopic imaging in progressive supranuclear palsy, Parkinson's disease and corticobasal degeneration. *Brain* 1997;120:1541–1552.
44. Fazzini E, Dogali M, Beric A, et al. The effects of unilateral ventral posterior medial pallidotomy in patients with Parkinson's disease and Parkinson's plus syndromes. In: Koller WC, Paulson G, eds. *Therapy of Parkison's disease.* New York: Marcel Dekker, 1995: 353–379.

Corticobasal Degeneration.
Advances in Neurology, Vol. 82,
edited by I. Litvan, C. G. Goetz, and A. E. Lang.
Lippincott Williams & Wilkins, Philadelphia © 2000.

9

Memory and Executive Processes in Corticobasal Degeneration

Bernard Pillon* and Bruno Dubois†

INSERM U 289 and †Department of Neurology, Hôpital de la Salpêtrière, 75013 Paris, France

INTRODUCTION

In this chapter, we will show that the symptomatology of corticobasal degeneration (CBD) cannot be restricted to motor and gesture disorders as was originally thought. Indeed, systematic evaluation of cognitive functions in CBD has regularly revealed impairments in the executive and memory domains and, in some cases, in visuospatial and linguistic functions. The same may apply for the pattern of cerebral lesions of CBD: It was first considered as relatively focal, involving specific cortical (fronto-parietal) and subcortical (thalamus, striatum, and substantia nigra) areas (1–4). Recent pathological studies have shown that the pattern of degeneration could be more diffuse (5,6).

Despite this relative heterogeneity, it is possible to postulate relationships between the clinical expression and the underlying lesions (Table 1) (7–23). Such is the case for memory disorders and executive dysfunction: In the absence of significant lesions of the hippocampus and medial temporal lobes structures in most cases, memory disorders may result from the disruption of the subcortico-frontal circuits that also account for the dysexecutive syndrome, as has been demonstrated in other degenerative diseases involving predominantly subcortical structures (23).

DISORDERS OF INSTRUMENTAL FUNCTIONS

CBD is typically defined by unilateral rigidity of one arm with praxis disorders, justifying the definition as "progressive asymmetric rigidity and apraxia syndrome" (24). Gesture disorders are so characteristic of the disease that the diagnosis can be suspected on the nature of the motor disturbances. They consist, at first, in the patient experiencing difficulty—or showing perplexity—in the performance of delicate and fine movements of the fingers of one hand. At this stage, patients complain of clumsiness and loss of manual dexterity, reminiscent of "limb apraxia," a disorder described as "kinaesthetic" in patients with lesions of the parietal cortex, or "kinetic" in patients with lesions of the premotor cortex (13,25,26). Asymmetric praxis disorders (difficulty in posture imitation, symbolic gesture execution, and object utilization) are also regularly observed, even at this stage. Ideomotor apraxia is frequent, especially in patients who have initial symptoms in the right limb, in agreement with the hypothesis of a predominant storage of "movement formulae" in the left hemisphere (9,27,28). In contrast with disturbances in all aspects of gesture execution, the ability to identify correctly the gestures performed by the examiner or seen on pictures is preserved, suggesting that mental representations and conceptual aspects of gestures are not involved (29). This finding is in agreement with the fact that conceptual apraxia (30–32) is usually reported only in the case of a severe cognitive impairment (i.e., with the existence of more diffuse lesions of the cerebral cortex) (27). The performance of complex gestures (posture reproduction, evocation and imitation of symbolic ges-

TABLE 1. *Proposed relationships between symptoms of CBD and localization of lesions*

Symptoms	Localization of lesions	Relationships established in CBD	Relationships established in focal lesions
Ideomotor and limb motor apraxia	Left parietal lobe	Kareken et al. (7) Otsuki et al. (8)	Heilman and Rothi (9)
Constructive disorders and neglect	Right parietal lobe	Rey et al. (10) Wenning et al. (11)	Hecaen et al. (12)
Dynamic motor disorders	Premotor cortex	NE	Freund and Hummelsheim (13)
Alien limb phenomenon	Supplementary motor area	NE	Goldberg et al. (14) Watson et al. (15)
Word finding difficulties	Left temporal lobe	Arima et al. (16) Ikeda et al. (17)	Goodglass (18)
Speech apraxia	Broca's area	Bergeron et al. (19)	Lecours and Lhermitte (20)
Dysexecutive syndrome	Subcortico-frontal circuits	Schneider et al. (5)	Stuss and Benson (21)
Encoding and recall deficits	Subcortico-frontal circuits	Beatty et al. (22)	Dubois et al. (23)

NE: nonestablished

tures, object use) can easily be related to the parietal and premotor lesions observed both in metabolic (33,34) and in postmortem studies (1,2). In advanced cases, however, dystonia, rigidity, and bradykinesia may be sufficiently severe to prevent the interpretation of gesture disorders, at least for the most impaired limb.

Other signs of cortical involvement have been described in CBD. Buccofacial apraxia is generally milder than limb apraxia, except in patients with progressive loss of speech output (35). Patients with initial lower extremity involvement complain of difficulty in walking, generally associated with stiffness or involuntary jerky movements of the leg (36). Constructive praxis disorders can be observed in patients with predominant right hemisphere lesions (37), in relation to the well-known influence of this hemisphere for visuospatial function. Reflexive horizontal saccade latency is markedly increased, as in focal lesions affecting the posterior parietal cortex, and this slowing has been correlated with the severity of apraxia (38). Alien limb phenomenon, in which a limb behaves in an uncooperative or foreign fashion, occurs in CBD, although its frequency is highly variable among studies. It is generally attributed to lesions affecting the supplementary motor area (14), and its occurrence, in the absence of a known callosal lesion, is highly suggestive of the diagnosis of CBD (39). Linguistic disturbances are found in some cases, consisting of decreased lexical fluency, transcortical motor aphasia, and progressive phonetic disintegration or word-finding difficulties (1–3,19,28,35,40). Neglect (3,10,41) as well as visuospatial deficits (2) have also been reported.

MEMORY

Temporospatial orientation, and remote and recent memories are generally preserved at least in the early stages of the disease (22,37), which favors overall maintained ability to store and retrieve information. The encoding and recall strategic processes are, however, dysfunctional, as shown by the impaired performance of patients with CBD on more demanding tasks, such as the logical memory, associate learning, and visual retention subtests of the Wechsler Memory Scale (29). Interestingly, the impairment is not as severe as that observed in patients with Alzheimer's disease (AD) at the same level of global intellectual deterioration (Table 2). For example, the percent of information retained from the Logical Memory stories over a 30-minute delay was 61.6% in average in CBD versus only 23.3% in AD (28). Taken together, these findings suggest that the impaired mechanisms are not the same in CBD and in AD.

To further examine this hypothesis, we need to study specific aspects of explicit memory

TABLE 2. *Performance on the Wechsler Memory Scale Revised of patients with CBD and AD*

	CBD ($N = 21$)	AD ($N = 21$)
Folstein MMSE	25.2 (4.5)	24.9 (3.0)
Logical memory		
Immediate recall	18.3 (7.6)	7.4 (4.4)*
Delayed recall	12.7 (7.3)	1.6 (2.2)*
Percent retention	61.6 (26.8)	23.3 (29.5)*
Paired associates		
Easy pairs	11.3 (1.2)	7.3 (3.2)*
Hard pairs	3.9 (2.3)	1.4 (2.1)*
Total	15.2 (3.1)	8.6 (4.5)*

* Significant difference ($p < 0.01$). Results are expressed as mean (SD). MMSE, MiniMental Status Examination. (From ref. 28, with permission.)

using tests that distinguish the inefficient encoding and retrieval processes observed in subcorticofrontal dysfunction from the true amnesic syndrome due to lesions of hippocampus and related medial temporal structures (42,43). The California Verbal Learning Test (CVLT) (44) allows to compare recall without (free recall) and with (cued recall) the help of semantic cues that may compensate for pure retrieval deficits. It measures the ability of the subject to self-elaborate efficient encoding and retrieval strategies by a spontaneous clustering of items belonging to the same implicit category. The CVLT includes the following seven steps:

1. Learning across five trials of a 16-item shopping list (list A) belonging to four embedded semantic categories (tools, spices and herbs, fruits, clothing);
2. One recall trial of an interference list of 16 shopping items (list B) belonging to four embedded semantic categories (fishes, spices and herbs, fruits, utensils), two of which are in common with list A;
3. Short-delay free recall of list A;
4. Short-delay cued recall of list A, providing the subject with each of the four category names to facilitate recall;
5. Long-delay free recall of list A (after a delay of 20 minutes);
6. Long-delay cued recall of list A; and
7. Recognition of list A items from a variety of foils, including items from list B from semantically similar and different categories.

In this test, where encoding is free, the performance of patients with CBD was lower when compared with control subjects in all subtests: Their difficulty was not limited to retrieval processes since they were also impaired at cued recall. Their pattern of performance was similar to that of patients with PSP but better than that of patients with AD in terms of short- and long-delay free recall and false positives at recognition.

In the Grober and Buschke's test (45), encoding is controlled by asking the examinee to point to and read aloud each of the 16 items to be remembered, presented four at a time, according to their semantic category. In contrast to the CVLT, this test allows measurement of the storage and retrieval abilities of information that has been truly encoded. Our adaptation of the procedure (46) used written printed words rather than labeled pictures. All 16 items had to be retrieved at immediate cued recall before starting memory assessment, which consisted of three consecutive series of free recall and cued recall with selective reminding. These series were separated by 20-second counting-backward periods, in order to obtain recall from secondary memory. Whenever a subject was unable to retrieve an item at cued recall, the examiner provided the correct answer. The numbers of correct answers retrieved by the subject at either free or cued recall for a given series were added to obtain a total recall score. Maximum total score for the three series was 48. Free recall, cued recall, and yes-no recognition performance were also measured after a delay of 20 minutes. The performance of patients with CBD was lower than that of control subjects in free recall, but did not differ from that of control subjects at total recall (Table 3). CBD patients, therefore, benefited from the semantic cues to recall those items that they were not able to retrieve spontaneously. This normalization of the recall performance by cueing indicates that the patients are able to store episodic information in the long term, even though they have difficulty in spontaneous retrieval. Their memory performance did not differ from that of patients with PSP, either at free or cued recall, but was better than that of patients with AD, particularly at cued recall, either immediate or delayed.

Therefore, patients with CBD have a pattern of memory impairment similar to that of other patients with subcortical dementia, suggesting inefficient strategies both of encoding and retrieval. For that reason, their performance may be compensated for when the same semantic cues are used both at encoding and retrieval memory stages (45) and not only at retrieval (CVLT [California Verbal Learning Test]). This memory profile is in agreement with Moscovitch hypothesis (47), according to which memory would have a medial temporal/hippocampal component that would mediate encoding, storage, and retrieval on associative cue-dependent explicit memory tests, and a frontal-lobe component "working memory" on strategic explicit tests. The former component is impaired in AD, but preserved in CBD and in other subcortico-frontal dementias; the last one would be particularly disturbed in CBD and in other subcortico-frontal dementias, but relatively preserved in the early stages of AD (29,42,43,48).

EXECUTIVE FUNCTIONS

In subcortico-frontal degenerative diseases, there are strong relationships between memory performance and executive functions (42,43). The similarity of memory pattern in CBD and PSP would imply the existence of a dysexecutive syndrome as severe in CBD as in PSP. This issue was addressed by assessing CBD and PSP patients with the same tests of executive functions: the simplified version of the Wisconsin Card Sorting Test (49), verbal fluency tests (category fluency: animal names in 1 minute; phonemic fluency: words beginning with "M" in 1 minute) (50), and a graphic series (26). Behavioral abnormalities (prehension, imitation, and utilization behaviors) (51) assessed the autonomy of the patient, that is, his ability to inhibit environmental adherence. To search for imitation behavior, for example, the examiner was seated in front of the subject and performed different gestures in front of him. Without saying anything or looking at the subject, the examiner touched the top of his head, scraped his chin, folded his arms, tapped twice on his shoulders, twice on his knees, stood up, and sat again. The behavior of the subject was scored using a scale with precise steps ranging from 4 (normal behavior) to 0 (very severe abnormality): (4) if he did not imitate the examiner or was perplexed by the examiner's ar-

TABLE 3. *Performance on the Grober and Buschke Verbal Learning Test of controls and patients with CBD, PSP, and SDAT*

	Controls	CBD	PSP	AD
Free recall				
Trial 1	7.3 ± 0.5	5.5 ± 0.8	**4.2 ± 0.5**	**3.2 ± 0.8**
Trial 2	8.7 ± 0.7	6.8 ± 0.8	**5.1 ± 0.4**	**2.4 ± 0.7**
Trial 3	9.9 ± 0.6	**6.6 ± 0.9***	**5.2 ± 0.5**	**2.1 ± 0.5**
Delayed trial	9.8 ± 0.6	7.5 ± 1.2	**5.2 ± 0.5**	**2.1 ± 0.7**
Total recall				
Trial 1	14.6 ± 0.3	13.6 ± 1.1	14.3 ± 0.5	**8.3 ± 0.9**
Trial 2	15.8 ± 0.1	14.5 ± 0.7	15.4 ± 0.3	**8.0 ± 0.8**
Trial 3	15.8 ± 0.1	14.4 ± 0.8	15.3 ± 0.3	**8.1 ± 1.0**
Delayed trial	15.9 ± 0.1	14.7 ± 0.6	15.7 ± 0.2	**8.1 ± 1.0**

* Bold characters indicate pathological scores. Results are expressed as mean ± SEM. (From ref. 29, with permission.)

bitrary gestures; (3) if he asked if he had to imitate; (2) if he imitated, but stopped when asked by the examiner not to imitate; (1) if he imitated again after a short distracting period; (0) if he continued to imitate while the examiner was saying not to do so. Previous studies have shown the reliability of these various tests, particularly when they are included in an extensive battery (52). From the performance on these tasks, a frontal score was defined that has been shown to be correlated with frontal hypometabolism in PSP (53). On all these tests of executive functions, the performance of patients with CBD differed significantly from that of control subjects, but not from that of patients with PSP (Table 4), except for utilization behavior: It was only observed in five out of 15 patients with CBD, as opposed to 11 out of 15 patients with PSP. The global frontal score was lower in patients with CBD than in patients with AD who presented with fewer behavioral abnormalities. Verbal fluency and evocation of verbal series were also impaired in patients with CBD in another study (28), with a trend for a lower performance in patients with right-side onset.

Different aspects of motor and gesture control, such as temporal organization, bimanual coordination, and interference inhibition, are also sensitive to frontal dysfunction (54). Unimanual and bimanual dexterity can be measured with the Purdue Pegboard Test (55). Tapping reproduction, rhythm reproduction, unimanual (fist-edge-palm) and bimanual (left hand fist—right hand fingers extended—switch hand positions simultaneously) motor series, graphic series (alternating squares and diamonds), go—no go (one tap—hand up; two taps—hand stay), and conflicting instructions (subject taps once when the examiner taps twice and vice versa) are assessed with tests adapted from Luria (26). Untouched hand up—touched hand stay evaluates the ability to respond to conflicting commands including the two hands (56). Using such frontal-related motor tasks, the performance of patients with CBD was worse than that of control subjects for all tests and that of patients with AD for the majority of them (29). In agreement with these results, unimanual and bimanual motor series were also more impaired in patients with CBD than in patients with AD in another study (28). In contrast, the performance of patients with CBD was similar to that of patients with PSP on nearly all tests of dynamic motor control and execution, except on unimanual and bimanual dexterity, where it was more impaired in CBD.

DEMENTIA

In most of the studies performed in CBD patients, the level of intellectual deterioration was mild or moderate until an advanced stage of the disease (1–4,37,57,58). For example, the mean

TABLE 4. *Performance of controls and patients with CBD, PSP, and AD on tests of global efficiency and executive function*

	Controls	CBD	PSP	AD
Global efficiency				
Mattis DRS	141.1 (3.0)	**110.7 (16.0)***	**110.8 (10.3)**	**112.9 (13.1)**
Raven PM 47 (IQ)	110.9 (13.8)	**89.9 (20.0)**	**101.3 (8.9)**	**94.5 (15.3)**
Executive function				
Wisconsin CST				
Criteria	5.6 (1.1)	**2.2 (1.7)**	**1.6 (1.0)**	**3.2 (2.0)**
Lexical fluency				
Animals (60 sec)	16.8 (4.7)	**10.7 (5.0)**	**9.9 (3.6)**	**10.2 (4.9)**
"M" (60 sec)	9.8 (4.0)	**4.7 (3.8)**	**3.3 (1.6)**	**6.3 (3.7)**
Graphic series	9.8 (0.4)	**0.0 (0.0)**	**3.3 (4.1)**	**5.5 (3.2)**
Prehension behavior	4.0 (0.0)	**2.3 (1.3)**	**1.5 (0.9)**	3.8 (0.6)
Imitation behavior	4.0 (0.0)	**2.1 (0.9)**	**1.3 (1.0)**	3.3 (1.0)
Utilization behavior	4.0 (0.0)	3.2 (1.3)	**2.2 (1.3)**	3.9 (0.5)
Global frontal score	58.5 (2.6)	**25.7 (12.1)**	**21.9 (6.7)**	**37.9 (13.9)**

* Bold characters indicate pathological scores. Results are expressed as mean (SD). (From ref. 29, with permission.)

verbal IQ on the Revised Wechsler Intelligence Scale (59) was 95.6 (SD: 16.7) in a group of 21 patients with a level of education of 13.2 (SD: 2.6) years (28). In some cases, however, patients with a severe dysexecutive syndrome associated with memory disorders and impaired instrumental activities may reach the threshold of dementia in which both cortical and subcortico-frontal components play a role. A mean score of 110/144 on the Mattis Dementia Rating Scale (60) was found in a group of 15 consecutive unselected patients with a mean disease duration of 3.4 ± 2.2 years, indicating a moderate level of dementia. It was similar in severity to that currently found in patients with PSP after 4 or 5 years of evolution or in AD at the early stage (Table 4). Thus, dementia is not infrequent in CBD. In 10 out of 13 cases with pathologically confirmed CBD, a dementia was noticed within 3 years of onset of symptoms (61). It is interesting to note that the clinical pattern of dementia in this study was relatively homogeneous, since most of the cases presented with early behavioral changes, whereas only one case was misdiagnosed as AD. Dementia may also be observed from the onset in unusual clinical presentations of CBD (19).

When are the cognitive disorders of CBD sufficiently severe to warrant the diagnosis of dementia? The answer depends on the criteria used to define dementia. For example, DSM III-R criteria may not apply to patients with CBD for at least two main reasons:

1. Specific memory disorders (i.e., isolated encoding and retrieval deficits) may be observed at an early stage but do not allow one to diagnose a true amnesic syndrome, as previously discussed.
2. The motor and gesture deficits may be severe enough to compromise by themselves the autonomy of patients whose judgment is preserved.

The DSM IV (62) is more appropriate to dementias with a "subcortico-frontal" cognitive and behavioral syndrome because it includes two important dimensions: the presence of a dysexecutive syndrome as a component of dementia, and the notion of decline from a previous level of functioning. It is thus possible to define dementia in these patients by the association of a dysexecutive syndrome and linguistic, praxis, or visuospatial dysfunction severe enough to induce a significant decline from a previous level. This cognitive decline may also be defined by a psychometric approach: by using a criterion of two standard deviations below the score of normal controls matched for age and cultural level (63) or one standard deviation below the level of a previous cognitive assessment.

No longitudinal study of the cognitive evolution of CBD has been reported to date, but it greatly differs from one patient to another. Some patients present only limb clumsiness and gesture disorders at the first examination, without any, or with few, cognitive or behavioral symptoms (8,64). Others begin with a subcortico-frontal cognitive and behavioral syndrome similar to that of PSP patients and their gesture disorders become manifest only after some years of evolution (61). Early subcortico-frontal syndrome would predict a shorter survival (11). Finally, a subgroup of patients with CBD may have a more global cognitive impairment that reflects a more diffuse cortical degeneration (27), affecting the anterior frontal lobe, amygdala, and enthorinal cortex (5,6), or more rarely the hippocampus (65). Furthermore, a damage of large-scale networks between cortical regions would lead to disconnection contributing to the disturbance of complex cortical functions in CBD (66) with a subsequent atrophy of the corpus callosum. This hypothesis is documented by a recent study (67), in which cognitive function was evaluated by the total score of subtests from the Wechsler Adult Intelligence Scale-Revised (59) sensitive to brain injury: Digit Span, Arithmetic, Picture Arrangement, Object Assembly, Block Design, and Digit Symbol. Interestingly, the degree of cognitive impairment and cortical hypometabolism on PET scan showed a stronger correlation with the severity of callosal atrophy than with the cortical atrophy or ventricular dilatation on MRI.

A CLINICAL CASE

The cognitive worsening with disease progression is best exemplified in the following case. This right-handed woman, a retired secretary with 10 years of education, was 66 years old when a carpal tunnel syndrome of the left-hand was diagnosed. After decompression of the median nerve at the wrist, the sensitive disturbances improved. Few months later, an extrapyramidal rigidity appeared progressively with a dystonic posture of the left wrist and hand. The patient was referred to the "Fédération de Neurologie" at Salpêtrière Hospital in Paris. There was no personal or familial history and no motor or sensory deficits. The CT scan showed a left parietal atrophy.

On the first neuropsychological assessment, about 18 months after the *onset of dystonia,* the patient had difficulty in separating her left fingers, as if they were stuck together. Consequently, she was unable to perform movements requiring selection of fingers with this hand. The rigidity of her left hand was so severe that she could not bend the hand and grasp objects. Although the global intention of symbolic gestures was preserved, even in evocation, the orientation of the hand during gestures was incorrect. In contrast, the right hand was normal at that time for motor dexterity, temporal organization, posture imitation, symbolic gesture evocation and imitation, and object use with pantomime or with real objects. Construction abilities were preserved with a normal visuospatial organization on the copy of the Rey complex figure reaching the score of 36/36. There was no impairment in global intellectual efficiency, orientation, memory, executive or linguistic functions, or behavior (Table 5).

On the second neuropsychological examination, 6 months later, the rigidity of the left side was markedly worsened, reaching the elbow, but sparing the shoulder and leg. Gesture disorders were noted in the right hand: loss of dexterity on the Purdue Pegboard Test, problems in finger

TABLE 5. *Longitudinal neuropsychological assessment of a clinical case*

	Symptom duration		
	18 Months	24 Months	42 Months
Global efficiency			
Folstein MMSE (30)	30	29	27
Mattis DRS (144)	137	**132**	**128**
Attention (37)	36	36	36
Initiation (37)	35	**30**	**28**
Construction (6)	6	6	**4**
Conceptualization (39)	36	36	36
Memory (25)	24	24	24
Memory			
Orientation (10)	10	10	10
Remote memories (10)	9	9	9
Recent memory (15)	14	14	**11**
Grober and Buschke			
Immediate cued recall (16)	16	16	16
Free recall (48)	28	25	**20**
Total recall (48)	48	48	47
Delayed free recall (16)	10	10	**8**
Delayed total recall (16)	16	16	16
Executive functions			
Wisconsin CST			
Criteria (6)	6	5	**4**
Errors	6	8	12
Perseverations	1	**4**	**8**
Abandons	0	**3**	**3**
Lexical fluency			
Animals (60 sec)	18	17	17
"M" (60 sec)	12	10	**7**
Graphic series (10)	10	9	**8**
Behavior (20)	20	**18**	**18**
Global frontal score (60)	55	51	**47**

* Bold characters indicate pathological scores.

selection for posture imitation, and clumsiness for object grasp and use. Evocation and imitation of symbolic gestures was normal, although some perplexity and spatial errors were noticed in object use pantomime. Construction abilities became altered, as shown by the copy of the Rey complex figure, with errors of proportion and spatial location and omission of details: The score was 22/36. There was also a mild decrease of performance on the Initiation subtest of the Mattis Dementia Rating Scale and on the Wisconsin Card Sorting Test, whereas temporospatial orientation, judgment, and linguistic activities were normal.

On the third neuropsychological assessment, 3½ years after the beginning of disease, the left hand was painfully contracted, with all the fingers fixed in a flexed dystonic posture, but there was still no clear abnormality of the shoulder or left leg. The gesture difficulties of the right hand were more severe than previously, with disturbances in motor series and symbolic gestures, and difficulties in finger selection. The clumsiness was aggravated, but there was still an automatic-voluntary dissociation: Pantomime was more severely impaired than real object use. The patient was able to independently eat food cut into little pieces, but had to be helped with personal hygiene and dressing. Assessment of visuospatial abilities revealed discrete signs of neglect in the left part of the Rey complex figure, although the score was similar to that of the previous exam (22/26). There was a mild worsening of the dysexecutive syndrome with the occurrence of an imitation behavior, in the absence of any other abnormal behavior (no prehension, utilization, inertia, or indifference). Free recall performance was decreased but normalized by cued recall, as shown by the total recall score (Table 5). Orientation, judgment, and linguistic activities were still normal. Autonomy was only impaired by gesture disorders. The patient was aware of her difficulties and concerned by the progression of the disease. This case shows a severe progressive gesture disorder associated with a mild dysexecutive syndrome in the absence of dementia in spite of an evolution of the disease of nearly 4 years.

DISCUSSION

Patients with CBD show a moderate cognitive deterioration in association with their motor and praxis disorders. Their neuropsychological pattern differs from that of patients with AD, characterized mainly by a true amnesic syndrome and linguistic disorders in relation with histologic changes in the hippocampus and the medial and temporal associative cortex. The fact that the hippocampus is relatively spared by CBD lesions (1–4) explains that the consolidation processes of explicit memory, normally controlled by the hippocampal system, are spared. The cortical lesions predominate in the sensorimotor and adjacent regions of the premotor cortex and parietal cortex, accounting for the motor and praxis disorders. The performance on motor and gesture organization is dramatically more impaired than in patients with AD at the same level of cognitive deterioration on nearly all tests, and also than in patients with PSP on tests of upper limb praxis, underlining the occurrence in CBD of praxis disorders not observed in PSP, and only at advanced stages in AD (68). One of the main characteristics of these praxis disorders is that they preserve the identification of gestures. They are described in detail in another chapter (see Chapter 10). Additional motor deficits are also found: (a) disorders of motor control and activation of simple movements, which account for the difficulties exhibited in unimanual and bimanual dexterity, are significantly more severe than those observed in patients with PSP; (b) disturbances of motor programming, which account for the impaired performance in temporal organization, bimanual coordination, control and inhibition of interfering motor activities, are also observed in PSP. These motor disorders imply that the dysfunction of premotor and prefrontal areas and basal ganglia also play a role in the gesture disorders of CBD.

The subcortical lesions, with their subsequent prefrontal dysfunction, are responsible for the additional cognitive changes in the domain of executive functions. This explains why the cognitive deterioration of CBD may also resemble the subcortico-frontal dysfunction currently reported in patients with neurodegenerative damage of the basal ganglia (23). Indeed, the dysexecutive syndrome of CBD may be as severe as that of patients with PSP and learning deficits can be alleviated by semantic cueing, as in other subcortical dementias (52). The environmental dependency syndrome (prehension, utilization, and imitation behaviors) is, however, less severe than in PSP, probably because its occurrence is related to the release of the parietal functions (51). Thus, the dysfunction of the parietal cortex in CBD would prevent the spontaneous expression of these behaviors.

In conclusion, a subcortico-frontal pattern of dementia associated with gesture disorders may be considered as relatively specific to CBD, because the former syndrome is unusual in AD and the latter one not found in degenerative diseases restricted to subcortical structures. Is this pattern representative of the majority of patients with CBD? The inclusion criteria generally used in most of the studies have a good specificity, but low sensitivity (69). They likely increase the homogeneity of the cognitive pattern. For instance, the introduction of praxis disorders as an inclusion criterion reinforces the clinical diagnosis, but may constitute a bias, since about 20% of patients with CBD do not have apraxia (27). Furthermore, CBD is neuropathologically and clinically relatively heterogeneous (5,6). It must be stated, therefore, that the cognitive pattern associating a moderate dysexecutive syndrome, retrieval deficits, and asymmetric gesture disorders probably characterizes a majority of patients with CBD, but not all of them. If such a pattern was confirmed by neuropathological verification, it could help in the differential diagnosis of CBD (23), since this disorder is frequently misdiagnosed during life as PSP, multiple system atrophy, Parkinson's disease, diffuse Lewy body disease, or other neurodegenerative disorders (69).

REFERENCES

1. Rebeiz JJ, Kolodny EH, Richardson EP. Corticodentatonigral degeneration with neuronal achromasia. *Arch Neurol* 1968;18:20–33.
2. Gibb WRG, Luthert PJ, Marsden CD. Corticobasal degeneration. *Brain* 1989;112:1171–1192.
3. Riley DE, Lang AE, Lewis A, et al. Corticobasal ganglionic degeneration. *Neurology* 1990;40:1203–1212.
4. Rinne JO, Lee MS, Thomson PD, Marsden CD. Corticobasal degeneration: a clinical study of 36 cases. *Brain* 1994;117:1183–1196.
5. Schneider JA, Watts RL, Gearing M. Corticobasal degeneration: neuropathologic and clinical heterogeneity. *Neurology* 1997;48:959–989.
6. Bergeron C, Davis A, Lang AE. Corticobasal ganglionic degeneration and progressive supranuclear palsy presenting with cognitive decline. *Brain Pathol* 1998;8: 355–365.
7. Kareken DA, Unverzagt F, Caldemeyer K, Farlow MR, Hutchins GD. Functional brain imagery in apraxia. *Arch Neurol* 1998;55:107–113.
8. Otsuki M, Soma Y, Yoshimura N, Tsuji S. Slowly progressive limb-kinetic apraxia. *Eur Neurol* 1997;37: 100–103.
9. Heilman KM, Gonzalez Rothi LJ. Apraxia. In: Heilman KM, Valenstein E, eds. *Clinical neuropsychology,* 2nd ed. Oxford: Oxford University Press, 1985:131–150.
10. Rey GJ, Tomer R, Levin BE, Sanchez-Ramos J, Bowen B, Bruce JH. Psychiatric symptoms, atypical dementia, and left visual field inattention in corticobasal ganglionic degeneration. *Mov Disord* 1995;10:106–110.
11. Wenning GK, Litvan I, Jankovic J, et al. Natural history and survival of 14 patients with corticobasal degeneration confirmed at postmortem examination. *J Neurol Neurosurg Psychiatry* 1998;64:184–189.
12. Hecaen H, Ajuriaguerra J de, Massonnet J. Les troubles visuoconstructifs par lésion pariéto-occipitale droite. *Encéphale* 1951;40:122–179.
13. Freund HJ, Hummelsheim H. Lesions of premotor cortex in man. *Brain* 1985;108:697–733.
14. Goldberg G, Mayer NH, Toglia JU. Medial frontal cortex infarction and the alien hand sign. *Arch Neurol* 1981; 38:683–686.
15. Watson R, Fleet S, Gonzalez Rothi LJ, Heilman KM. Apraxia and the supplementary motor area. *Arch Neurol* 1986;43:787–792.
16. Arima K, Uesugi H, Fujita I, et al. Corticonigral degeneration with neuronal achromasia presenting with primary progressive aphasia: ultrastructural and immunocytochemical studies. *J Neurol Sci* 1994;127:186–197.
17. Ikeda K, Akiyama H, Iritani S, et al. Corticobasal degeneration with primary progressive aphasia and accentuated cortical lesion in superior temporal gyrus: case report and review. *Acta Neuropathol* 1996;92:534–539.
18. Goodglass H. Disorders of naming following brain injury. *Am Scientist* 1980;68:647–655.
19. Bergeron C, Pollanen MS, Weyer L, Black SE, Lang AE. Unusual clinical presentations of cortico-basal ganglionic degeneration. *Ann Neurol* 1996;40:893–900.
20. Lecours AR, Lhermitte F, eds. *L'aphasie.* Paris: Flammarion Medecine Sciences, 1979.
21. Stuss DT, Benson DF. *The frontal lobes.* New York: Raven Press, 1986.
22. Beatty WW, Scott JG, Wilson DA, Prince JR, Williamson DJ. Memory deficits in a demented patient with probable corticobasal degeneration. *J Geriatr Psychiatry Neurol* 1995;8:132–136.
23. Dubois B, Pillon B. Cognitive and behavioral aspects of movement disorders. In: Jankovic J, Tolosa E, eds. *Parkinson's disease and movement disorders,* 3rd ed. Baltimore: Williams & Wilkins, 1998:837–858.

24. Lang AE, Maragonore D, Marsden CD, Tanner C. Movement Disorder Society Symposium on corticobasal ganglionic degeneration (CBGD) and its relationship to other asymmetrical cortical degeneration syndromes. *Mov Disord* 1996;11:346–357.
25. Habib M, Alicherif A, Balzamo M, Milandre L, Donnet A, Khalil R. Caractérisation du trouble gestuel dans l'apraxie progressive primaire apport diagnostique et nosographique. *Rev Neurol* 1995;151:541–551.
26. Luria AR. *Higher cortical functions in man.* New York: Basic Books, 1966.
27. Leiguarda R, Lees AJ, Merello M, Starkstein S, Marsden CD. The nature of apraxia in corticobasal degeneration. *J Neurol Neurosurg Psychiatry* 1994;57:455–459.
28. Massman PJ, Kreiter KT, Jankovic J, Doody RS. Neuropsychological functioning in cortical-basal ganglionic degeneration: differentiation from Alzheimer's disease. *Neurology* 1996;46:720–726.
29. Pillon B, Blin J, Vidailhet M, Deweer B, Sirigu A, Dubois B, Agid Y. The neuropsychological pattern of corticobasal degeneration. Comparison with progressive supranuclear palsy and Alzheimer's disease. *Neurology* 1995;45:1477–1483.
30. De Renzi E, Luchelli F. Ideational apraxia. *Brain* 1988; 114:1173–1185.
31. Ochipa C, Rothi LJ, Heilman KM. Conceptual apraxia in Alzheimer's disease. *Brain* 1992;115:1061–1071.
32. Roy EA, Square PA. Common considerations in the study of limb, verbal and oral apraxia. In: Roy EA, ed. *Neuropsychological studies of apraxia and related disorders.* Amsterdam: North-Holland, 1985:111–161.
33. Blin J, Vidailhet MJ, Pillon B, Dubois B, Feve JR, Agid Y. Cortico-basal degeneration: decreased and asymetrical glucose consumption as studied with PET. *Mov Dis* 1992;7:348–354.
34. Eidelberg D, Dhawan V, Moeller JR, et al. The metabolic lanscape of corticobasal ganglionic degeneration: regional asymmetries studied with positron emission tomography. *J Neurol Neurosurg Psychiatry* 1991;54: 856–862.
35. Lang AE. Cortical basal ganglionic degeneration presenting with "progressive loss of speech output and orofacial dyspraxia." *J Neurol Neurosurg Psychiatry* 1992; 55:1101.
36. Watts RL, Mirra SS, Richardson EP. Corticobasal ganglionic degeneration. In: Marsden CD, Fahn S, eds. *Movement disorders,* 3rd ed. Oxford: Butterworth-Heinemann, 1994:282–299.
37. Leger JM, Levasseur M, Benoit N, et al. Apraxie d'aggravation lentement progressive: étude par IRM et tomographie à positons dans 4 cas. *Rev Neurol* 1991; 147:183–191.
38. Vidailhet M, Rivaud S, Gouider-Khouja N, et al. Eye movements in parkinsonian syndromes. *Ann Neurol* 1994,35:420–426.
39. Cohen S, Freedman M. Cognitive and behavioral changes in the Parkinson-Plus syndromes. In: Weiner WJ, Lang AE, eds. Behavioral neurology of movement disorders. *Advances in neurology; Vol. 65.* New York: Raven, 1995:139–157.
40. Lippa CF, Cohen R, Smith TW, Drachman DA. Primary progressive aphasia with focal neuronal achromasia. *Neurology* 1991;41:882–886.
41. Stark ME, Clark K, Grafman J, Litvan I. Evidence from a multimodal disruption of space in cortical-basal ganglionic degeneration. *Mov Disord* 1996;11:353.
42. Pillon B, Deweer B, Agid Y, Dubois B. Explicit memory in Alzheimer's, Huntington's and Parkinson's diseases. *Arch Neurol* 1993;50:374–379.
43. Pillon B, Deweer B, Michon A, Malapani C, Agid Y, Dubois B. Are explicit memory disorders of progressive supranuclear palsy related to damage of striato-frontal circuits? Comparison with Alzheimer's, Parkinson's, and Huntington's diseases. *Neurology* 1994;44:1264–1270.
44. Delis DC, Kramer JH, Kaplan E, Ober BA. *California Verbal Learning Test:* research edition. New York: Psychological Corporation, 1987.
45. Grober E, Buschke H. Genuine memory deficits in dementia. *Dev Neuropsychol* 1987;3:13–36.
46. Ergis AM, Van Der Linden M, Boller F, Degos JD, Deweer B. Mémoire visuospatiale à court et à long terme dans la maladie d'Alzheimer débutante. *Neuropsychologia Latina* 1995;1:18–25.
47. Moscovitch M. Memory and working with memory: evaluation of a component process model and comparisons with other models. In: Schacter DL, Tulving E, eds. *Memory systems.* Cambridge, MA: MIT Press, 1994:269–310.
48. Tounsi H, Deweer B, Ergis AM, et al. Sensitivity to semantic cuing: An index of episodic memory dysfunction in early Alzheimer's disease. *Alzheimer disease and associated disorders* 1999:13;38–116.
49. Nelson HE. A modified Card Sorting Test sensitive to frontal lobe defect. *Cortex* 1976;12:313–324.
50. Benton AL. Differential behavioral effects in frontal lobe disease. *Neuropsychologia* 1968;6:53–60.
51. Lhermitte F, Pillon B, Serdaru M. Human autonomy and the frontal lobes. Part I: Imitation and utilization behaviors: a neuropsychological study of 75 patients. *Ann Neurol* 1986;19:326–334.
52. Pillon B, Dubois B, Agid Y. Testing cognition may contribute to the diagnosis of movement disorders. *Neurology* 1996;46:329–333.
53. Blin J, Baron JC, Dubois B, et al. Pet study in progressive supranuclear palsy: brain hypometabolic pattern and clinico-metabolic correlations. *Arch Neurol* 1990;47: 747–752.
54. Le Gall D, Truelle JL, Joseph PA, et al. Gestural disturbances following frontal lobe lesions: a qualitative analysis. *J Clin Exp Neuropsychol* 1992;14:375.
55. Lezak MD. *Neuropsychological assessment.* Oxford: Oxford University Press, 1995.
56. Verfaellie M, Heilman KM. Response preparation and response inhibition after lesions of the medial frontal lobe. *Arch Neurol* 1987;44:1265–1271.
57. Sawle GV, Brooks DJ, Marsden CD, Frackoviack RJ; Corticobasal degeneration. A unique pattern of regional cortical oxygen hypometabolism and striatal fluorodopa uptake demonstrated by positron emission tomography. *Brain* 1991;114:541–556.
58. Watts RL, Brewer RP. Cortical-basal ganglionic degeneration: classical clinical features and natural history. *Mov Disord* 1996;11:346.
59. Wechsler DA. *Wechsler Adult Intelligence Scale-Revised.* New York: Psychological Corporation, 1981.
60. Mattis S. *Dementia Rating Scale.* Odessa, FL: Psychological Assessment Resources, 1988.
61. Grimes DA, Lang AE, Bergeron C. Dementia is the most common presentation of corticobasal ganglionic degeneration. *Neurology* 1998;50(S4):A96.
62. American Psychiatric Association. *Diagnostic and Statistical Manual of Mental Disorders,* 4th ed. DSM-IV™. Washington, DC: American Psychiatric Association, 1994.

63. Pillon B, Dubois B. Cognitive and behavioral impairments. In: Litvan I, Agid Y, eds. *Progressive supranuclear palsy.* Oxford: Oxford University Press, 1992: 223–239.
64. Moreaud O, Naegelé B, Pellat J. The nature of apraxia in corticobasal degeneration. A case of melokinetic apraxia. *Neuropsychiatry Neuropsychol Behav Neurol* 1996;9: 288–292.
65. Matsuyama Y, Masuda K, Inoue T, Koono M, Kora S, Nakamura T. Primary progressive dementia with swollen chromatolitic neurons. *Dementia* 1992;3: 223–231.
66. Mesulam MM. Large-scale neurocognitive networks and distributed processing for attention, language and memory. *Ann Neurol* 1990;28:597–613.
67. Yamauchi H, Fukuyama H, Nagahama Y, et al. Atrophy of the corpus callosum, cortical hypometabolism, and cognitive impairment in corticobasal degeneration. *Arch Neurol* 1998;55:609–614.
68. Rapcsack SZ, Croswell SC, Rubens AB. Apraxia in Alzheimer's disease. *Neurology* 1989;39:664–668.
69. Litvan I, Agid Y, Goetz C, et al. Accuracy of clinical diagnosis of corticobasal degeneration. *Neurology* 1997;48:119–125.

Corticobasal Degeneration.
Advances in Neurology, Vol. 82,
edited by I. Litvan, C. G. Goetz, and A. E. Lang.
Lippincott Williams & Wilkins, Philadelphia © 2000.

10

Apraxia in Corticobasal Degeneration

*Ramón Leiguarda, Marcelo Merello†, and Jorge Balej†

Departments of Neurology and Movement Disorders†, Raúl Carrea Institute of Neurological Research, FLENI, Buenos Aires, Argentina*

INTRODUCTION

Limb apraxia is the most striking and disabling neurocognitive deficit in corticobasal degeneration (CBD) (1–4). It is an early sign of the disease and present in roughly 80% of patients (5,6). As such, it constitutes a hallmark clinical finding for the proper diagnosis of the disorder (7).

In the present chapter we will first briefly consider the current approach to limb praxic disorders, to discuss thereafter the nature of limb apraxia in CBD as disclosed by clinical and three-dimensional motion analysis, the differences in apraxia profile with other related disorders as well as the underlying pathophysiological mechanisms.

CURRENT APPROACH TO LIMB PRAXIS DISORDERS

Limb apraxia comprises a wide spectrum of cognitive-motor disorders owing to acquired brain disease affecting the performance of skilled, learned, purposeful movements with or without preservation of the ability to perform the same movement outside the clinical setting in the appropriate situation, context, or environment, which cannot be accounted for by elementary motor or sensory deficits (8–10).

Skilled, learned movements differ from the novel ones because their performance is characterized by preprogrammed processes; individual differences increase with the degree of skill; and they are context-dependent (11–13).

The performance of familiar, everyday action routines and overlearned movements in the appropriate context would largely depend on the supplementary motor area (SMA), premotor (PM), primary sensorimotor cortices, basal ganglia, and cerebellum of either hemisphere and independent of neocortical commissures, whereas the performance of a nonroutine movement or a routine one outside its usual context would primarily need the additional participation of the parietal and other frontal association cortices (14–17).

The left hemisphere in right-handed subjects appears to be dominant for context-independent performance (i.e., pantomiming transitive movements) and in learning novel movements, whereas either hemisphere may control the execution of context-dependent, familiar, automatic motor acts (i.e., transitive movements using the tool and object, intransitive movements) (18,19). Pantomiming the use of a tool or object without actually handling it is an unfamiliar and "abstract" task that is rarely being performed outside the clinical setting. By contrast, performance with the tool or object calls for the execution of "concrete" well-practiced familiar actions (everyday action routines) similar to performance in a natural setting (20). However, apraxia as tested by the imitation of gestures and object use pantomime has been found in about 50% of patients with left hemisphere damage and in less than 10% of those with right hemisphere damage, which means that in many subjects higher-order motor functions have bilateral hemisphere representations (9).

Therefore, there is no meaningful interpretation of a limb praxis deficit if all of the following factors are not taken into account: (a) the possible lateralization of motor representation as inferred from handedness; (b) the type of movement requested (i.e., transitive vs. intransitive); and (c) the pathway through which a movement is evoked (i.e., verbal, visual, tactile) (8–10, 21).

Roy and Square (8) have recently proposed a model for the organization of actions based on the operation of a two-part system involving a conceptual component that encompasses an abstract knowledge base for actions and a production component that provides the mechanisms for movements. According to these authors, the conceptual system (or action semantics) incorporates three types of knowledge relevant to limb praxis: knowledge of the functions that tool and object may serve, knowledge of actions independent of tools and objects, and knowledge relevant to the organization of single actions into sequences. On the other hand, the production system involves the sensorimotor component of action knowledge that includes the information contained in action programs and the translation of these programs into actions. Thus, acting in the world would depend on the interaction of abstract knowledge related to tools, objects, and actions and the structural information contained in motor programs (8). The dysfunction of the praxis production system causes ideomotor (IMA) and limb-kinetic (LKA) apraxias, whereas damage to the conceptual system gives rise to ideational (IA) or conceptual (CA) apraxias. The identification of these praxis disorders requires a comprehensive assessment of the different praxis functions as well as a proper analysis of praxis error types (Table 1).

Ideomotor apraxia is defined as an "impairment in the timing, sequencing and spatial organization of gestural movements" (22). Patients with IMA commit mainly temporal (i.e., irregular speed, sequencing abnormalities) and spatial errors (i.e., abnormal amplitude, improper spatial orientation of objects and movements, abnormal hand and limb configuration during movements, use of body parts as objects) (23). Unilateral damage to the motor dominant hemisphere produces bilateral deficits, usually less severe in the left than in the right limb. Transitive movements are more affected than intransitive ones on pan-

TABLE 1. *Limb praxis assessment*

Evaluation of the praxis production system		Evaluation of the praxis conceptual system	
Intransitive movements	Nonrepresentational (e.g., touch your nose, wiggle your fingers)	Multiple step tasks	(e.g., prepare a letter for mailing)
	Representational (e.g., wave goodbye, hitchhike)	Tool selection tasks	To select the appropriate tool to complete a task such as a hammer for a partly driven nail
Transitive movements	(e.g., use a hammer, use a screwdriver) under verbal, visual, and tactile modalities	Alternative tool selection tasks	To select an alternative tool such as pliers to complete a task as pounding a nail, when the appropriate tool (i.e., hammer) is not available
Imitation of meaningful and meaningless movements, postures, and sequences		Gesture recognition tasks	To assess the capacity to comprehend gestures, either verbally (to name gestures performed by the examiner), as well as nonverbally (to match a gesture performed by the examiner with cards depicting the tool/objects corresponding to the pantomime)
		Gesture discrimination tasks	To assess the capacity to differentiate an accurately performed gesture from an altered gesture, either temporally or spatially

(From refs. 9, 10, and 27, with permission.)

tomiming to commands. Performance may improve on imitation and handling the tools or objects is carried out better than pantomiming their use, but in most instances it is not normal. Quite commonly, there is a voluntary-automatic dissociation, which means that there are no complaints about the disorder, since it is not apparent in the natural setting and only appears in the clinical setting when the patient has to represent explicitly the content of an action outside the situational props. IMA is associated with damage to the parietal association areas, small premotor cortex, and intrahemispheric white matter bundles that interconnect them, as well as with involvement of basal ganglia and thalamus (9,10,24).

Limb-kinetic apraxia is confined to the limbs contralateral to the lesion, regardless of its hemispheric side. Finger and hand movements are predominantly affected. Manipulative behavior is particularly involved at the beginning of the disease, but later on even simple movements are abnormal. All movements, either complex or routine, independently of whether the patient creates or imitates them, are coarse, awkward, and mutilated; the starting point of the movement may not even be found; the motion becomes amorphous and frequently contaminated by extraneous movements. Unsuccessful attempts usually precede deranged movements. The difficulties produced by the disorder interfere with the patients' daily activities and they complain about them, which means that there is no voluntary-automatic dissociation. This form of apraxia is observed mainly with damage to the premotor cortex with or without associated parietal cortex or basal ganglia involvement. IMA and LKA may coexist in the same patient and both were originally considered by Liepmann as motor apraxias (18).

Dysfunction of the praxis conceptual system causes IA or CA (25–28). Abnormal performance in these patients is primarily characterized by content and tool selection errors (23,27). Content errors include perseverations, pantomime-related errors (an accurately produced pantomime associated in content to the target such as pantomime playing a trombone for a target of a bugle), non–pantomime-related errors (a pantomime not associated in content with the target such as pantomime hammering for a target of shaving) (23). Patients may not use the tool at all (no response) or produce unrecognizable movements. They also have difficulties to select the appropriate tool to complete a partially completed task and to sequence correctly a series of acts (25,27). The deficits affect everyday activities. Disruption of the praxis conceptual system may also give rise to action recognition abnormalities (8). Since there has been much confusion about the term ideational apraxia, Ochipa et al. have suggested reserving it to denote an inability to sequence correctly a series of acts leading to an action goal, as originally described by Pick (25), whereas the term conceptual apraxia should be used to describe the loss of different types of tool-action knowledge (27). However, the distinction is not so clear, because patients with IA are also often impaired in demonstrating the use of single objects (29).

Ideational or conceptual apraxias are more commonly seen in patients with dementia of the Alzheimer type (27), but they can also be induced by lateralized lesions in the parietal, frontal, and temporal regions and even in the basal ganglia of the left dominant hemisphere in right-handed patients (28,29). CA and IMA may coexist in the same patient (28).

THE NATURE OF APRAXIA IN CBD

Patients with CBD usually exhibit an asymmetric apraxic syndrome mainly characterized by spatial, temporal, and sequencing errors that reflect disruption of the action production system. In advanced stages of the disease some patients may also display manifestations attributable to a coexisting conceptual defect.

Up to now, we have studied for the presence of apraxia in 14 right-handed patients, aged 58 to 78 years, who met accepted clinical criteria for the diagnosis of CBD (5,30,31). Disease duration ranged from 2 to 6 years. To minimize confounding effects imposed by the elementary motor disorder, the original 10 patients were assessed in the less affected limb, whereas in the last four, both limbs were evaluated. Eleven patients exhibited ideomotor apraxia; spatial and temporal errors were more frequently observed when performing transitive than intransitive movements, either to command, imitation, and even with the use of the real object or tool. Spatial errors such as incorrect positioning of the hand to grasp the tool (internal configuration errors), difficulty in orienting the hand with respect to the body and the tool with respect to the object receiving the tool's action in extrapersonal space (external configuration errors), abnormal movement trajectories, and body-part-as-object errors were observed in decreasing order of frequency. Sequencing and timing errors were also found. All these patients have difficulties when imitating meaningful and meaningless postures and movements and those with the most severe praxic disturbances also exhibit errors (i.e., omissions, intrusions) when performing sequential arm movements. In addition to spatial and temporal errors, three patients committed errors reflecting disruption of the conceptual system, such as mislocations, misuse, and absent or unrecognizable response, which were particularly evident when they performed multiple step tasks. These patients also showed deficits on gesture recognition that further support a conceptual defect.

The praxis disorders were more frequent in patients who had initial symptoms in the right limb (left hemisphere dysfunction) than in the left limb (right hemisphere dysfunction) in agreement with the fact that most right handers develop ideomotor as well as ideational apraxia with left but not right hemisphere lesions. Although there was a tendency for limb apraxia to be more severe in patients with longer disease duration, no significant correlation was found between apraxia scores and duration of illness.

Ideomotor and ideational apraxia scores significantly correlated with MMSE scores. Ideomotor apraxia scores also correlated with a task sensitive to frontal lobe dysfunction, and alien limb behavior (usually produced by frontomesial lesions) was only seen in patients with ideomotor apraxia. On the other hand, primitive reflexes were particularly evident in patients with ideational apraxia.

We found no LKA in our original 10 patients, most likely owing to the fact that we only assessed the less affected limb (5), as also happened with Jacobs' study (32). Two out of the last four patients we evaluated with the classical clinical picture of CBD presented a clear-cut unilateral limb-kinetic type of praxic deficit in addition to bilateral IMA (30,31). Both patients showed slow, awkward, and mutilated finger and hand movements and complained about difficulties using the affected hand, which means there was no voluntary-automatic dissociation. Manipulative behavior and sequence of finger movements were more deranged at early stages of the disease but thereafter even simple movements, either on command or imitation, were amorphous and contaminated by extraneous movements. For example, when asked to imitate throwing pebbles, the patients only rubbed the index finger once with the thumb, then kept both fingers in tight contact and immobile, while the patients looked at their hands claiming impotence to improve their performance. Fruitless attempts, which finally brought the wrong muscles into play, often preceded most movements. Imitation of finger postures were abnormal and some patients used the other hand to move the abnormal one to reproduce the requested posture. Sometimes, the fingers and hand remained in an abnormal posture while the patients performed other tasks with the contralateral hand. Patients were aware of poor performance but were unable to correct their errors.

Jacobs et al. (32) studied six patients with clinical diagnosis of CBD of brief duration. Testing the less affected upper extremity, they found ideomotor types of praxis errors on gesture to command as well as imitation with relative preservation on gesture recognition. Pillon et al. (33) evaluated 15 right-handed patients with probable CBD (mean age ± SD, 67.8 ± 8 years) and disease duration less than 10 years. They found a bilateral though asymmetric praxis disorder that they identified as an ideomotor type of apraxia. Recognition of gesture and object use was largely spared in this group of patients. Finally, Blondel et al. (34) found in three right-handed patients with clinical diagnosis of CBD a severe and selective impairment of the action production system mainly categorized as ideomotor apraxia with "some traits of limb-kinetic apraxia."

The limb-kinetic type of apraxia has also been frequently reported in CBD (35–38) and some authors have claimed that it represents the most common type of apraxia in this disorder (35). However, most studies lack a proper description of the praxic abnormalities to allow clear discrimination from elementary motor disorders as well as from IMA. Okuda et al. (36) described two patients with presumed CBD who had difficulty making fine finger movements, imitating finger patterns, and manipulating objects. Three patients in the Pillon et al. (33) study had a unilateral limb type of deficit that "might correspond to limb-kinetic apraxia." Tsuchiya et al. (37) reported that two out of five patients with pathological proven CBD had LKA but they failed to describe the clinical aspects of the praxic deficit. Denes et al. (38) recently reported five patients (three with presumed CBD) with a type of limb apraxia, whose characteristics perfectly fit the definition of LKA originally proposed by Liepmann; three also had IMA and one oral apraxia.

Ideational apraxia has been scarcely reported in patients with CBD. Martinez-Lage and Kertesz (39) studied 24 patients with CBD, including two cases originally diagnosed as frontal lobe dementia and progressive supranuclear palsy (PSP) because autopsy showed CBD. Half the patients presented with a motor disorder and half with cognitive behavioral manifestations, particularly a language disorder. Limb apraxia, usually ideational and ideomotor, was the most common feature (23/24) of CBD, in addition to unilateral akinesia and rigidity.

Orofacial apraxia is not so frequent in CBD. Pillon et al. (33) found orofacial apraxia in their patients, although milder than limb apraxia. We only demonstrated orofacial apraxia in three out of 14 patients, but Jacob et al. (32) and Blondel et al. (34) failed to mention it in their studies. However, orofacial apraxia together with loss of speech output have been reported as the presenting manifestations of the disease (40).

In summary, patients with CBD usually have severe impairment of the action production system that expresses itself as a bilateral ideomotor type of apraxia, which in many cases coexists with unilateral or less frequently bilateral limb-kinetic praxis deficits. Disruption of the action conceptual system is unusual but occasionally observed in demented patients in advanced stages of the disease or in those with atypical presentation such as with language disorders.

KINEMATIC ANALYSIS OF LIMB PRAXIS

Three-Dimensional Motion Analysis of a Gestural Movement

When studying patients with limb apraxia one problem has been the lack of an objective method to analyze the spatial and temporal aspects of a nonrestricted multijoint limb movement, which is essential to disclose the exact nature of the underlying motor disorder. In a recent series of landmark papers. Poizner and coworkers described the application of new technological advances in movement analysis to the study of patients with limb apraxia. Using three-dimensional motion analysis they demonstrated that patients with apraxia owing to focal cortical lesions as well as a patient with primary progressive apraxia show deficits in the spatio-temporal attributes of the wrist trajectory and in the coordination of the joint motion (41–44). We further demonstrated similar abnormalities in patients with ideomotor apraxia in the context of CBD (30).

Up to now, we have studied four right-handed patients aged 68 to 80 years who met diagnostic criteria for CBD (5,30,31). Duration of the illness ranged from 1 to 5 years. All patients had bilateral IMA and two also had LKA.

Patients were requested to perform the gesture of slicing a loaf of bread to verbal command with the less affected hand. The gesture consisted of a series of self-paced cyclic back-and-forth movements of the hand. The slicing gesture was evaluated during two periods lasting 10 sec each.

A Selspott II System was used for three-dimensional data acquisition, processing, and reconstruction. Kinematic analysis was performed on the trajectories of the wrist, and on the angular motion of the shoulder and elbow joints. Kinematic analysis includes temporal and spatial variables as well as measurements of spatiotemporal relationships and interjoint coordination (40–42).

The kinematic analysis of the gesture of slicing a loaf of bread in patients with CBD showed deficits in spatial accuracy, timing, spatiotemporal relationships, and interjoint coordination (30).

Disruption of Spatial Accuracy and Phase Reversal Abnormalities

Figure 1 shows lateral views of the reconstructed trajectories of the limb segments during the slicing gesture performed by a control subject and a patient with CBD. Stick figure representations of the arm, forearm, wrist, and hand show successive limb positions at 20-ms intervals. When produced by a control subject the gesture consisted of a stereotyped sequence of forward and backward movements of the hand; the trajectory paths of the wrist were located perpendicular to the object with minimal horizontal and vertical displacement, and were also aligned in the sagittal plane. The patient showed an abnormal pattern owing to less excursion of the elbow and marked vertical displacement of the wrist and hand. Figure 2 shows that in control subjects the direction of wrist movements reverses sharply, so that inward and outward phases are closely aligned. In contrast, the patient showed a pronounced widening of the wrist path during the reversal phase with a resulting spatial separation of inward and outward irregular paths, which corresponds with anomalous peaks in wrist velocity and acceleration.

Decoupling of Space-Time Relationships

Complex trajectories are planned through the proportional control of speed and spatial path of the movement. When the speed of the wrist decreases, the degree of bending or curvature of the path increases (45,46). Velocity curvature relationship is measured as the temporal difference between each minimum wrist tangential velocity and the minimum radius of curvature. Time differences approaching zero indicate a tight spatiotemporal coupling (control subject), whereas larger time differences reflect spatiotemporal decoupling. Patients showed greater than zero time differences, demonstrating significant velocity-curvature decoupling.

Deficits in Interjoint Coordination

The kinematic abnormalities of the wrist may reflect deficits in interjoint coordination, since the trajectory of the wrist results from the combined motion of the shoulder and elbow joints. Kinematic studies in control subjects demonstrated a smooth and linear relationship between elbow flexion or extension and lateral displacement of the upper arm (yaw). As the elbow extended, the upper arm elevated and moved laterally across the body in a coordinated pattern. This normal relationship helps to keep the wrist in the sagittal plane. In contrast, patients showed a distorted angle to angle relationship owing to dissimilar elbow or flexion extension and upper arm yaw movements. They also exhibited asynchronous intersegmental joint velocities (Fig. 3).

Figure 4 shows the variation in arm angle over time for a control subject and a patient with CBD. Sinusoidal oscillations in a control subject were regular and smooth, whereas patients produced less sinusoidal, irregular, and distorted oscillations.

Thus, the kinematic abnormalities observed in the orientation of the movement, shape of wrist trajectory, and timing, as well as joint coordination during the performance of a gestural movement in patients with CBD constitute objective evidence of the praxis production errors observed on clinical examination.

Kinematic Analysis of Reaching, Grasping, and Manipulating

Three-dimensional motion analysis of a gestural movement such as slicing a loaf of bread allowed the disruption of the temporal and spatial aspects of wrist trajectory and deficits on interjoint coordination to be confirmed and their nature accurately depicted. Now, to understand better which components of the action system are particularly involved and how they are integrated with the perceptual attributes of objects, as well as their location, thus providing a further approach to the identification of the specific neural mechanism underlying the praxic disorder, we studied the kinematics of pointing, reaching, grasping and manipulation in two right-handed patients, aged 68 and 70 years, with CBD (31); disease duration was 1 and 5 years and both had IMA and LKA.

Pointing to a small ball revealed a highly irregular wrist trajectory in both patients with

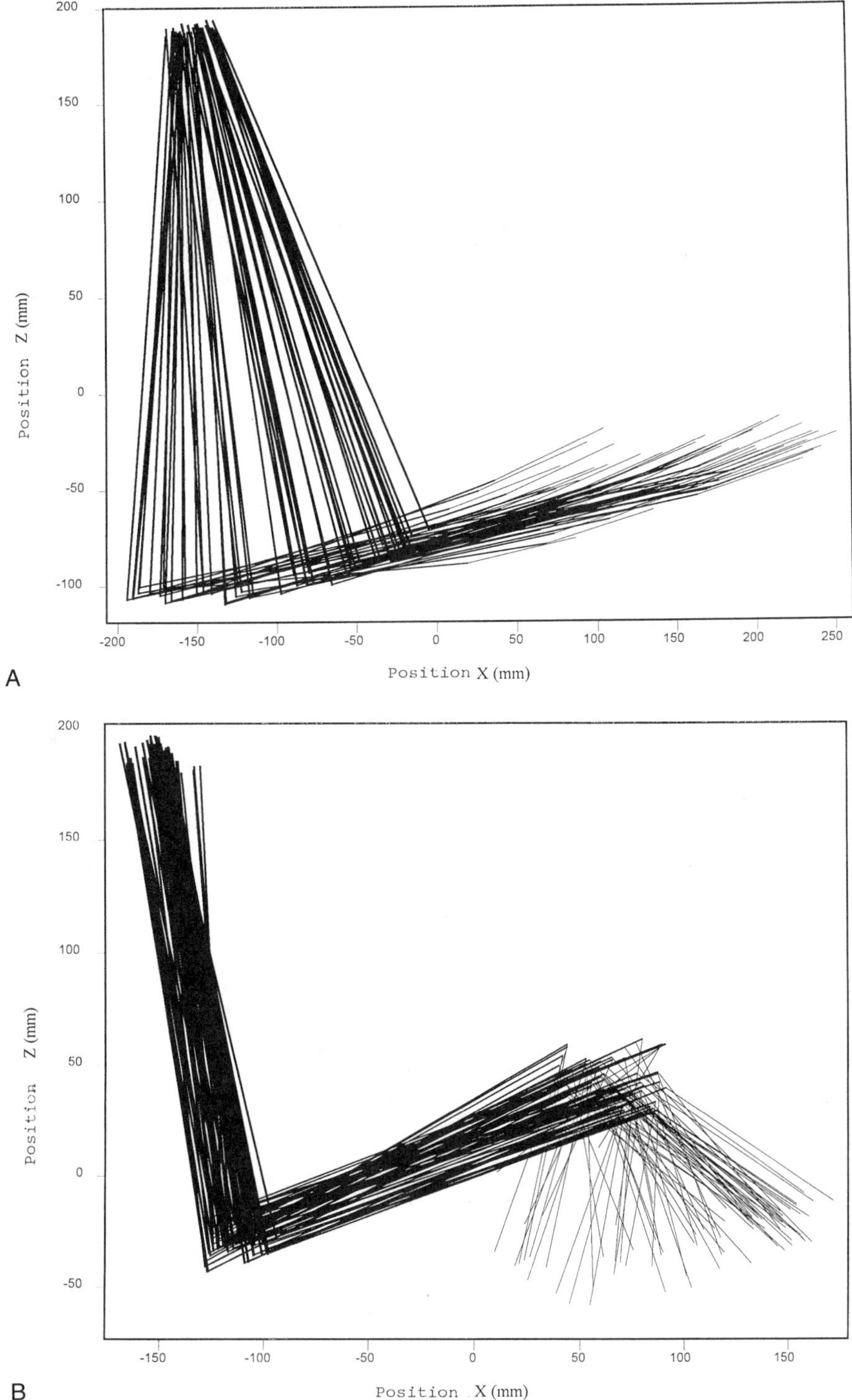

FIG. 1. Lateral view of the reconstructed trajectories of limb segments during the slicing gesture performed by a control subject (**A**) and patient with CBD (**B**). Wrist trajectories in the control subject are located perpendicular to the goal object and aligned in the sagittal plane with a slight vertical and horizontal displacement, whereas the patient's wrist path exhibited abnormal upward and downward movements and less forward and backward displacement.

PHASE REVERSAL - Control Subject

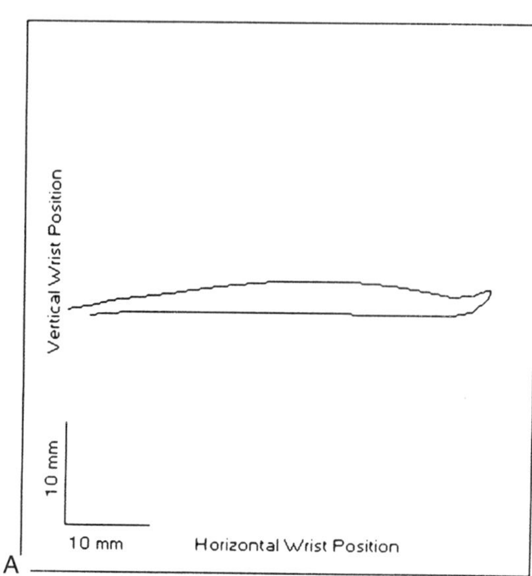

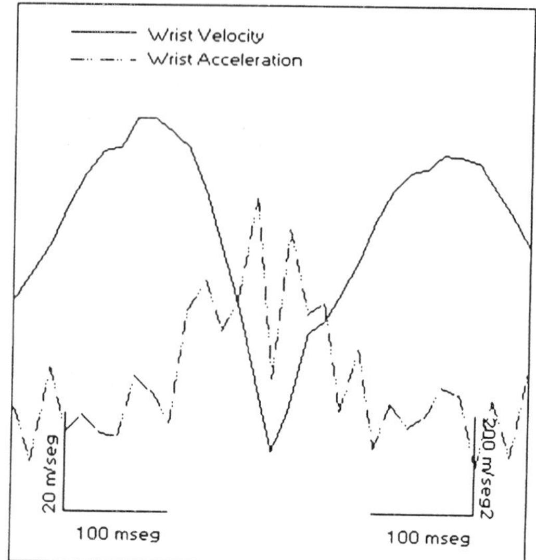

PHASE REVERSAL - CBD Patient

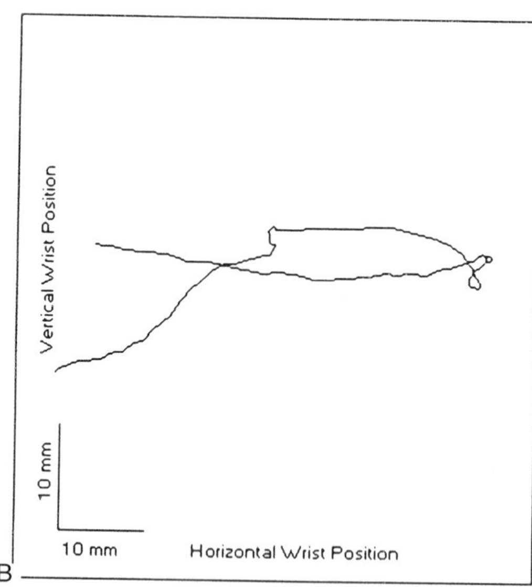

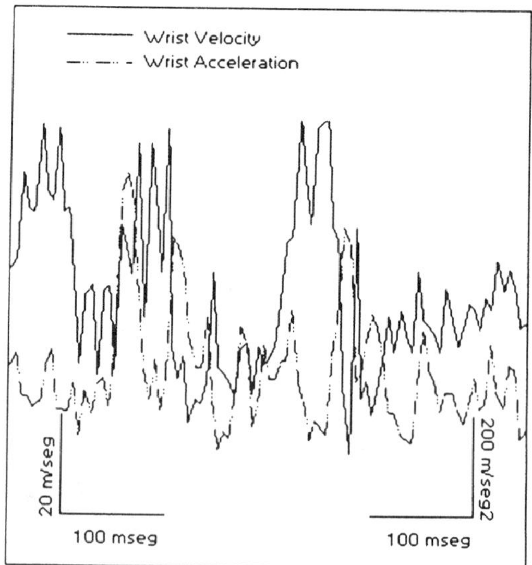

FIG. 2. Phase reversal in a control subject (**A**) and in a patient with CBD (**B**). The patient showed an abnormal widening of the wrist path during the reversal phase with a resulting spatial separation of inward and outward paths, both of which are also irregular. The spatial distortion corresponds with a grossly disrupted relationship between wrist velocity and wrist acceleration.

CBD but end-point errors were only observed in one case. The analysis of the kinematic parameters for *reaching* and *grasping* a glass revealed several abnormalities (Table 2). Patients showed a total movement time that almost doubled that of control subjects. The transport component of the movement was severely disrupted in both patients; peak velocity was reached later during the movement than in control subjects; therefore peak deceleration had to be achieved faster. Both

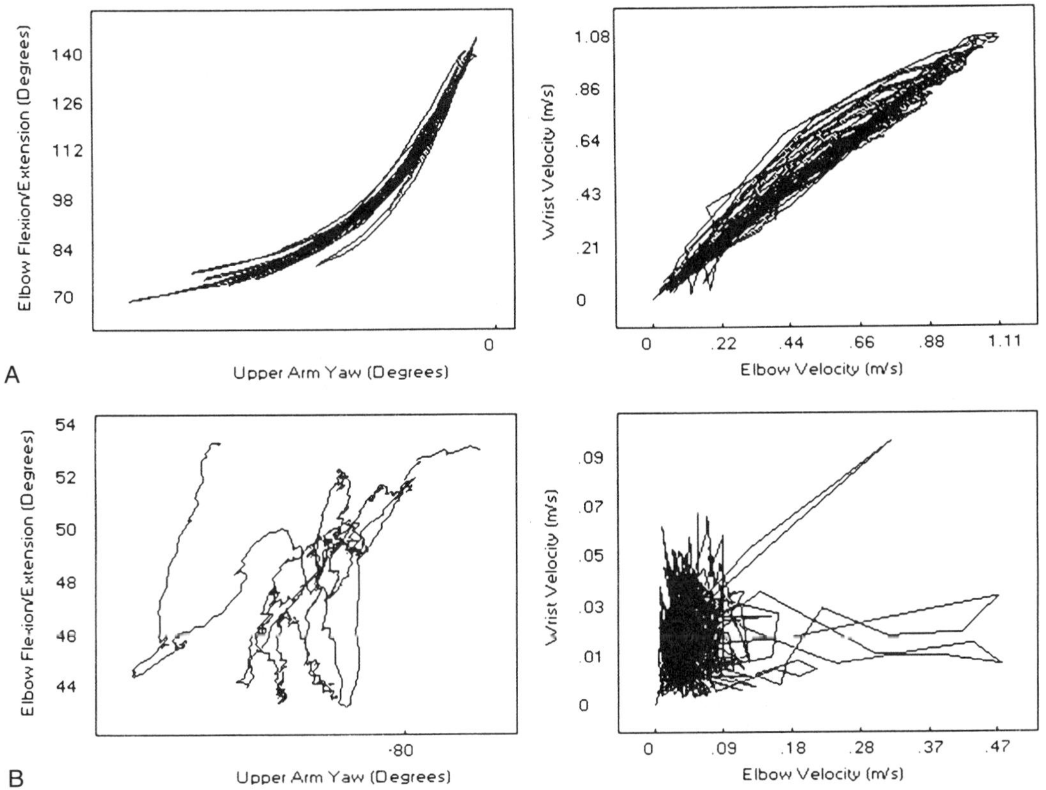

FIG. 3. Interjoint coordination in a control subject (**A**) and a patient with CBD (**B**). The control subject showed a smooth and linear relationship between elbow flexion/extension and upper arm yaw. As the elbow extended, the upper arm moves laterally across the body in a well-coordinated pattern. In contrast the patient showed distorted angle/angle relationships owing to poor coordination between elbow flexion/extension and upper arm yaw as well as asynchronous intersegmental joint velocities.

patients began grip aperture at a correct moment but they took a longer time to reach maximal grip aperture. Maximal grip aperture was wider than controls but significantly abnormal only in the patient with longer disease duration (Fig. 5).

Manipulatory finger movements were recorded during exploration of a ball between the thumb, index, and middle finger. The task was to discover whether the ball has a small hole or not. Kinematic analysis disclosed that the work-space of the scanning movements was much larger and more irregular in patients than in controls, whereas the temporal profile of vertical movement trajectories showed breakdown of the regular sinusoidal movements observed in controls (Fig. 6).

Caselli et al. also kinematically assessed proximal (transport) and distal (grasping) upper limb control in five patients with progressive apraxia, one of whom had autopsy-confirmed CBD. Compared to controls, patients exhibited slower transport and grasping kinematics, greater lateral deviation from the linear prehension trajectory, motor programming disturbances, and transport-grasping uncoupling (47).

DIFFERENCES IN APRAXIA PROFILE BETWEEN CBD AND OTHER RELATED DISORDERS

CBD is presumed to be a distinct clinicopathological entity. However, unusual cases of CBD exhibiting atypical clinical features (e.g., progressive aphasia, dementia of the frontal lobe type) as well as other disorders that may mimic the classical clinical syndrome of CBD (e.g., Alzheimer's disease, progressive supranuclear palsy) have been increasingly reported (48). Furthermore, the unusual syndrome of progressive

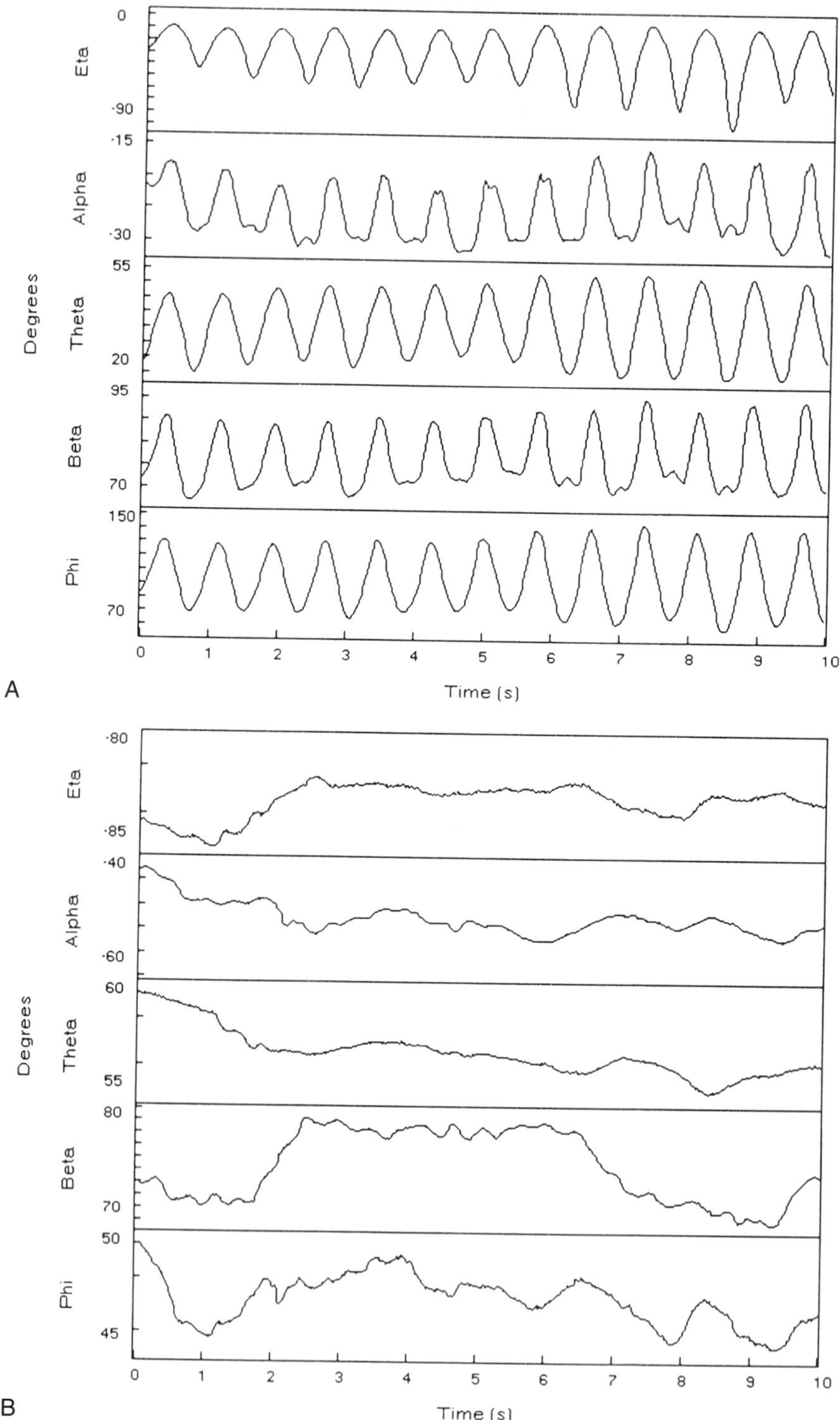

FIG. 4. Variation in arm angle over time for a control subject (**A**) and a patient with CBD (**B**). The control subject exhibited regular and smooth sinusoidal oscillations, whereas the patient showed less sinusoidal, irregular, and distorted oscillations.

TABLE 2. *Kinematic parameters for reaching and grasping a glass*

	Control subjects (*mean* ± *SD*)	Patients (*mean* ± *SD*)	
Movement time (msec)	870 ± 50	1626 ± 430	($p < 0.02$)
Transport component			
Time to peak velocity (%)	51 ± 12	81 ± 8	($p < 0.03$)
Time to peak acceleration (%)	42 ± 7	77 ± 12	($p < 0.005$)
Time to peak deceleration (%)	75 ± 5	93 ± 15	($p < 0.005$)
Grasping component			
Onset of grasping component (%)	5 ± 2	7 ± 3	($p < 0.1$)
Time to maximal grip aperture (%)	64 ± 8	58 ± 18	($p < 0.04$)
Maximum grip aperture (mm)	83 ± 20	95 ± 32	($p < 0.75$)

apraxia, characterized by a severe disruption of the action production system, may have several underlying pathologies, including features overlapping both CBD and Pick's disease (49) and Alzheimer's disease (50). Thus, the absence of apraxia at presentation does not exclude the possibility of CBD and the presence of an apraxic disorder "typically" encountered in patients with CBD may occasionally be a manifestation of a different disease. Nevertheless, in most cases the profile of praxic disorders exhibits some features that allow the presumptive diagnosis of the disease to be made.

Patients with PSP may have limb apraxia, particularly of the ideomotor type (51–55). We have found bilateral IMA for transitive movements in eight out of 12 patients with PSP; five of them also had IMA for intransitive movements. Performance improved on imitation and with tactile cues provided by the tool or object. Spatial errors (i.e., external and internal configuration, body-part-as-object and trajectory errors) were more prominent than temporal (i.e., hesitation, delay); sequencing errors occurred rarely. In addition to the ideomotor type of praxis errors, five patients also showed an abnormal motor behavior compatible with LKA. Content errors were not observed and none of the patients failed on pantomime comprehension (53).

Few studies on apraxia in Parkinson's disease (PD) have been published (53,56–58). Sharpe et al. (56) found that PD patients performed at a lower gestural level on representational tasks and made significantly more spatial errors on the nonrepresentational tasks than normal controls. Goldenberg et al. (57) studied 42 patients with moderate to severe PD; execution of movement sequence and a "total apraxia score" were worse in patients than in controls, and such deficits appeared to correlate with visuospatial disabilities. We have found bilateral IMA for transitive movements, which improved on imitation and became almost normal with the use of tools or objects in 12 out of 45 PD patients. Spatial errors (i.e., external configuration, body-part-as-object, internal configuration, and trajectory errors) were the most frequently found, whereas hesitation, occurrence and sequence errors were unusual and content errors were not observed. Comprehension of pantomimes was normal. Since we have found that IMA scores correlated with deficits in frontal lobe-related neuropsychological tasks in PD patients and with cognitive decline in PSP patients, we have suggested that apraxia in both of these conditions reflects combined corticostriatal dysfunction (53).

No apraxia was observed in any of our patients with multiple system atrophy. However, Monza et al. did find ideomotor apraxia in two of 19 patients with MSA, as well as in three of 15 patients with PSP (55).

Apraxia is found in 70% to 80% of patients in advanced stages of Alzheimer's disease (AD). IMA is not an usual early feature of the disease and pantomime to command may be found equally or more affected than gesture imitation (59). On the other hand, CA is a frequent finding in patients with the Alzheimer type of dementia, and may or may not be associated with IMA (27). Ochipa et al. evaluated 32 AD patients on language skill and praxis, systematically assessing tool use, the association of tools with objects and mechanical problem solving. They found double dissociation on language performance and ideomotor and concep-

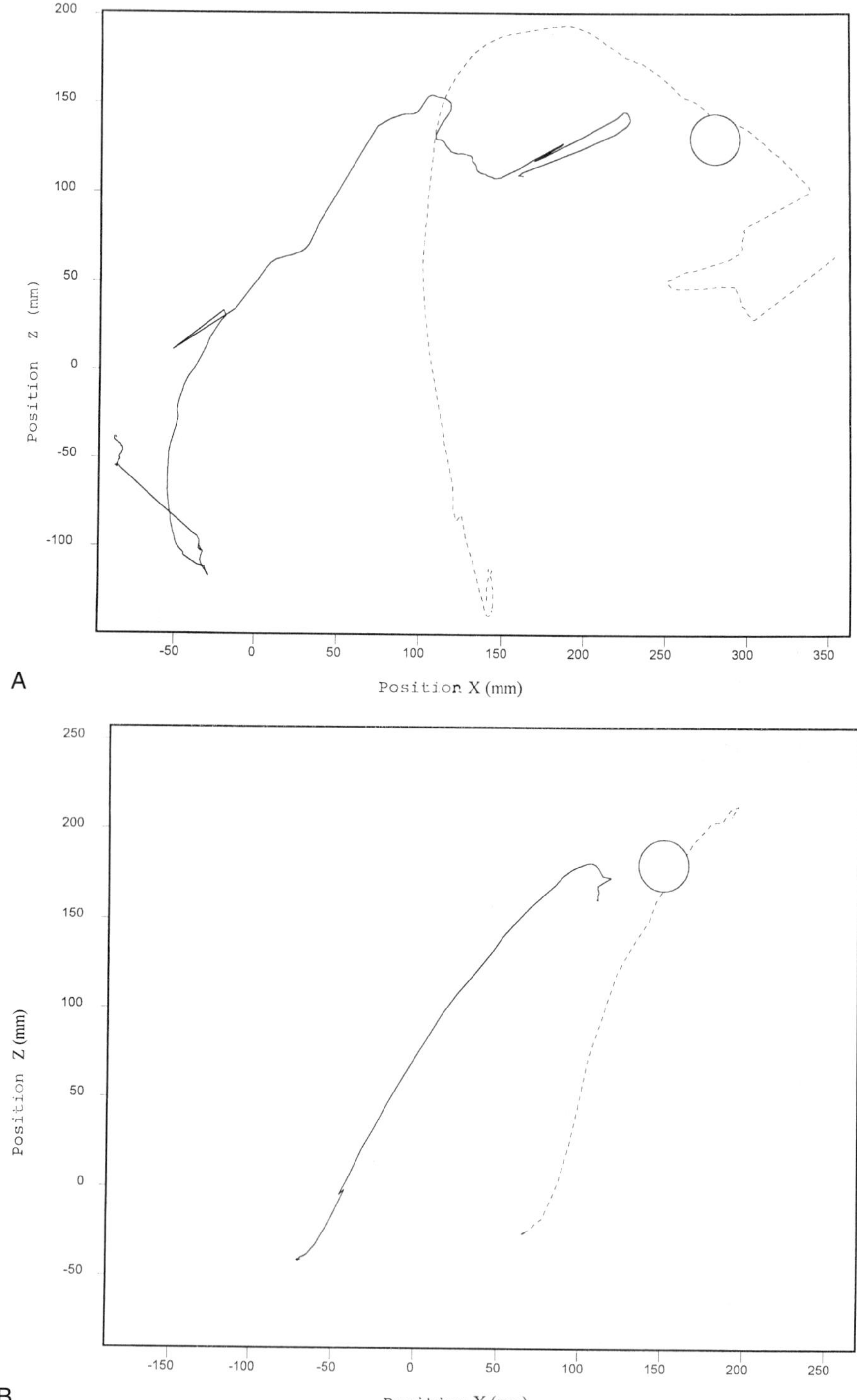

FIG. 5. Grasping in a patient with CBD (**A**) showing abnormal grip widening with grossly distorted thumb and index finger trajectory compared with a control subject (**B**).

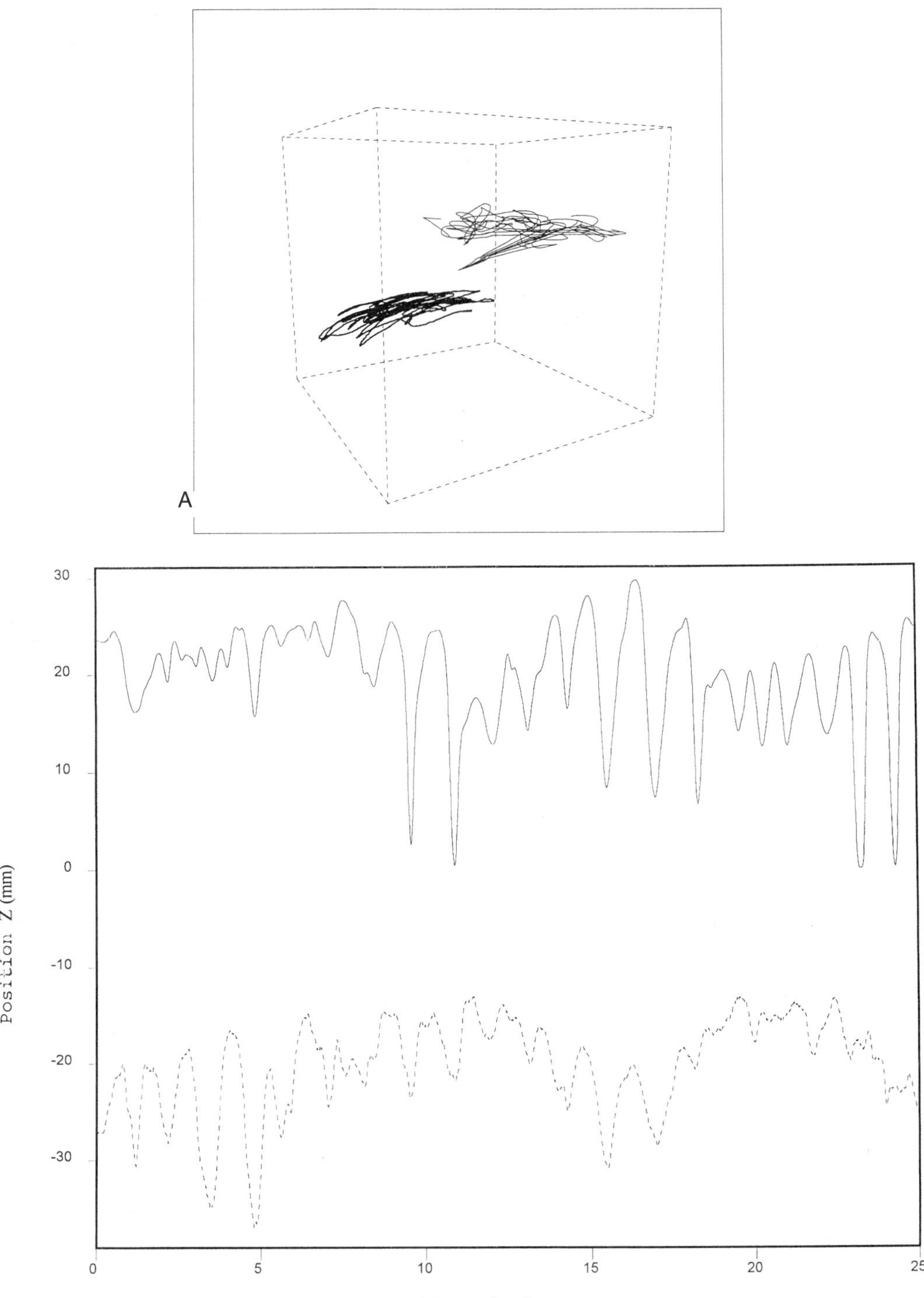

FIG. 6. Spatial and temporal characteristics of exploratory finger movement in a control subject (**A,B**) and in a patient with CBD (**C,D**). **A:** Movements trajectories of the thumb and index fingers are shown as viewed from the front, so that the vertical and horizontal movement components are displayed. **B:** Temporal profile of the vertical movements trajectories. Patient's movements showed a deranged trajectory formation and altered temporal characteristics distinctly different from the normal movement pattern.

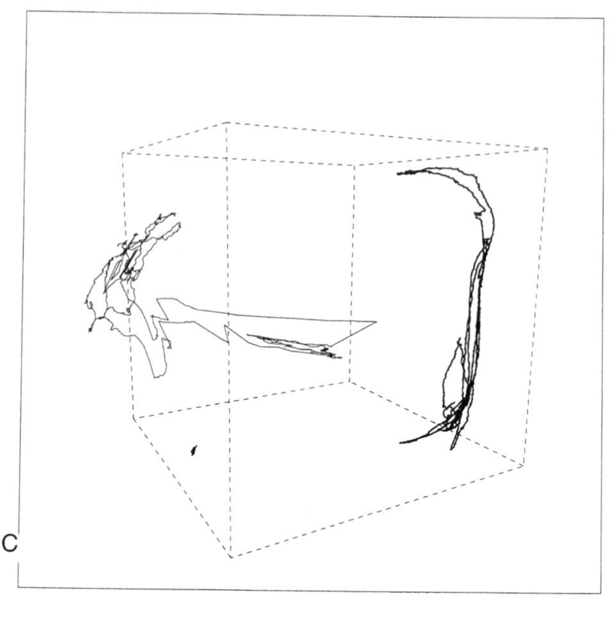

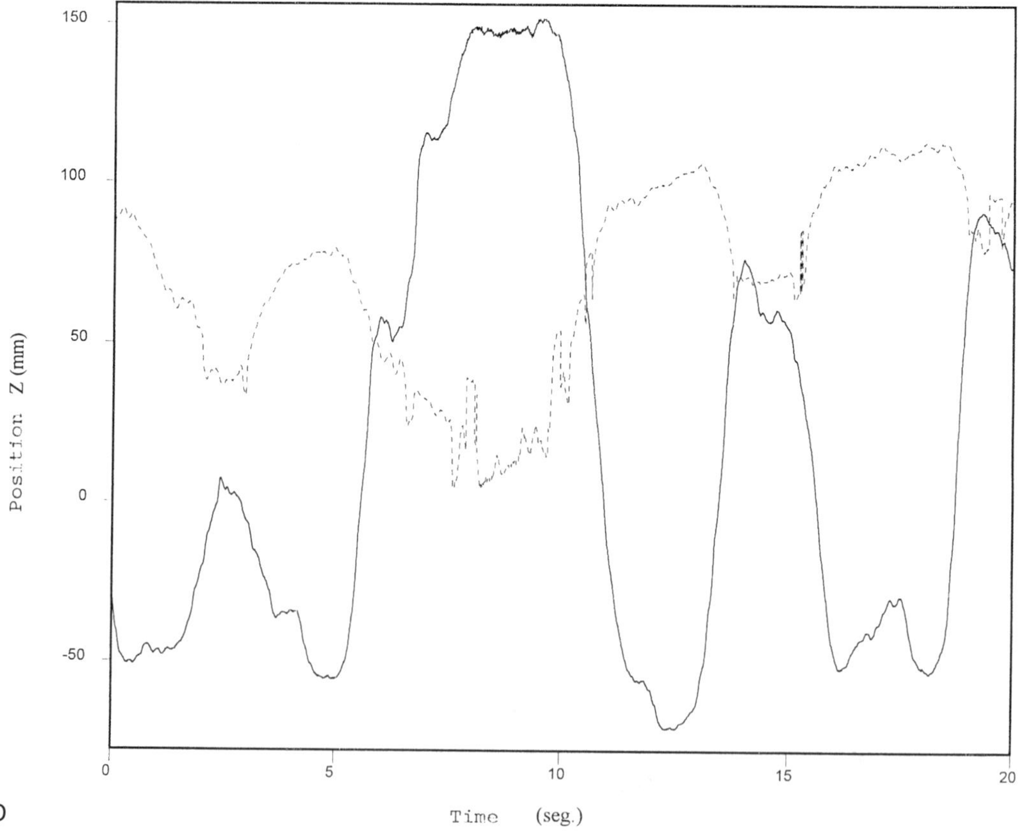

FIG. 6. (*Continued*)

tual apraxia (27). A PET study has demonstrated that deficits in pantomime performance correlated with language abnormalities and left frontal and temporal hypometabolism, whereas imitation deficits correlated with visual-spatial defects and right parietal hypometabolism (60).

Apraxia is not a clinical feature of frontotemporal dementia (FTD); mild praxis deficits owing to dysfunction of the action production system have been occasionally found only in advanced stages of the disease, perhaps revealing the distribution of the pathological changes within the frontal lobe and the association with striatal or late parietal involvement (30).

Both IMA and orofacial apraxia are common findings in patients with nonfluent primary progressive aphasia (PPA), whereas patients with fluent PPA may show IMA as well as IA. Although in most PPA patients IMA is mild and slowly progressive, PPA patients with more severe apraxic deficits may later develop a CBD. On the other hand, the presence of IA may herald progression toward an Alzheimer type of dementia (30).

PATHOPHYSIOLOGY

As described, most patients with CBD present a quite distinct apraxic syndrome characterized by an asymmetric ideomotor and limb-kinetic type of deficits owing to impairment of the action production system.

The praxis production system seems to be represented in a distributed brain network that is essentially centered in the dorsal (parieto-frontal) system devoted to object-oriented actions and functionally interconnected systems such as the frontostriatal and fronto-cerebellar ones (Fig. 7). The dorsal system can be divided into two main processing channels or subsystems. The medial subsystem is responsible for the transport phase of the movement and is mainly represented in the superior parietal lobe (SPL) and dorsal premotor cortex (PMd) connections, whereas the lateral subsystem subserves the grasping and manipulating phases and is primarily represented in the inferior parietal lobe (IPL) and ventral premotor cortex (PMv) connections (61).

In the parietal cortex the process of multisensory integration required for the composition of motor commands is planned. Different areas in the superior parietal cortex are engaged in the representation of target location and limb position for the early elaboration of movement trajectories toward an object in the extrapersonal space (62). A similar mechanism seems to operate in the IPL, where different populations of neurons encode egocentric distance to the target as well as the intrinsic properties of the objects (e.g., size, shape) and the pattern of hand movements required to manipulate them (hand manipulation neurons) (63). Thus, the parietal cortex

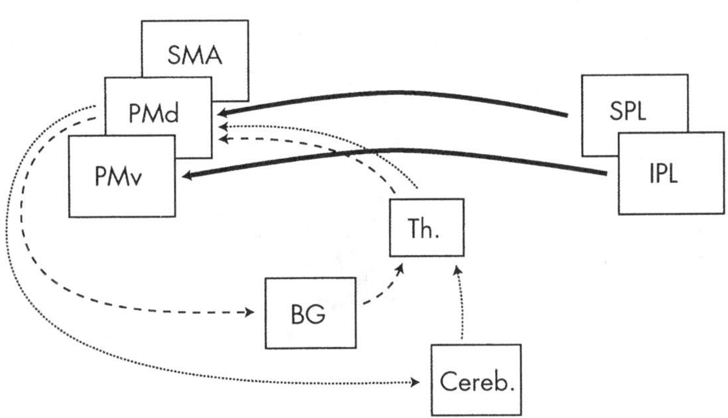

FIG. 7. Schematic diagram of the dorsal (*parieto-frontal*) system (→) subserving reaching, grasping and manipulation and functionally interconnected systems (*fronto-striatal* - -→ *and fronto-cerebellar* ···→) participating in timing and sequencing of of actions. These systems are specifically involved in CBD (*see text for abbreviations*).

would signal "where" and "how" an object is as well as the potential motor actions on it (62).

The dorsal premotor cortex (PMd), which is intimately connected with the SPL, is a crucial structure of the neural network subserving reaching. It plays a prominent role in movement preparation, in the retrieval of movement on the basis of stimulus characteristics (associate learning), and in the selection of the kinematic parameters of movement (e.g., amplitude, velocity) necessary for trajectory planning (64). The ventral premotor cortex (PMv) receives afferents mainly from the IPL. It seems to form a system together with area 7b and the putamen for the representation of peripersonal space somatotopically (65) and plays a prominent role in online control of movements. Area F5 lies in the rostral part of inferior area 6; it is connected with the hand area of MI, and therefore is specifically related to distal arm movements. In this area, diverse neuron populations encode different motor acts (schemas) that represent general categories of action (e.g., grasp, hold), how objects are to be grasped (e.g., held, torn) and the effectors (fingers) appropriate for the actions as well as schemas concerned with the temporal coordination among them (66). The motor schemas form a basic "vocabulary" from which many dextrous movements can be constructed as coordinated control programs (63). The final updating of the motor (or motor-sensory) schemas related to an object's physical properties seems to be based on afferent information about specific mechanical events at the skin-object contact areas occurring during manipulation (67). Thus, whereas parietal neurons encode elementary hand actions, F5 neurons are more related to a particular segment of the action; the ultimate fragmentation of the movement finally takes place in MI. It has been proposed that reaching and grasping functions are coordinated through timing (63).

Interval timing (reproduction and perception) seems to be directly mediated by the fronto-striatal and fronto-cerebellar loops, whereas the prefrontal-inferior parietal network primarily contributes to temporal perception through time dependent attention and working memory. The SMA, PM, and primary sensorimotor cortices, basal ganglia, and cerebellum are also engaged in the execution of simple, automatic, overlearned sequential movements that in this system appear to be structured temporally or rhythmically. On the other hand, the prefrontal, premotor, and inferior parietal system would mainly process complex or new learned sequences on the basis of spatial attention, integration of multimodal information, and visuospatial working memory (68,69).

The basal ganglia may participate in object-oriented action: (a) through the selection of kinematic parameters of movement (e.g., acceleration, velocity, amplitude) (70); (b) as an integral part of brain systems involved in timing and representation of action sequences (71); (c) by signaling the spatial location of visual stimuli relative to body parts may contribute, together with area 7b and premotor cortex, to transformation from extrinsic to intrinsic coordinates to guide movements directed to objects in peripersonal space (65; and (d) by encoding behavioral context (fronto-striatal circuits) (13).

Damage to the medial and lateral subsystems of the dorsal system, including its subcortical-basal ganglia connections, underlie the disruption of the action production system and praxic errors observed in patients with CBD. Dysfunction of the medial subsystem causes errors in limb position, configuration, and orientation as well as wrist trajectory errors, whereas errors in shaping the hand, grasping, and manipulating result from involvement of the lateral subsystem. The entire action is affected by an extensive lesion of the parietal cortex. On the other hand, damage to the frontal lobe primarily disrupts particular segments of the actions and the specificity for different hand and finger configurations (dexterity). Furthermore, some processes, such as timing and sequencing of motor events, are mediated by neural subsystems (e.g., fronto-striatal, fronto-cerebellar) that are functionally interrelated with the dorsal system.

The main pathologic changes in CBD are typically asymmetric and confined to the frontal and parietal cortices, the basal ganglia (substantia nigra, caudate, and lenticular nuclei) thalamus, and dentate nucleus (1–3,37). In the frontal lobe, pathology predominates in the premotor and SMA, although minor changes are usually found in the prefrontal and precentral regions. In the parietal cortex, the brunt of involvement lies in the superior region, although PET studies have disclosed hypometabolism in the inferior parietal lobe (72). However, atypical cases are not so uncommon and may show severe changes in the anterior portion of the frontal lobe as well as in the perisylvian region, including the first temporal gyrus (37).

In patients with CBD, parieto-frontal and basal ganglia damage may affect the reaching and grasping phases of movement. When left (dominant) hemisphere involvement predominates, a bilateral ideomotor type of praxis deficit supervenes. The deficit in the right upper limb may be masked by the associated elementary motor and sensory abnormalities; hence, the left upper limb should be evaluated for the presence of this type of apraxia. However, if the pathological process primarily involves the premotor cortex, the manipulating phase of the movement is mainly affected; the "motor vocabulary" necessary for the proper selection of skilled finger and hand movements is disrupted, and then a limb-kinetic type of praxis deficit appears in the hand contralateral to the more affected hemisphere, regardless of the pattern of cerebral dominance. An associated sensory deficit in addition interferes with the information necessary for the final updating of the finger and hand schemas to the object's physical characteristics, further undermining the process of manipulation. This "adextrous" hand is aggravated by the presence of akinesia and rigidity as a result of basal ganglia dysfunction. The concomitant damage of those subsystems involved in timing and sequencing further contributes to the apraxic deficits. Therefore, the severe impairment of the action production system observed in patients with CBD is the result of the particular cortical and subcortical distribution of the pathological changes that predominantly affect the structures integrating the dorsal as well as the fronto-striatal and fronto-cerebellar systems.

The complexity of limb praxis disorders requires a multidisciplinary approach that should encompass expertise from clinical neurology and neuropsychology to basic neuroscience. Future studies exploring normal praxis functions with functional neuroimaging as well as kinematics analysis of praxis errors and reaching, grasping, and manipulating components of object-oriented actions in patients with different types of limb praxis deficits will likely allow specific underlying neural mechanisms to be identified and limb praxis disorders to be classified within the framework of neurophysiological principles.

REFERENCES

1. Rebeiz JJ, Kolodny EH, Richardson EP. Corticodentatonigral degeneration with neuronal achromasia. *Arch Neurol* 1968;18:20–33.
2. Riley DE, Lang AE, Lewis A, et al. Corticobasal ganglionic degeneration. *Neurology* 1990;40:1203–1212.
3. Gibb WR, Luthert PJ, Marsden CD. Corticobasal degeneration. *Brain* 1989; 112:1171–1192.
4. Rinne J, Lee M, Thompson P, Marsden C. Corticobasal degeneration: a clinical study of 36 cases. *Brain* 1994;117:1183–1196.
5. Leiguarda R, Lees AJ, Merello M, Starkstein S, Marsden CD. The nature of apraxia in corticobasal degeneration. *J Neurol Neurosurg Psychiatry* 1994; 57:455–459.
6. Kampoliti K, Goetz CG, Boeve BF, et al. Clinical presentation and pharmacological therapy in corticobasal degeneration. *Arch Neurol* 1998; 55:957–961.
7. Litvan I, Agid Y, Goetz C, et al. Accuracy of the clinical diagnosis of corticobasal degeneration: a clinicopathologic study. *Neurology* 1997; 48:119–125.
8. Roy EA, Square PA. Common considerations in the study of limb, verbal, and oral apraxia. In: Roy EA, ed. *Neuropsychological studies of apraxia and related disorders.* Amsterdam: North-Holland 1985:111–161.
9. De Renzi E. Apraxia. In: Boller F, Grafman J, eds. *Handbook of neuropsychology.* Elsevier Science Publishers, Amsterdam, 1989;2:13:245–263.
10. Rothi LJ, Heilman K. *Apraxia, the neuropsychology of action.* Psychology Press, East Sussex, 1997.
11. Halsband U, Freund H. Motor learning. *Curr Op Neurobiol* 1993;3:940–949.
12. Schlang G, Knorr U, Seitz RJ. Intersubject variability of cerebral activation in acquiring a motor skill: a study with PET. *Exp Brain Res* 1994;98:523–534.
13. Dominey P, Boussaoud D. Encoding behavioral context in recurrent networks of the fronto-striatal system: a simulation study. *Cog Brain Res* 1997;6:53–65.
14. Roland PE, Larsen B, Lassen NA, Skinhöj E. Supplementary motor area and other cortical areas in organization of voluntary movements in man. *J Neurophysiol* 1980;43:118–136.
15. Seitz RJ, Roland E, Bohm C, Gretiz T, Stone-Elander S. Motor learning in man: a positron emission tomographic study. *Neuroreport* 1990;1:57–60.
16. Seitz RJ, Roland PE. Learning of sequential finger movements in man: a combined kinematic and positron emission tomography (PET) study. *Eur J Neurosci* 1992; 4:154–165.
17. Passingham R. Functional organization of the motor system. In: Frackowiak RSJ, Friston KJ, Frith CD, Dolan

RJ, Mazziotta JC, eds. *Human Brain Function.* Academic Press, San Diego, 1997:243–274.
18. Liepmann H. Apraxia. *Ergeb Gesamten Medizin* 1920;1: 516–543.
19. Haaland KY, Flaherty D. The different types of limb apraxia errors made by patients with left vs. right hemisphere damage. *Brain Cognition* 1984;3:370–384.
20. Rapcsak SZ, Ochipa C, Beeson PM, Rubens A. Apraxia and the right hemisphere. *Brain Cognition* 1993;23: 181–202.
21. De Renzi E, Faglioni P, Sorgato P. Modality-specific and supramodal mechanisms of apraxia. *Brain* 1982;105: 301–312.
22. Rothi LJG, Ochipa C, Heilman KM. A cognitive neuropsychological model of limb praxis. *Cog Neuropsychol* 1991;8(6):443–458.
23. Rothi LJG, Mack L, Verfaellie M, Brown P, Heilman KM. Ideomotor apraxia: error pattern analysis. *Aphasiology* 1988;2:381–388.
24. Faglioni P, Basso A. Historical perspectives on neuroanatomical correlates of limb apraxia. In: Roy EA, ed *Neuropsychological studies of apraxia and relates disorders.* Amsterdam: North-Holland, 1985:3–44.
25. Pick A. *Studien über Motorische Apraxie und ihre Mahestenhende Erscheinungen: ihre Bedeutung in der Symptonatologie Psychopathologischer Symptomenkomplexe.* Leipzig: Deuticke, 1905.
26. Poeck K. Ideational apraxia. *J Neurol* 1983;230:1–5.
27. Ochipa C, Rothi LJG, Heilman KM. Conceptual apraxia in Alzheimer's Disease. *Brain* 1992;115:1061–1071.
28. Heilman KM, Maher LH, Greenwald L, Rothi LJ. Conceptual apraxia from lateralized lesions. *Neurology* 1997;49:457–464.
29. De Renzi E, Lucchelli F. Ideational Apraxia. *Brain* 1988; 113:1173–1188.
30. Leiguarda R, Starkstein S. Apraxia in the syndromes of Pick complex. In: Kertesz, A, Muñoz DG, eds. *Pick's disease and Pick complex.* Wiley Liss, New York, 1998:129–143.
31. Leiguarda R, Merello M, Balej J, et al. Disruption of the medial and lateral processing channels of the dorsal stream in corticobasal degeneration: impairment of reaching, grasping and manipulation. *Mov Disord* 1998; 13(suppl 2):76.
32. Jacobs DH, Boston MA, Adair JC, Macauley BL, Gold M, Gonzalez Rothi LJ, Heilman KM. Apraxia in corticobasal degeneration. *Neurology* 1995;45(suppl 4):A266–A267.
33. Pillon B, Blin J, Vadailhet M, Deweer B, Sirigy A, Dubois B, Agid Y. The neuropsychological pattern of corticobasal degeneration: comparison with supranuclear palsy and Alzheimer's disease. *Neurology* 1995;45:1477–1483.
34. Blondel A, Eustache F, Schaeffer S, Marie R, Lechvalier B, Sayette V. Etudie clinique et cognitive de l'apraxie dans l'atrophie cortico-basale. *Rev Neurol (Paris)* 1997; 153:737–747.
35. Okuda B, Tachibana H. The nature of apraxia in corticobasal degeneration (letter; comment). *J Neurol Neurosurg Psychiatry* 1994; 57:1548–1549.
36. Okuda B, Tachibana H, Kawabata K, Takeda M, Sugita M. Slowly progressive limb-kinetic apraxia with a decrease in unilateral cerebral blood flow. *Acta Neurol Scand* 1992;86:76–81.
37. Tsuchiya K, Ikeda K, Uchihara T, Oda T, Shimada H. Distribution of cerebral cortical lesions in corticobasal degeneration: a clinicopathological study of five autopsy cases in Japan. *Acta Neuropathol* 1997;94:416–424.
38. Denes G, Mantovan MC, Gallana A, Cappelletti JV. Limb-kinetic apraxia. *Mov Disord* 1998;13:468–476.
39. Martinez-Lage P, Kertesz A. Behavioral and language involvement in corticobasal degeneration. *J Neuropsychol* 1997;9:649(abstract).
40. Lang AE. Cortical basal ganglionic degeneration presenting with progressive loss of speech output and orofacial dyspraxia. *J Neurol Neurosurg Psychiatry* 1992; 55:1101.
41. Poizner H, Mack L, Verfaellie M, Rothi LJG, Heilman KM. Three-dimensional computergraphic analysis of apraxia. *Brain* 1990;113:85–101.
42. Clark MA, Merians AS, Kothari A, et al. Spatial planning deficits in limb apraxia. *Brain* 1994;117:1093–1106.
43. Poizner H, Clark MA, Merians AS, et al. Joint coordination deficits in limb apraxia. *Brain* 1995;118:227–242.
44. Rapscak SZ, Ochipa C, Anderson KA, Poizner H. Progressive ideomotor apraxia: evidence for a selective impairment of the action production system. *Brain Cognition* 1995;27:213–236.
45. Viviani P, Stucchi N. Biological movements look uniform: evidence for motor-perceptual interactions. *J Exp Psychol Hum Percept Perform* 1992;18:603–623.
46. Morasso P. Three-dimensional arm trajectories. *Biol Cybernetics* 1983;48:187–194.
47. Caselli RJ, Stelmach GE, Caviness JV, et al. A kinematic study of progressive apraxia with and without dementia. *Mov Disord* 1998;12(suppl 2):25.
48. Boeve BF, Maraganore DM, Parisi JE, et al. Disorders mimicking the classical syndrome of cortical-basal ganglionic degeneration: report of nine cases. *Mov Disord* 1996;11:351 (abst.).
49. Jeudroska K, Rossor MN, Mathias CJ, Daniel SE. Morphological overlap between corticobasal degeneration and Pick's disease: a clinicopathological report. *Mov Disord* 1995;10:111–114.
50. Green RC, Goldstein FC, Mirra SS, Alarzaki NP, Baxt JL, Bakay RAE. Slowly progressive apraxia in Alzheimer's disease. *J Neurol Neurosurg Psychiatry* 1995;59: 312–315.
51. Cambier J, Masson M, Viader F, Limodin J, Strube A. Le syndrome frontal de la paralysie supranucléaaire progressive. *Rev Neurol (Paris)* 1985;141:528–536.
52. Collins SJ, Ahlskog JE, Parisi JE, Maraganore DM. Progressive supranuclear palsy: neuropathologically based diagnostic clinical criteria (see comments). *J Neurol Neurosurg Psychiatry* 1995;58:167–173. Comment in: *J Neurol Neurosurg Psychiatry* 1995;59:106, Comment in: *J Neurol Neurosurg Psychiatry* 1995;59:343.
53. Leiguarda R, Pramstaller P, Merello M, Starkstein S, Lees AJ, Marsden CD. Apraxia in Parkinson's disease, progressive supranuclear palsy, multiple system atrophy, and neuroleptic induced parkinsonism. *Brain* 1997;120: 75–90.
54. Soliveri P, Piacentini S, Monza D, et al. Differences in the cognitive profile in corticobasal degeneration and progressive supranuclear palsy. *Mov Disord* 1998;13 (suppl 2):116.
55. Monza D, Soliveri P, Radice D, et al. Cognitive dysfunction and impaired organization of complex mobility in degenerative parkinsonian syndromes. *Arch Neurol* 1998;55:372–378.
56. Sharpe MH, Cermak SA, Sax DS. Motor planning in Parkinson patients. *Neuropsychologia* 1983;21:455–462.
57. Goldenberg G, Wimmer A, Auff E, Schnaberth G. Impairment of motor planning in patients with Parkinson's

disease: evidence for ideomotor apraxia testing. *J Neurol Neurosurg Psychiatry* 1986;49:1266–1272.
58. Grossman M, Carvell S, Gollomp S, Stern MB, Vernon G, Hurtig HI. Sentence comprehension and praxis deficits in Parkinson's disease. *Neurology* 1991;41:1620–1626.
59. Luchelli F, Lopez O, Faglioni P, Boller F. Ideomotor and ideational apraxias in Alzheimer's disease. *Int J Ger Psych* 1993;8:413–417.
60. Foster NL, Chase TN, Patronas N, Gillespie M, Fedio P. Cerebral mapping of apraxia in Alzheimer's disease by position emission tomography. *Ann Neurol* 1986;19: 139–143.
61. Jeanneroad M. Cortical coding of visual object attributes during object-oriented behaviour. In Caminitti R, Hoffman KP, Lacquanti F, Altman J, eds. Vision and movements mechanisms in the cerebral cortex. *HFSP Strasbourg* 1966;15–23.
62. Kalaska JF, Scott SH, Cisek P, Sergio LE. Cortical control of reaching movements. *Curr Opin Neurobiol* 1997;7:849–859.
63. Jeannerod M, Arbid MA, Rizzolatti G, Sakata H. Grasping objects: the cortical mechanisms of visuomotor transformation. *Trends Neurosci* 1995;18:314–320.
64. Roland Pe, Zilles K. Functions and structures of the motor cortices in humans. *Curr Opin Neurobiol* 1996;6: 773–781.
65. Graziano MSA, Gross CG. The representation of extrapersonal space: A possible role for bimodal visual-tactile neurons. In Gazzaniga MS, ed. *The cognitive neurosciences.* Cambridge, MA, 1996:1021–1034.
66. Gallese V, Fadiga L, Fogassi L, Rizzolatti G. Action recognition in the premotor cortex. *Brain* 1996;119: 593–609.
67. Lemon R. Mechanisms of cortical control of hand function. *Neuroscientist* 1997;3:389–398.
68. Gibbon J, Malapani C, Dale C, Galiste CR. Toward a neurobiology of temporal cognition: advances and challenges. *Curr Opin Neurobiol* 1997;7:170–184.
69. Harrington DL, Haaland KY, Knight J. Cortical networks underlying mechanisms of time perception. *J Neurosci* 1998;18:1085–1095.
70. Mitchell SJ, Richardson RT, Baker FH, De Long MR. The primate globus pallidus: neuronal activity related with the direction of movements. *Exp Brain Res* 1987;68:491–505.
71. Graybiel AM. Building action repertoires: memory and learning functions of the basal ganglia. *Curr Opin Neurobiol* 1995;5:733–741.
72. Eidelberg D, Dhawan V, Moeller JR, et al. The metabolic landscape of corticobasal ganglionic degeneration: regional asymmetries studied with positron emission tomography. *J Neurol Neurosurg Psychiatry* 1991;54: 856–862.

Corticobasal Degeneration.
Advances in Neurology, Vol. 82,
edited by I. Litvan, C. G. Goetz, and A. E. Lang.
Lippincott Williams & Wilkins, Philadelphia © 2000.

11

Aphasia in Corticobasal Degeneration

Sandra E. Black

Division of Neurology, Sunnybrook and Women's College Health Sciences Centre, Toronto, Ontario, M4N 3M5, Canada

INTRODUCTION

Aphasia has been frequently included in accounts of the clinical syndrome of corticobasal degeneration (CBD), but its frequency, clinical characteristics, and neuropathological correlations have been little studied. Aphasia is not considered a "core" feature of CBD, but rather serves as an indictor of the heterogeneity of the clinical syndrome. CBD pathology in turn represents one of the neuropathological substrates of primary progressive aphasia (PPA). To understand the relative importance of aphasia in CBD, a definition and neurological classification of aphasia is provided and the syndrome of PPA is discussed. A brief overview of the relevant clinical-pathological characteristics of CBD, including neuroimaging and neuropsychological profile, is then given to put in context the current knowledge of aphasia in CBD as derived from group and single-case studies. The evidence suggests that aphasia is more common than is usually recognized in most CBD series and should be routinely assessed in suspected CBD cases. Likewise, PPA cases should be neurologically followed for the possible development of an asymmetric akinetic-rigid syndrome. Further research is needed on the clinical characteristics and pathological correlations of aphasia in the context of CBD.

Neurogenic Communication Disorders: Aphasia, Verbal Apraxia, Dysarthria

Aphasia refers to loss of language formulation or comprehension skills caused by dysfunction in the brain regions specialized for language processing, which is in the left hemisphere in more than 99% of right-handed and approximately 2/3 of left-handed individuals (1). Language involves the use of symbols to transfer and receive information from one human being to another. The neurological classification of aphasic disorders is based primarily on the effects of sudden ablation of function, most commonly from occlusive or hemorrhagic stroke in the left middle cerebral artery territory (2). When the inferior frontal region including Broca's area is damaged, a nonfluent speech pattern results, which is marked by anomia, phonological, and syntactic difficulties, whereas comprehension is partially preserved. When the posterior-superior temporal and inferior parietal regions are damaged, fluent speech output is produced with disturbed lexical-semantic processing and poor comprehension, the constellation called Wernicke's aphasia. Damage to both anterior and posterior regions of the perisylvian language cortex results in global aphasia with severely impaired comprehension and speech output. When damage occurs outside the perisylvian region, the so-called transcortical aphasias can occur in which repetition is relatively preserved since Wernicke's and Broca's areas and the association fibers connecting them are intact (1,2). Transcortical motor aphasia, a nonfluent disorder, can result if damage involves dorsolateral or medial frontal cortex (including the supplementary motor area) (3). If the posterior occipital-temporal region is damaged, a fluent disorder similar to Wernicke's aphasia but with intact repetition, transcortical sensory aphasia, is produced. If anterior and posterior regions are injured with sparing of the perisylvian cortex, mixed transcortical aphasia results, in which repetition is relatively spared, but both speech output and comprehension are severely affected. Aphasic disturbances have also been associated with lesions confined to the subcortical regions, including the basal ganglia and thalamus (4,5). A neurodegenerative disorder that adversely affects function in any of these regions in the left hemisphere could therefore be expected to be associated with aphasia, the nature of which would depend on the region(s) damaged.

It is important to recognize that aphasia is multimodal, producing deficits in language output, in the form of speech, sign language, or writing, or deficits in comprehension of spoken, written, or gestural language. It is therefore important that language impairment be assessed in a standardized fashion that samples all modalities. Neurolinguistic studies have revealed that word type, word frequency, and word length as well as phonological, syntactical, and semantic aspects of language should all be considered in a comprehensive language assessment (6). In North America, frequently used standardized aphasia assessments include the Boston Diagnostic Aphasia. Assessment (7) and the Western Aphasia Battery (WAB) (8), which sample all oral modalities as well as reading and writing, but do not specifically manipulate linguistic features such as word frequency, spelling regularity, or lexicality. The use of standardized assessment to investigate aphasia in CBD would be an important advance since the neurolinguistic profile has not been well studied. In most of the autopsy and clinical series, the diagnosis of aphasia is usually based on a brief neurological screening that may be sufficient to recognize that language dysfunction is present, but not to define it in any detail. Only a few recent case reports have used standardized assessments, as will be discussed in the following.

Another impediment is that the high prevalence of hypokinetic dysarthria in CBD often confounds the assessment of communication ability. Speech may become unintelligible because of the extrapyramidal syndrome, and the presence of a nonfluent language disturbance may be difficult to recognize, since comprehension may be relatively intact in either condition. Dysarthria refers to a motor speech deficit related to neuromuscular or central nervous system dysfunction in the control of the muscles involved in respiration, phonation, resonance, articulation, and prosody (9). Hypophonic dysarthria commonly results from the rigidity and bradykinesia of extrapyramidal disease. Another possible confounding factor is verbal apraxia, a disorder of motor programming in the production of the sequences of speech sounds that constitute words (9,10). With verbal apraxia, as with dysarthria, comprehension and written expression are intact, and there should be no word-finding difficulty. Verbal apraxia in CBD has been even less studied than aphasia. Given the pathological topography of CBD and the predominance of ideomotor limb apraxia, however, it would certainly not be surprising if verbal apraxia was frequent in CBD. Verbal apraxia usually localizes to the inferior frontal cortex and underlying white matter extending to the basal ganglia. One can speculate that the stuttering speech substitutions frequently described in CBD patients could reflect verbal apraxia, which may also contribute significantly to eventual mutism. In fact it is very likely that the mutism seen in many cases of endstage CBD is a combined deficit with aphasia, verbal apraxia, and dysarthria all contributing. Given the topography of neurodegeneration in CBD, therefore, neurogenic communication disorders, including aphasia should be common in CBD, especially if there is preferential asymmetric involvement of the left hemisphere. In fact, CBD is one of the recognized pathological substrates for PPA as will now be briefly discussed.

Primary Progressive Aphasia

Clinical Syndrome

When aphasia occurs in the context of a neurodegenerative disorder, there is a gradual rather than sudden deterioration of language function, which can unfold over several years (11–13). An aphasic disturbance was quite prominent in the index cases described by both Alzheimer and Pick in the diseases named after them (14). Over subsequent years, however, the emphasis changed with behavioral alteration and dysexecutive syndrome being emphasized in Pick's disease and memory loss in Alzheimer's disease (AD) (14). In 1982 Mesulam described six patients in whom gradual language dissolution was the predominant finding, whereas other cognitive functions were relatively intact and independence in activities of daily living was well maintained (11). He described initial word-finding difficulty characterized by hesitant output and reduced speech rate in the presence of normal phrase length and grammar, a profile he called "logopenia" (11). Comprehension difficulty gradually developed in some cases. He proposed the term PPA to bring attention to this clinical syndrome and emphasized the relative preservation of cognitive functions (15). He further noted that phonemic paraphasias are more common (62%) in PPA versus AD (8%), whereas semantic substitutions are more frequent along with the other cognitive deficits particularly loss of memory and visual-spatial ability in AD. In a later review of the syndrome, Mesulam and Weintraub (1992) continued to emphasize that progressive language deterioration occurred early in the course of PPA with preserved episodic memory, visual-spatial skills, insight, and comportment, although more generalized deterioration could arise later on in the disease (16,17). Nonfluent aphasia was present in 44%; the remainder had fluent aphasia, but often with "logopenia." Neuroimaging usually revealed left perisylvian dysfunction or atrophy. Mesulam and Weintraub suggested that isolated language disturbance should be present for at least 2 years to warrant the diagnosis of PPA (16,17). A review of 161 literature and 27 additional cases of PPA in 1996 confirmed a presenile onset (mean age 59) with relatively isolated aphasic syndrome, most frequently nonfluent, lasting an average of 5 years (12). Westbury and Bub (1997) have further reviewed the neurolinguistic and clinical-pathological features (13).

Neuropathology of Primary Progressive Aphasia

The pathological substrate in over half of the 40 available autopsied cases of PPA reviewed by Black (1996), was neuronal loss, gliosis, and spongiosis in the outer layers of frontal and temporal cortices with or without ballooned cells and Pick bodies (12). This neuropathological configuration was called frontal-temporal dementia (FTD) by the Lund-Manchester group, who published clinical and pathological criteria in 1994 (18,19). Primary progressive non-fluent aphasia was regarded as the clinical phenotype when left frontal-temporal degeneration predominated early on in the disease (20). A fluent manifestation of PPA arising from bilateral anterior temporal degeneration called "semantic dementia" was also described (21), including loss of access to representations for word and object meaning (semantics) with relative preservation of phonology (21). In this disorder, the meaning of words, objects, and faces gradually dissolves. Reading and writing are also affected, such that regularization errors are frequent in reading and writing of irregularly spelled words, reflecting loss of word recognition with intact phonological processing (letter-sound correspondences). Thus, progressive fluent aphasia comprises fluent speech output with semantic paraphasias initially, with relative preservation of phonology and severe impairment of comprehension. In progressive nonfluent aphasia, semantic processing is relatively preserved, at least early on, whereas phonological processing is impaired. The aphasic disturbance in AD is also characterized by fluent spontaneous speech early on with anomia and eventually comprehension impairment (22). There is loss of access to semantics in AD, although this usually occurs later on in the disease as opposed to being an early manifestation in semantic dementia. In the neurodegenerative aphasias, the aphasic subtype corresponds to the regional pathology. Thus, in progressive nonfluent aphasia the left inferior frontal and anterior temporal region is affected. In semantic dementia the anterior temporal regions are affected bilaterally. AD has a predilection for the posterior temporal-parietal region. In typical cases of PPA owing to FTD a personality and behavioral disorder usually supervenes as the disease spreads anteriorly and bilaterally. In contradistinction to AD, however, patients with PPA owing to FTD usually have relative retention of spatial skills and remain independent in activities of daily living until more advanced stages. A small subset of

PPA patients turn out to have AD and as the course unfolds, episodic memory and spatial impairments as well as problems in activities of daily living, become quite apparent (12).

CBD frequently involves perisylvian cortex, including inferior dorsolateral frontal, medial frontal and inferior parietal regions and when the left hemisphere is preferentially involved, aphasia may be evident early in the course of disease. Thus, some cases of PPA followed to autopsy have turned out to have pathology typical for CBD (23,24).

In summary, PPA can arise from several pathological conditions, most commonly from the so-called Pick complex diseases, including FTD without Pick bodies, with or without motor neuron disease, classic Pick's disease and CBD (14,25). It can also be caused by AD, but if nonfluency or logopenic speech is a key feature, then Pick complex diseases would be more common as a cause than would AD. With standardized assessment these aphasic disorders can be classified into different subtypes depending on the anatomical region most involved initially. Thus, transcortical motor, transcortical sensory, Broca's, Wernicke's, or mixed aphasia, have all been described, although the application of this neurological classification system does not always properly capture the syndromes seen in the neurodegenerative conditions. An aphasic disturbance would not be unexpected in CBD, especially when there is predominant involvement of the left hemisphere.

The characteristics of the aphasic disturbance in a given individual will reflect the degree of involvement of language-eloquent, left perisylvian regions such as the inferior frontal, posterior temporal, and parietal regions. Nonfluent aphasia would usually be associated with left inferior frontal predilection and fluent aphasia with posterior-temporal and parietal CBD. Involvement of the supplementary motor area could give rise to a transcortical motor aphasia. Global aphasia could result if both anterior and posterior language areas are affected, usually at a later stage of the disease. Transcortical sensory aphasia would be less likely since it usually arises from more posterior regions than are usually affected in CBD. Having considered the neuronal substrates for aphasia, what then is the evidence for aphasia in CBD? Before examining this evidence, it is first necessary to put aphasia into the context of the typical clinical profile of the CBD syndrome.

Corticobasal Degeneration

Clinical-Pathological Syndrome

CBD is an asymmetric akinetic-rigid syndrome frequently associated with dystonic posturing of the arm, with limb and oculomotor apraxia, cortical sensory loss, and myoclonus (26,27). Also common are hypokinetic dysarthria, gait imbalance, and alien limb syndrome, in which the affected arm takes up postures or carries out movements that are not intended. CBD is frequently underdiagnosed and recent studies applying clinical criteria indicate a low sensitivity (34% to 48%) but high specificity (99.6%) when expert neurologists blindly assessed clinical scenarios (27). Pathologically, it has a typical brain topography usually associated with swollen achromatic neurons and widespread white matter pathological changes (28), but there can be overlap with other pathologies and clinical syndromes such as FTD, Pick's disease, and PSP (29,30). Immunohistochemistry may help further clarify whether these are fundamentally different biological disorders that share some neuropathological and clinical features, as suggested by Feany and Dickson (31) or whether they are better considered as a family of tauopathies that are more similar than different (25) These nosological issues arise because the typical clinical phenotype can be mimicked by other disorders, (32) particularly Pick's disease, and because the typical pathological phenotype can be found at autopsy in individuals who did not manifest the typical clinical syndrome (30). A way through the nosological dilemmas posed by the CBD syndrome is to combine clinical and pathological criteria to arrive at a final diagnosis (27). Clinical characteristics and diagnostic criteria are thoroughly addressed in Chapters 2, 3, 17, and 21.

Functioning Imaging Patterns

Neuropathological studies provide important information on the end-stage distribution of pathology in CBD, but modern neuroimaging techniques can be used to track the disease topography over time, and in the case of functional imaging can help to distinguish different neurodegenerative conditions. A number of positron emission tomography (PET) and single photon emission control tomography (SPECT) studies have been conducted in CBD, although usually with small samples (often five or six patients) because of the rarity of the condition (33–36). Despite attempts to find distinct patterns for CBD, abnormalities are unpredictable in individual cases. Thus, not surprisingly, given the heterogeneity of CBD, the abnormalities reported have varied in different studies. Lateral and medial prefrontal hypoperfusion or hypometabolism are frequently reported as well as decreases in the inferior frontal, pre- and postcentral gyri and inferior parietal lobule as well as caudate and putamen (36–38). Some studies have found superior temporal involvement (38) and others have not (36). Dopaminergic imaging has consistently shown both presynaptic and postsynaptic striatal dysfunction (36,38).

A typical and important finding in CBD is asymmetry with greater hypoperfusion or hypometabolism in the hemisphere contralateral to the more affected limb (33–36). In patients with right arm dystonia and aphasia, for example, left hemisphere abnormalities predominate. Hence, greater decrease in the left hemisphere in a patient with right side predominance in the akinetic-rigid syndrome should prompt careful assessment of language function. (For further details on neuroimaging in CBD, see Chapters 20 and 21.)

Neuropsychological Profile

The neuropsychological profile of CBD is less well characterized than its motor symptomatology (39–41). So far there is only one group study that has investigated the neuropsychological pattern in CBD with a detailed standardized battery. Included were 15 patients clinically diagnosed as CBD, 19 age-matched controls, 15 patients with probable AD, and 15 with PSP (41). The patients with CBD showed moderate global deterioration with a dysexecutive syndrome similar to PSP and worse than AD, memory retrieval deficits comparable to PSP with relatively intact encoding in contrast to AD, and a disorder of motor control with asymmetric apraxia, more severe than that observed in PSP or AD. A combination of dysexecutive syndrome and asymmetric apraxia was felt to be a distinguishing neuropsychological profile in CBD (39,41). A number of neuropsychological tasks were performed in this study, but there was no separate evaluation of language, although it was noted that phonemic and semantic word list generation was significantly reduced compared to normal in the CBD patients. Thus, although this is the most comprehensive neuropsychological study so far conducted in CBD, little information is forthcoming concerning the language profile apart from the decrease in the verbal fluency task. For further insight into language breakdown in CBD, it is necessary first to note the frequency of aphasia in group studies of CBD and then to review single case studies in which aphasia has figured prominently. (See Chapter 14 for further detail on neuropsychiatric aspects of CBD.)

Aphasia as Documented in Group Studies of CBD

As stated, progressive language loss can be the presenting sign or occur in the course of several neurodegenerative disorders, reflecting dysfunction in the perisylvian cortex in the left hemisphere. The clinical syndrome of CBD has a typical profile, which can be distinguished by history and examination, and possibly aided by neuroimaging, and this has given rise to a number of group studies. In the context of these studies, the frequency and characteristics of aphasia can be determined in the setting of the recognizable clinical syndrome of CBD and compared to other clinical phenomenology.

So far there have been three major clinical series reporting on the clinical phenotype first described by Rebeiz et al. (1968) (42), as well as three pathological series. The clinical series include two single-center series with a review of previous cases (26,43) contributing 15 and 36 new patients, respectively, and one multicenter study of 147 subjects (44). Patients were given a tentative diagnosis of CBD based on the clinical picture; autopsy confirmation was available in 15 of the 198 cases in these series (26,43,44). Most of these group studies were collected through referrals to movement disorder clinics with a resulting predominance in the extrapyramidal syndrome and motor deficits. The cognitive profile has been less well studied. Indeed, since memory is often only mildly impaired in CBD subjects, the generalization has been made that higher mental functions are relatively spared in CBD with the prominent exception of ideomotor apraxia (43). Furthermore, because of the extrapyramidal syndrome, cognitive testing becomes difficult with disease progression. This is particularly true of aphasia because dysarthria or verbal apraxia can independently impede speech fluency and make the presence of an aphasic output disturbance difficult to disentangle. In most clinical series, only the presence or absence of aphasia was noted without further characterization. It is likely, therefore, that there has been a tendency to underestimate the cases with language disturbance in CBD, but at the same time when aphasia was recorded as present, it was usually clinically significant. Furthermore, clinical series are often cross-sectional, providing a point prevalence of aphasia in patients at different stages of the disease.

With these caveats, what can be learned from the published case series on aphasia in CBD? The first large series included 15 patients with clinically diagnosed CBD (two with autopsy confirmation), three of whom (cases 10, 14, and 15) had aphasia, giving a frequency of 20% (26). A case description was provided for case 10. Three years into the course of the illness that began at age 65, slow, slurred speech with frequent stuttering and occasional literal and verbal paraphasia was noted. Repetition was mildly impaired and comprehension appeared to be intact. There was generalized rigidity most severe in the right arm, apraxia, dystonia, alien limb phenomenon in the left arm, and bilateral myoclonus. Rinné et al. (1994) reported aphasia without further details in 10 of their 36 patients who had typical features of CBD (seven autopsied) (43). They also reviewed 28 previous cases, counting 10 out of 64 cases with aphasia for an overall frequency of 16%. More recently Kompoliti et al. (1998) analyzed 147 patients (seven autopsied) compiled from eight major movement disorder clinics over a period of 5 years (44). In contrast to previous observations, they described higher cortical dysfunction in 93% of this CBD series. In the clinical cases, aphasia was reported in 15 patients (10%), but in the autopsy-confirmed cases one had aphasia, giving a frequency 14%. Again the aphasia was not further characterized.

One group study took a different approach. Noting that the frequency of clinical characteristics, particularly the typical CBD extrapyramidal syndrome and the presence of cognitive deficits, tends to reflect the focus of the clinic to which the patient was initially referred, these authors carefully reviewed 24 cases of CBD, some of whom presented with the extrapyramidal syndrome and were being followed through a movement disorder clinic and some of whom had cognitive deficits and were being followed through a behavioral neurology clinic (45). They found that cognitive and behavioral deficits were actually present in 11/12 cases presenting with the typical extrapyramidal syndrome, seven of whom had progressive aphasia, and four of whom had a frontal syndrome. Furthermore, a typical CBD extrapyramidal syndrome developed in 12 cases presenting with PPA or FTD with aphasia prominent in 9/12 and behavior and personality change in 3/12 (45). They noted in the aphasia cases that the asymmetric rigidity involved predominantly the right hand, which also frequently demonstrated an alien hand syndrome. Thus, a neurobehavioral disorder was detectable in 23/24 of these cases. Apraxia was also equally frequent in both extrapyramidal and cognitive presentations (23/24 cases). There was no difference in age or in the eventual clinical features that developed in these two types of presentations. Two of their autopsied cases were diagnosed as FTD and PSP *in vivo*. The clinical phenotype of CBD has been defined primarily in relation to the extrapyramidal disorder, so it is not surprising, as these authors suggest, that there is relative under-recognition of the cognitive and behavioral presentations. The authors emphasized that CBD pathology can be associated with behavioral-personality change or progressive aphasia that may occur before, after, or concomitantly with the extrapyramidal syndrome (45). Although CBD is now known to be a potential anatomical substrate of PPA, it is less frequently included in the differential diagnosis of a frontal lobe syndrome, although this is starting to be recognized (27,30,45).

A clinical series recently completed set out to assess aphasic disturbance prospectively in the CBD syndrome using the Western Aphasia Battery as the standardized test (46). The authors found definite aphasia in 53% of the sample of 15 patients meeting clinical criteria for CBD. Although full details are still awaited, most of the aphasic patients had a nonfluent aphasia with the exception of one, who had a mild anomic aphasia with word-retrieval difficulty in the context of fluent speech. This study suggests that a systematic screening for aphasia will more than double case finding in patients with the CBD syndrome.

The higher incidence of aphasia noted by these authors in vivo tends to be supported by autopsy studies in which the patients usually have had the opportunity to run the course of the disease in its full spectrum over several years. The problem with autopsy series remains, however, that the clinical details may be even skimpier than in the clinical series. The confounding effects of dysarthria, verbal apraxia, and aphasia are problematic as indicated in the preceding, because they may be difficult to distinguish in the absence of special expertise. As the disease progresses patients may become mute from one or a combination of these neurogenic communication disorders. Thus, Schneider reported that 8/11 autopsy cases of CBD had speech disturbance leading to mutism, but the authors do not specify how many cases had aphasia (47). Wenning et al. (1998) analyzed 14 autopsy cases from a multicenter trial and tracked different clinical features from time of presentation to the time of last visit (48). In this autopsy series, aphasia was present in 29% at the first visit and by the last visit over 50% of the patients were noted to have an aphasic disturbance, which was not further specified. In the same series ideomotor apraxia was present initially in 64% and by last visit in 75%. Dysarthria was present initially in 29% and 75% at last visit with aphonia and anarthria present in 33%. Cortical dementia was noted in 36% initially and 42% by last visit. In comparison, extrapyramidal symptoms, including limb rigidity, bradykinesia, postural instability, or gait disorder were present in over 93% of the subjects with autopsy-confirmed CBD.

In summary, autopsy series suggest that over half of the patients with CBD syndrome suffer from a language disturbance, presumably owing in part to the fact that postmortem examination captures the full spectrum of the disease as it runs its course in different individuals. Clinical series report a frequency of aphasia of 10% to 20%, but with more systematic evaluation the frequency of aphasia is closer to 50% (45,46). This is not surprising given the predilection of CBD for language-related cortex, including the inferior frontal, supplementary motor, and parietal cortices. This 50% prevalence is similar to the frequency of aphasia in acute left hemisphere stroke in which MCA territory infarctions often involve the language-specialized cortex, including frontal, parietal, and temporal regions (2). Since most of the large CBD case series lacked any systematic assessment of aphasia, the aphasia profile(s) in CBD remains poorly characterized. For more detail concerning the language profile, one needs to turn to the few single-case studies in which aphasia is the focus of clinical-pathological correlations.

Aphasia as Documented by Small Series or Single-Case Studies of Pathologically Confirmed CBD

A historical case of probable CBD was recently brought to light from a report in 1925 in the *Revue Neurologique* (49). Lhermitte described a 67-year-old carpenter who developed clumsiness of the right hand that progressed to dystonic posturing with alien limb features and altered cortical sensation. Apraxia was the main symptom in this patient, but he was noted to have dysarthria and mild aphasic errors in complex comprehension as well as word-finding difficulties without alexia and agraphia. No pathology was available, but it is of note that in this first presumed case of the CBD syndrome an aphasic disturbance was recorded in conjunction with apraxia and the extrapyramidal syndrome. In the original cases described by Rebeiz et al., case one was noted to have hesitant speech early in the course and 4 years later had stammering, monosyllabic speech and decreased fluency, suggesting an aphasic disturbance, although this term was not actually used (42). Other reports followed: For example, a 61-year-old man presented with dysarthria, anomia, and problems in episodic memory and developed right arm rigidity and apraxia over 6 years. CBD was confirmed at pathological examination (50). Two cases of dementia associated with swollen achromatic neurons in the cortex had speech difficulty early on in the course and became mute over a 4- and 7-year course, respectively (51). Aphasic features were also prominent in several other case descriptions (30,40,50,52–54).

In most of these cases the language disturbance began with anomia and nonfluent speech output and progressed to mutism in the context of an evolving akinetic rigid syndrome. In other cases the aphasia predominated with less evidence of the extrapyramidal syndrome. For example, a 53-year-old patient presented with anomia and gradually progressed over several years to a severe expressive and comprehension deficit. Autopsy revealed spongiform change, neuronal loss, gliosis, balloon cells, and tau positive immunoreactivity in the left middle and inferior temporal, right anterior, and inferior temporal and left temporal-parietal regions (55,56). Likewise, Kertesz et al. (1994) described a series of 12 PPA patients, three of whom at autopsy showed balloon cells, tau positive reactivity in neurons, and the absence of Pick bodies in the hippocampus (24). Two out of three had Pick bodies in the frontal cortex, leading this group, as discussed, to propose the concept of Pick complex disease (14,25).

In summary, these case reports described an aphasic disturbance of more or less prominence in the clinical course of patients who fit the clinical picture or had autopsy findings consistent with CBD. In many cases, however, with the exception of Kirshner et al. (56) and Kertesz et al. (24) the aphasic disturbance was not described in any detail. The first detailed description of PPA associated with pathological changes consistent with CBD was reported in 1991 by Lippa and colleagues, who described a 66-year-old physician presenting with a 1-year history of language difficulty and hesitant speech (57). Over the next year he developed increased tone and posturing of the right arm. His speech became telegraphic and by the third year he could only utter "yes" and "no" and write his name. He could no longer read, although comprehension was still relatively spared. He died suddenly of a choking episode at age 68. Serial neuropsychological testing showed a progressive impairment in his verbal IQ on the Wechsler Adult Intelligence Scale (WAIS) with a verbal IQ score of 113 initially; 104 4 months later, and 96 10 months later. Word list generation using phonemic and semantic cuing was 28 and 12 respectively when seen early in the illness, and 13 and 6 4 months later. Since at final testing his repetition and comprehension were still relatively intact and speech production was severely reduced, he was classified as transcortical motor aphasia. At pathology, he showed involvement of the superior, middle, and inferior frontal region with typical neuronal achromasia. What was particularly interesting was that this patient did not develop an extrapyramidal syndrome and had no involvement of the substantia nigra. The authors pointed out the obvious clinical and pathological similarities with Pick's disease (57,58). In 1996 Ikeda et al. reported a 58-year-old woman with progressive sensory aphasia running a 10-year course (59). Interestingly, in addition to problems with both oral and written language comprehension, the patient had a more generalized hearing loss implying bilateral involvement of the primary auditory cortex. Initially, speech output consisted of fluent semantic jargon with meaningless phrases. Over time this deteriorated to stereotyped phrases with poor comprehension and eventually global aphasia supervened. About 6 years into the illness she developed agitation and problems with self-care, then a shuffling gait with axial and limb rigidity, and she eventually died of pneumonia. The case was initially published as an example of atypical Pick's disease, but the authors reconsidered the diagnosis based on advances in immunohistochemistry (59). Specifically, the patient had bilateral involvement of the posterior two-thirds of the superior temporal lobe and the pars opercularis. Less severely involved were the insular cortex, pre- and postcentral gyri, superior and inferior parietal regions, as well as the rest of the temporal lobe and posterior frontal region (59). Subcortical involvement included the substantia nigra, thalamus, globus *pallidus,* corpus striatum, amygdala, and the locus ceruleus. Microscopically, the cortical regions involved revealed spongiosis and gliosis throughout all layers. Achromatic neurons were detected in the absence of amyloid plaques, Pick bodies or Lewy bodies, and there were few neurofibrillary tangles. Anti-tau staining was positive in both neurons and glia. Neuropil threads were scattered throughout gray and white matter in both affected and unaffected regions. Oligodendroglial coils and astrocytic plaques were also abundant. This was one of the best documented cases of a progressive fluent aphasia owing to CBD with presumed initial bilateral involvement of the superior temporal region, explaining the fluent speech disorder (59). Thus, a variant of CBD involving superior temporal cortex and sometimes initially presenting as fluent aphasia should be considered in the differential diagnosis of progressive fluent aphasia. A few other Japanese cases with superior temporal involvement from CBD have also been described (60). (Also see summary Table in Ikeda et al., 1996) (59). One of these patients presented with progressive nonfluent aphasia, dysarthria, buccal-facial apraxia, and hearing loss, and was found at autopsy to have typical histopathological and immunohistochemical changes of CBD in Broca's, Wernicke's, and supplementary motor areas (60).

Finally, another detailed case study was published by Sakurai et al., (1996) who described a 64-year-old patient who developed hesitant speech and anomia, but was able to work for another 18 months (61). On examination, speech was decreased but fluent with paragrammatism. Performance IQ on the WAIS was 74. Four years into the illness the patient could write but could no longer speak and had developed bilateral hearing loss. Performance IQ dropped to 62. On the WAB, the speech pattern was now nonfluent with decreased output and frequent phonemic paraphasias, which produced jargon speech. His subscores were 0 on both the information and fluency subtests of the WAB. Naming (0.5/10) and repetition (0/10) were severely impaired with auditory comprehension (6/10) and reading (7/10) less affected. He also had buccal-facial apraxia, mild constructional apraxia, problems with calculation and attention, but episodic memory was relatively intact. Prior to complete mutism the patient spoke in phonemic jargon and had logoclonia. Seven years into a 9-year course, mild Parkinsonism developed with behavioral change, including disinhibition and wandering. The patient became bedridden and died of pneumonia. Serial CT scanning showed progressive atrophy, left more than right, which eventually became symmetrical. A PET scan 7 years into the course showed bilateral frontal temporal decrease with involvement also of the right parietal region (61). At pathology there was bilateral involvement of the superior frontal, lower inferior precentral lobule, as well as the frontal operculum, superior temporal, and angular gyri. Neuronal loss and spongiosis were seen in the upper layers of these regions along with fibrillary gliosis and tau positive argyrophilic inclusions in the neurons. Although at autopsy the patient showed bilateral cerebral involvement, the clinical picture was dominated by progressive aphasia, which initially had fluent features and eventually deteriorated into global aphasia (61).

CONCLUSION

In summary, CBD is now a recognized substrate of the syndrome of PPA, but the prevalence and characteristics of the aphasic disturbance in CBD vary depending on the referral base, the availability of pathological correlation and the topographical distribution of pathology in the individual case. What seems clear is that diagnosis relying only on the typical extrapyramidal phenotype will underascertain cognitive presentations, including progressive aphasia. The presence of the clinical syndrome of asymmetric rigidity with prominent ideomotor apraxia is highly predictive of the pathological entity designated as CBD, but it is likely that there are many cases unrecognized in life because of the lack of these typical features, including cases presenting with progressive aphasia or with behavior-personality change. Even with autopsy confirmation controversy continues as to the distinctiveness of the CBD syndrome with some authors suggesting it is part of the Pick complex (25) and others indicating that it is a separate entity that will be increasingly identifiable with immunohistochemical staining (31). In clinical series the prevalence of aphasia ranges from 10% to 20%, but when aphasia is more systematically assessed the prevalence is closer to 50%, which is in keeping with autopsy series. The prevalence of aphasia reflects the topographical distribution of CBD pathology, which frequently affects language-specialized cortex in the left hemisphere including the inferior frontal, supplementary motor, parietal, and sometimes superior temporal regions. Nevertheless, CBD is a heterogeneous disorder, as are other neurodegenerative conditions, and the characteristics of the aphasic disturbance reflect its variable topography. Although most of the cases reported have a nonfluent aphasia presumably reflecting inferior frontal or supplementary motor area involvement, there has been at least one well-documented case of predominant involvement of the superior temporal region with progressive fluent aphasia. Few studies, however, have conducted thorough aphasia assessments and there are no neurolinguistic studies so far reported. The series to date do indicate, however, that assessment of language function should be part of the routine examination of patients suspected in the clinic to have CBD. Likewise, PPA cases should be carefully followed neurologically for the development of an extrapyramidal syndrome. It is also clear given the paucity of information currently available, that further characterization of the aphasic disturbance in CBD would be a fruitful topic for further research.

ACKNOWLEDGMENTS

I would like to acknowledge personal financial support from the Research Program in Aging and Department of Medicine at Sunnybrook & Women's College Health Sciences Centre, as well as research support from the Medical Research Council of Canada, and to thank Tatiana Christensen and Kira Barbour for their help in preparing this manuscript.

REFERENCES

1. Damasio AR. Aphasia. *New Engl J Med* 1992;326: 531–539.
2. Kertesz A, Black SE. Cerebrovascular disease and aphasia. In: Darby J, ed. *Speech evaluation in neurology.* New York: Grune & Stratton, 1984.
3. Freedman M, Alexander MP, Naeser MA. Anatomic basis of transcortical motor aphasia. *Neurology* 1998;34: 409–417.
4. Naeser MA, Alexander MP, Helm-Estabrooks N, Levine HL, Laughlin SA, Geschwind N. Aphasia with predominantly subcortical lesion sites. *Arch Neurol* 1982;39:2–14.
5. Damasio AR, Damasio H, Rizzo M, Nils V, Gersh F. Aphasia with nonhemorrhagic lesions in the basal ganglia and internal capsule. *Arch Neurol* 1982;39:15–20.
6. Caplan D. *Neurolinguistics and linguistic aphasiology: an introduction.* Cambridge, MA: Cambridge University Press, 1987.
7. Goodglass H, Kaplan E. *The assessment of aphasia and related disorders.* Philadelphia. Lea & Febiger, 1972.
8. Kertesz A. *Western Aphasia Battery.* New York: Grune & Stratton, 1982.
9. Darley FL, Aronson AE, Brown JR. *Motor Speech Disorders.* Philadelphia: WB Saunders, 1975.
10. Square-Storer P. *Acquired apraxia of speech in aphasic adults.* Philadelphia: Taylor & Francis, 1989.
11. Mesulam MM. Slowly progressive aphasia without generalized dementia. *Ann Neurol* 1982;11:592–598.
12. Black SE. Focal cortical atrophy syndromes. *Brain Cogn* 1996;31:188–229.
13. Westbury C, Bub D. Primary progressive aphasia: A review of 112 cases. *Brain Lang* 1997;60:381–406.
14. Kertesz A, Munoz D. Clinical and pathological characteristics of primary progressive aphasia and frontal dementia. *J Neural Transm* 1996;47:133–141.
15. Mesulam MM. Primary progressive aphasia—differentiation from Alzheimer's disease. *Ann Neurol* 1987;22: 533–534.
16. Mesulam MM, Weintraub S. Primary progressive aphasia: sharpening the focus on a clinical syndrome. In: Boller F, Forcette F, Khachaturian Z, Poncet M, Christen Y, eds. *Heterogeneity of Alzheimer's disease.* Berlin: Springer-Velag, 1992:43–66.
17. Mesulam MM, Weintraub S. Spectrum of primary progressive aphasia. *Baillieres Clin Neurol* 1992;1(3): 583–609.
18. Brun A, Englund B, Gustafson L, et al. Lund-Manchester group consensus on clinical and neuropathological criteria for frontal-temporal dementia. *J Neurol Neurosurg Psychiatry* 1994;57:416–448.
19. Neary D, Snowden JS, Gustafson L, et al. Frontotemporal lobar degeneration: a consensus on clinical diagnostic criteria. *Neurology* 1998;51:1546–1554.
20. Snowden JS, Neary D, Mann DMA, Goulding PJ, Testa HJ. Progressive language disorder due to lobar atrophy. *Ann Neurol* 1992;31:174–183.
21. Hodges JR, Patterson P, Oxbury S, Funnell E. Semantic dementia: progressive fluent aphasia with temporal lobe atrophy. *Brain* 1992;115:1783–1806.
22. Kertesz A, Appell J, Fisman M. The dissolution of language in Alzheimer's disease. *Can J Neurol Sci* 1986;13: 415–418.
23. Lippa CF, Smith TW, Saunders AM, Hulette C, Pulaski-Salo D, Roses AD. Apolipoprotein E-epsilon 2 and Alzheimer's disease: genotype influences pathologic phenotype. *Neurology* 1997;48:515–519.
24. Kertesz A, Hudson L, Mackenzie IRA, Munoz DG. The pathology and nosology of primary progressive aphasia. *Neurology* 1994;44:2065–2072.
25. Kertesz A, Munoz DG. *Pick's disease and Pick complex.* New York: Wiley, 1998.
26. Riley DE, Lang AE, Lewis A, et al. Cortical basal ganglionic degeneration. *Neurology* 1990;40:1203–1212.
27. Litvan I, Agid Y, Goetz C, et al. Accuracy of the clinical diagnosis of corticobasal degeneration: a clinicopathologic study. *Neurology* 1997;48:119–125.

28. Feany MB, Dickson DW. Widespread cytoskeletal pathology characterizes corticobasal degeneration. *Am J Pathol* 1995;146:1388–1396.
29. Jendroska K, Rossor MN, Mathias CJ, Daniel SE. Morphological overlap between corticobasal degeneration and Pick's disease: a clinicopathological report. *Mov Disord* 1995;10:111–114.
30. Bergeron C, Pollanen MS, Weyer L, Black SE, Lang AE. Unusual clinical presentations of cortical-basal ganglionic degeneration. *Ann Neurol* 1996;40:893–900.
31. Feany MB, Dickson DW. Neurodegenerative disorders with extensive tau pathology: a comparative study and review. *Ann Neurol* 1996;40:139–148.
32. Tsuchiya K, Ikeda K, Uchihara T, Oda T, Shimada H. Distribution of cerebral cortical lesions in corticobasal degeneration: a clinicopathological study of five autopsy cases in Japan. *Acta Neuropathol* 1997;94:416–424.
33. Blin J, Vidailnet MJ, Phillon B, Dubois B, Feve JR, Agid Y. Corticobasal degeneration: decreased and asymmetrical glucose consumption as studied with PET. *Mov Disord* 1992;7:348–354.
34. Eidelberg D, Dhawan V, Moeller JR, et al. The metabolic landscape of Corticobasal ganglionic degeneration: regional asymmetries studied with positron emision tomography. *J Neurol Neurosurg Psychiatry* 1991;54: 856–862.
35. Frisoni GB, Pizzolato G, Zanetti O, Bianchetti A, Chierichetti F, Trabucchi M. Corticobasal degeneration: neuropsychological assessment and Dopamine D2 receptor SPECT analysis. *Eur Neurol* 1995;35:50–54.
36. Markus HS, Lees AJ, Lennox G, Marsden CD, Costa DC. Patterns of regional cerebral blood flow in corticobasal degeneration studies using HMPAO SPECT; comparison with Parkinson's disease and normal controls. *Mov Disord* 1995;10:179–187.
37. Okuda B, Tachibana H, Takeda M, Kawabata K, Sugita M, Fukuchi M. Focal cortical hypoperfusion in corticobasal degeneration demonstrated by three-dimensional surface display with 123I-IMP: a possible cause of apraxia. *Neuroradiology* 1995;37:642–644.
38. Sawle GV, Brooks DJ, Marsden CD, Frackowiak RSJ. Corticobasal degeneration. A unique pattern of regional cortical oxygen hypometabolism and striatal fluoropoda uptake demonstrated by positron emmision tomography. *Brain* 1991;114:541–556.
39. Cohen S, Freedman M. Cognitive and behavioral changes in the Parkinson-plus syndromes. In: Weiner WJ, Lang AE, eds. *Advances in neurology.* Vol. 65. New York: Raven, 1995;139–156.
40. Beatty WW, Scott JG, Wilson DA, Prince JR, Williamson DJ. Memory deficits in a demented patient with probable corticobasal degeneration. *J Geriatr Psychiatry Neurol* 1995;8:132–136.
41. Pillon B, Blin J, Vidailhet M, et al. The neuropsychological pattern of corticobasal degeneration: comparisons with progressive supranuclear palsy and Alzheimer's disease. *Neurology* 1995;45:1477–1483 (abstract).
42. Rebeiz JJ, Kolodny EH, Richardson EP. Corticodentatonigral degeneration with neuronal achromasia. *Arch Neurol* 1968;18:20–33.
43. Rinne JO, Lee MS, Thompson PD, Marsden CD. Corticobasal degeneration. A clinical study of 36 cases. *Brain* 1994;117:1183–1196.
44. Kompoliti K, Goetz CG, Boeve BF, et al. Clinical presentation and pharmacological therapy in corticobasal degeneration. *Arch Neurol* 1998;55:957–961.
45. Martinez-Lage P, Kertesz A. Behavioral and language involvement in corticobasal degeneration (CBD). *J Neuropsychiat* 1997;9:649–650, (abstract).
46. Frattali CM, Grafman J, Patronas N, Maclhouf F, Litvan I. Characterizing language and cognitive disturbances in corticobasal degeneration, submitted.
47. Schneider JA, Watts RL, Gearing M, Brewer RP, Mirra SS. Corticobasal degeneration: neuropathologic and clinical heterogeneity. *Neurology* 1997;48:959–969.
48. Wenning G, Litvan I, Jankovic J, et al. Natural history and survival of 14 patients with corticobasal degeneration confirmed at postmortem examination. *J Neurol Neurosurg Psychiatry* 1998;64:184–189.
49. Ballan G, Tison F. A historical case of probable corticobasal degeneration? *Mov Disord* 1997;12:1073–1074.
50. Scully RE, Mark EJ, McNeely BU. Case records of the Massachusetts General Hospital. Weekly clinicopathological exercises. Case 38-1985. *New Engl J Med* 1985; 313:739–748.
51. Clark AW, Manz HJ, White CL, Lehmann J, Miller D, Coyle JT. Cortical degeneration with swollen chromatolytic neurons: its relationship to Pick's disease. *J Neuropathol Exp Neurol* 1986;45;268–284.
52. Gibb WRG, Luthert PJ, Marsden CD. Corticobasal degeneration. *Brain* 1989;112:1171–1192.
53. Goulding PJ, Northern B, Snowden JS, MacDermott N, Neary D. Progressive aphasia with right-sided extrapyramidal signs: Another manifestation of localized cerebral atrophy. *J Neurol Neurosurg Psychiatry* 1989;52:128–130.
54. Lang AE. Cortical basal ganglionic degeneration presenting with "progressive loss of speech output and orofacial dyspraxia." *J Neurol Neurosurg Psychiatry* 1992;55:1101
55. Kirshner HS, Webb WG, Kelly MP, Wells CE. Language disturbance. An initial symptom of cortical degenerations and dementia. *Arch Neurol* 1984;41:491–496.
56. Kirshner HS, Tanridag O, Thurman L, Whetsell WO Jr. Progressive aphasia without dementia: two cases with focal spongiform degeneration. *Ann Neurol* 1987;22: 527–532.
57. Lippa CF, Cohen R, Smith TW, Drachman DA. Primary progressive aphasia with focal neuronal achromasia. *Neurology* 1991;41:882–886.
58. Lippa CF, Smith TW, Fontneau N. Corticonigral degeneration with neuronal achromasia. A clinicopathologic study of two cases. *J Neurol Sci* 1990;98:301–310.
59. Ikeda K, Akiyama H, Iritani S, et al. Corticobasal degeneration with primary progressive aphasia and accentuated cortical lesion in superior temporal gyrus: case report and review. *Acta Neuropathol* 1996;92:534–539.
60. Arima K, Uesugi H, Fujita I, et al. Corticonigral degeneration with neuronal achromasia presenting with primary progressive aphasia: ultrastructural and immunocytochemical studies. *J Neurol Sci* 1994;127:186–197.
61. Sakurai Y, Hashida H, Uesugi H, et al. A clinical profile of corticobasal degeneration presenting as primary progressive aphasia. *Eur Neurol* 1996;36:134–137.

Corticobasal Degeneration.
Advances in Neurology, Vol. 82,
edited by I. Litvan, C. G. Goetz, and A. E. Lang.
Lippincott Williams & Wilkins, Philadelphia © 2000.

12

Alien Limb Sign

Philip A. Hanna* and Rachelle S. Doody†

**New Jersey Neuroscience Institute, JFK Medical Center, Edison, New Jersey 08818; and †Department of Neurology, Baylor College of Medicine, Houston, Texas 77030*

DEFINITION AND HISTORICAL BACKGROUND

Definition of Alien Limb

Alien limb is defined as a "feeling that one limb is foreign or 'has a will of its own,' *together with* observable involuntary motor activity" (1). Thus, both subjective sensory impressions and motor manifestations need to be present at some time in the illness. The syndrome is not limited to involvement of the hand, although the upper extremity is the most frequently affected limb. Any limb or combination of limbs may fulfill the alien limb definition (1). The alien limb sign includes the failure to perceive ownership of one's limb in the absence of visual cues, an impression that the limb is foreign, personification of the affected limb, and autonomous motor activity deemed by the patient as beyond voluntary control.

Historical Background

Brion and Jedynak have been credited with the first description of the term alien hand sign, "le signe de la main etrangere" (translated as "strange hand sign" in the English abstract of their article) in their report of three patients with tumors of the corpus callosum (2). They used this term in reference to a sense of strangeness or unawareness of one side of the body as evidenced by the patients' inability to recognize ownership of the affected (alien) limb when that limb was held by the normal limb in the absence of visual input, such as with the arms placed behind the patient's back (the behind-the-back test). Their patients had difficulty transferring sensory information and functions between the hemispheres, including the inability to name objects felt by the left hand (tactile anomia). Some patients demonstrated left (unilateral) agraphia, difficulty imitating hand postures of one hand by the other (cross-replication of hand postures), verbal apraxia of the affected limb (left-sided) in response to verbal commands, and right-hand constructional apraxia. One patient indicated that certain activities, particularly writing, were performed autonomously. Wilson et al. modified the translation of the term from the Brion and Jedynak article to the "stranger's hand sign" (3). These authors defined the term as a feeling of the patient that the affected hand no longer belonged to him or her.

Bogen, in an extensive discussion of callosal syndromes, modified the word "strange" to "alien" and considered the sign as "related to intermanual conflict." Intermanual conflict, in which the hands act at cross purposes to each other, is according to Bogen, "the dissociative phenomenon most clearly identifiable with hemispheric disconnection" (4). One example cited by Bogen was a complete commissurotomy patient (handedness was not specified) in which "one hand was buttoning up his shirt and the other hand was coming along right behind it undoing the buttons!" In another example (patient 7 of one series) the patient's hands would struggle with each other while each attempted to answer the telephone (1).

Tanaka et al. expanded on the term "diagonstic dyspraxia" in describing a 51-year-old right-handed man who displayed abnormal motor behavior in the left hand "triggered by voluntary activities of the right hand" along with complaints that "my left hand will not do what I want it to do." They defined diagonistic dyspraxia as "abnormal motor behavior of one hand *triggered* by voluntary activities of the other hand" (5).

Feinberg et al. proposed two distinct alien hand syndromes (AHS): a frontal AHS that is "associated with reflexive grasping, groping, and compulsive manipulation of tools" and a callosal variant (callosal AHS) with intermanual conflict as the primary characteristic. Frontal AHS typically affects the dominant hand and is, according to this schema, owing to damage to the dominant SMA, anterior cingulate gyrus, medial prefrontal cortex, and the anterior corpus callosum, whereas the callosal AHS is hypothesized to require only an anterior callosal lesion (6).

Sign vs. Syndrome

Throughout the history of the description of the alien limb phenomenon, authors have used both the terms "sign" and "syndrome" in reference to the alien limb phenomenon. Kety illustrated that in human illness, when symptoms are recognized to occur in fairly consistent clusters, they may be described as syndromes (7). In a number of articles regarding alien limb, a given neuroanatomical lesion (e.g., frontal vs. callosal) or etiology (corticobasal degeneration (CBD) or stroke) has been associated with signs and symptoms including alien limb. Yet, there has not been a clearly defined syndrome that includes "all cases with a given neuroanatomical lesion or fully characterizes clinical phenomena so well that the underlying etiology (stroke vs. CBD vs. tumor, etc.) can be predicted" (8). Alien limb is, therefore, better referred to as a sign reflecting a brain response to diverse insults. It may occur within selected syndromes, such as CBD, as discussed in the following.

CORE AND ASSOCIATED SIGNS AND SYMPTOMS

Autonomous motor activities, core features of alien limb, display a range from seemingly non–goal-directed behavior, such as groping and grasping (1,6,9–15), (often with an associated grasp reflex [1,6,9–14,16] or perseveration [1,9,10,13,15]), to goal-directed activities, such as the compulsive manipulation of tools (utilization behavior) (9), or self-destructive actions (1). Nearly all patients display difficulty with bimanual coordination that may include intermanual conflict (6,9–13,17,18), and mirror movements (where one limb involuntarily imitates the activity of the other) (1,17,19). Alien limb grasping movements are vividly depicted in the patient of Banks et al. in which "the left hand would tenaciously grope for and grasp any nearby object, pick and pull at her clothes and even grasp her throat during sleep" (12). Patients may also display "self-restriction" (9,13), in which the unaffected limb attempts to control the behavior of the alien limb. Patients may clasp their hands or hold the alien limb with the unaffected hand, often unknowingly. Personification of the limb may be present in a subset of patients, such as in case 6 of one series who believed that her left arm was a baby named Joseph whose actions (pinching her nipples) were "mischievous behaviors" (1). A related phenomenon termed autocriticism ("l'autocritique interhemispherique" by Brion and Jedynak [20]), reflects the observation that patients may express bewilderment at the ability of the alien limb to behave independently. The patient may blame the affected limb for the behavior instead of acknowledging responsibility. See Gasquoine (21) for a comprehensive review of 20 published cases of alien hand sign.

In addition to these core features, alien limb sometimes occurs with associated motor or sensory signs and symptoms. Motor signs such as hemiparesis, cortical reflex myoclonus, apraxia, motor forms of aphasia, athetosis, pseudoathetosis, action dystonia, hemiballismus, and hemiataxia therefore arise in the differential diagnosis of alien limb (1). Apraxia is defined as a "disorder of skilled movement not caused by weakness, akinesia, deafferentation, abnormal tone or posture, movement disorders (such as tremors or chorea), intellectual deterioration, poor comprehension, or uncooperativeness," and is "defined by exclusion" (22). Hesitancy or difficulty with speech initiation, a component of transcortical aphasia (which may be seen in association with a lesions of the supplementary motor area [23]) has been reported in a number of cases (9–11,13–17). Three patients with CBD had slow, paraphasic speech and another patient with CBD had dysnomia in one series, but none had true transcortical motor aphasia (1).

Patients with the alien limb phenomenon may also have associated sensory findings, which include sensory neglect, opticosensory ataxia (24,25), impaired somaesthetic transfer, astereognosis, and agraphesthesia. Levine and Rinn described a patient with a right posterior cerebral artery distribution infarct (involving right temporo-occipital and right thalamic VPL nucleus) who, in addition to left homonymous hemianopia and left hemianesthesia, suffered from left-sided ataxia (likely sensory) and crossed optic ataxia. This 79-year-old right-handed female attributed "hostile motivations" to the left arm, such as attempts to choke her. The authors reported that the patient "soon came to treat it as a misbehaving child, fondling it and talking to it. . . ." (personification) (24). Ay et al. described an 81-year-old right-handed woman with left alien hand and "triple ataxia" (sensory, optic, and cerebellar ataxia) of the left arm without hemiparesis or motor neglect. Imaging demonstrated a "subacute infarction in the right thalamus, hippocampus, inferior temporal lobes, splenium of the corpus callosum, and occipital lobe due to right posterior artery occlusion" (25). In one series, complex sensory functions such as graphesthesia, stereognosis, and somaesthetic transfer (cross-localization of fingertip stimulation) were frequently noted (1). Bogen described the impairment of interhemispheric transfer of sensory modalities such as touch, pressure, and proprioception in patients following brain bisection (4).

THE ALIEN LIMB IN CBD

There are some particular difficulties encountered in evaluating for alien limb in patients with CBD. These patients frequently have concomitant dystonia of the same limb. If the dystonia is severe or has resulted in contractures, autonomous movements may not be manifest secondary to limitation of movement of the affected limbs. Similar limitation may be seen if the limb has severe rigidity. The history is therefore critical in establishing the previous presence of this definitional behavior. Furthermore, apraxia of the limb may be misinterpreted as groping or grasping. Many patients with parkinsonian syndromes (and hyperkinetic movement disorders) complain of difficulty controlling a limb, stating that a limb "won't obey" them, but failure of function secondary to rigidity, bradykinesia, or a hyperkinetic disorder needs to be distinguished from truly autonomous movements. Posturing and levitation have been associated with alien limb in CBD in a number of cases, seemingly more commonly than in other etiologies (1,26).

HISTORY AND EXAMINATION

A suggested comprehensive history and physical examination has been previously suggested (1) (Table 1). Here, we will emphasize certain key aspects. The examiner should seek information regarding the temporal onset of alien limb phenomenon and other aspects of the illness, the location, sequence, and timing of various limb involvements, relationship to hand dominance, and whether the alien limb is ipsilateral or contralateral to associated signs and pathology. The examiner should also seek to determine the presence and timing of the following features: evidence of grasp; denial of ownership of the affected limb or autocriticism or personification of the limb; autonomous motor activity and whether such activity is non–goal-directed (grasping or groping) or goal-directed (utilization behavior or self-destructive behavior); impairment of bimanual coordination, intermanual conflict, diagonistic dyspraxia, or mirror movements; and a history of self-restriction by the unaffected hand such as persistent clasping of the hands. The examination should include testing for a grasp reflex; cortical reflex myoclonus; alternating motor sets (such as fist-palm-side alternation); graphesthesia and stereognosis; tactile naming with each hand; somaesthetic transfer; recognition of ownership of the limb when held behind the patient's back; sequential movements (touching each finger to the thumb in order); bimanual coordination (e.g., buttoning); verbal praxis (ability to carry out verbal commands with each limb); observing for mirror movements or intermanual

TABLE 1. *Suggested evaluation for alien limb*

Historical information
- Assess for subjective impression that the limb is foreign, alien, and/or "has a mind of its own."
- Note temporal onset, location, sequence, and timing of various limb involvements, relationship to hand dominance, and whether the alien limb is ipsilateral or contralateral to associated signs and pathology.
- Note denial of ownership, autocriticism, or personification of the limb.
- Are autonomous motor activities present and are these non–goal-directed (grasping or groping) or goal-directed (utilization behavior or self-destructive behavior)?
- Is there impairment of bimanual coordination, intermanual conflict, diagonistic dyspraxia, or mirror movements?
- Self-restriction of the affected limb by the unaffected hand such as persistent clasping of the hands.

Physical examination—evaluate
- Grasp reflex
- Cortical reflex myoclonus
- Alternating motor sets (such as fist-palm-side alternation)
- Sequential movements (touching each finger to the thumb in order)
- Bimanual coordination (e.g., buttoning)
- Graphesthesia and stereognosis
- Tactile naming with each hand
- Somaesthetic transfer
- Recognition of ownership of the limb when held behind the patient's back
- Verbal praxis (ability to carry out verbal commands with each limb)
- Mirror movements or intermanual conflict
- Aphasia, especially transcortical motor aphasia

conflict; and language testing to assess for aphasia, especially transcortical motor aphasia.

ETIOLOGIC AND ANATOMICAL ISSUES

Vascular Etiologies

Several etiologies have been associated with the alien limb sign (Table 2). The most commonly reported pathophysiology involves ischemic vascular lesions, especially infarctions affecting the anterior cerebral artery (ACA) territory (3,6,9,10, 14,16,18,27–31). Alien limb has also been reported in the context of hemorrhagic lesions, often as a result of aneurysmal rupture and typically in the ACA or anterior communicating artery (ACom) distribution (5,11,12,17,32,33).

There have been cases of alien limb sign in patients with ischemia or hemorrhage not involving damage to the corpus callosum or medial frontal cortices (Table 3). Ventura et al. reported a 58-year-old woman with a left alien hand in the context of a right capsulothalamic hemorrhage with mesencephalic extension without involvement of the corpus callosum (34). Dolado described an 80-year-old right-handed man who developed a left alien hand in the context of bilat-

TABLE 2. *Etiologic and anatomic correlates with alien limb*

- Ischemic strokes
  - Anterior cerebral artery distribution (6,9,10,13,14,16,18,27,28–31)
  - Posterior cerebral artery distribution (1,24,25,35)
- Hemorrhagic strokes
  - Anterior cerebral artery and anterior communicating artery rupture (5,11,12,17,32,33)
  - Capsulothalamic (34)
- Surgical lesions
  - Corpus callosectomy and/or supplementary motor area (4,36,37)
  - Thalamotomy (38)
- Corticobasal degeneration (1,26,39–42)
- Tumors of the corpus callosum (2)
- Creutzfeldt-Jakob disease (43)
- Alzheimer's disease (44)
- Seizure vs. TIA (45,46)

eral dorsoparieto-occipital ischemic lesions (an acute right hemispheric infarct along with an old left-sided lesion) (35). Case 6 of one series had radiographical evidence of infarction of the right posterior temporo-occipital, parietal lobe, posterior limb of the internal capsule, right basal ganglia, as well as left caudate and left cerebellar infarcts (1). The case by Levine and Rinn was also a result of a predominantly posterior (posterior cerebral artery distribution) infarct, yet they proposed that there was likely involvement of the splenium of the corpus callosum to help explain some of the findings in their patient (24). The patient reported by Ay et al. demonstrated left alien hand and "triple ataxia" in the context of a subacute infarction in the right posterior cerebral artery distribution (25).

Surgical Etiologies

In addition to vascular lesions, alien limb sign with or without associated features has been described in conjunction with surgical lesions, particularly callosectomy (4,36). A primate study by Brinkman evaluated the behavioral effects of unilateral supplementary motor area (SMA) lesions in five monkeys. All monkeys had an initial few weeks of bilateral forelimb clumsiness and two who were studied for 1 year postoperatively demonstrated a "deficit of bimanual coordination where the two hands tended to behave in a similar manner instead of sharing the task between them." The author proposed that the intact SMA influences the motor outflow of both the ipsilateral hemisphere and the contralateral one through the corpus callosum. Indeed, callosal sectioning eliminated this deficit of bimanual coordination (37). Walker and Hunt described two patients with autonomous movements of dystonic limbs, one of whom had undergone bilateral thalamotomies, and since surgery, "her right hand has become mischievous—pinching her unexpectedly, pulling down the neck of her blouse, or grabbing strangers" (38).

Corticobasal Degeneration

Alien limb syndrome is a well established part of the CBD syndrome (1,26,39,40–42). Kumar et al. report that nearly 50% of patients with CBD develop the alien limb phenomenon (39). Based on their review, alien limb is "rare" as an initial presentation, but is "common" (approximately 30% to 40%) in the early course (<3 years), and approximately 50% in the late course (>3 years). In a review of 36 cases by Rinne et al., 14 patients described a classical "alien limb." They reported that the alien limb typically developed after 1 year (median) from the onset of symptoms (40). Kompoliti et al. in a review of 147 cases of CBD reported 42% of patients had alien limb, although clinical details were not provided (41). A few patients with pathologically proven CBD and alien limb have been reported (26,42). One patient reported in Gibb et al. postmortem examination depicted cell loss in the locus ceruleus, substantia nigra, and nucleus ambiguous with corticobasal inclusion bodies, and with minimal cortical involvement (42). In two other patients reported by Riley et al., one patient had typical changes of CBD primarily affecting the left medial cortex, ipsilateral to the side of initial and most prominent clinical findings, whereas the changes in the second patient were primarily in the central frontoparietal cortex contralateral to the side of onset (26). There was notable involvement of the substantia nigra in both patients.

Our experience at Baylor College of Medicine (unpublished) with alien limb in CBD is summarized below. Sixty-six patients (44W, 22M) who satisfied the clinical or pathological criteria for the diagnosis of CBD, evaluated between 1988 and 1998 were included in the analysis. Of these 66 patients, 33 (50%) had either definite (23/33) or probable (10/33) (subjective or motor symptoms but not both) alien limb (according to Doody and Jankovic criteria (1). Of the 33 patients with alien limb, 26 were female. Mean age at presentation to our clinic for patients with alien limb was 68.4 ± 7.5 (range: 50 to 79), similar to the mean age of 68.4 ± 7.1 (range: 52–79) for those without alien limb. All patients were right-handed except one (ambidextrous). The alien limb was limited to one arm in 26 patients (12 L, 14 R), unilateral (arm greater than leg) in three patients, bilateral (asymmetrical) in two patients, and it involved one leg in two patients. The alien limb features either stabilized or diminished with time as increasing immobility limited the autonomous motor mani-

TABLE 3. *Selected previously published reports of alien limb syndrome by etiology*

References	Number of pts	Age	Sex	Site of lesion	Alien hand	Principal motor symptom	Other features
Ischemic strokes							
Goldberg et al. (9)	2	63	F	L medial frontal cortex	Right	Grasping/IMC	Self-restriction
		76	F	L medial frontal cortex	Right	Utilization behavior	Self-restriction
Levine and Rinn (24)	1	79	F	R temporo-occipital cortex, thalamus, CC	Left	Grasping/choking	Personification
Watson et al. (16)	1	65	M	L medial frontal cortex	Right	Not described	Grasp reflex
McNabb et al. (10)	3	75	F	L medial frontal/parietal cortex, CC	Right	Grasping/IMC	Self-restriction
		58	F	L ACA distribution	Right	IMC	Perseveration
		68	F	L ACA distribution	Right	IMC	Self-restriction
Kuhn et al. (14)	1	75	M	B medial frontal cortices, CC (head injury)	Right	Grasping	Self-restriction
Goldberg and Bloom (13)	4	53	F	R medial frontal cortex, CC	Left	Grasping/IMC	Self-restriction
		76	F	L medial frontal cortex,	Right	Grasping	Self-restriction
		61	M	R medial frontal cortex	Left	Grasping	Self-restriction
		75	F	L medial frontal cortex	Right	Grasping	Self-restriction
Mark et al. (27)	1	52	M	R medial frontal cortex	Bilateral	IMC	Left-handed
Hanakita and Nishi (18)	1	43	M	L medial frontal cortex, CC	Left	IMC	—
Feinberg et al. (6)	1	68	M	L medial frontal cortex, CC	Right	Grasping/IMC	Grasp reflex
Doody and Jankovic (1)	2 (of 7)	85	F	R temporo-parieto-occipital cortex, post. limb of internal capsule, R basal ganglia, L caudate, and cerebellum	Left	Utilization behavior	L hemi-inattention
		63	M	B subcortical white matter (adjacent to CC), R putamen, R parietal, and L parieto-temporal New R frontal, parietal, and L parieto-temporal	Bilateral	IMC	R grasp (ambidextrous)
Trojano et al. (29)	1	65	F	R ACA distribution	Left	IMC, utilization behavior	Groping
Giroud et al. (28)	2 (of 8)	62	F	CC	NS	Grasp reflex, perseveration	
		69	M	CC	NS	Grasp reflex, perseveration	
Dolado et al. (35)	1	80	M	B dorsal parieto-occipital	Left	?	
Kischka et al. (30)	1	66	M	L ACA, including the CC	Right	Grasping, groping	
Nicholas et al. (31)	1	67	M	R ACA distribution	Left	Grasping, groping	

Ay et al. (25)	1	81	F	R PCA (thalamus, hippocampus, inf. tempora lobes, CC, occipital lobe)	Left	Grasping, self-destructive behavior	Ataxia (sensory optic, cerebellar)
Hemorrhagic strokes							
Watson and Heilman (32)	1	43	F	CC	Left	IMC	
Starkstein et al. (11)	1	35	M	Anterior Communicating artery aneurysm, CC	Left	IMC	
Banks et al. (12)	2	39	F	Bifrontal cortex, CC	Left	Grasping	
		40	M	Bimedial frontal cortex, CC	Left	IMC	
Leiguarda et al. (17)	3	57,51 35	M	CC	Left	IMC	
Tanaka et al. (5)	1	51	M	R>L medial frontal cortex, CC	Left	Diagonistic dyspraxia	
Papagno and Marsile (33)	1	40	F	R medial frontal, CC	Left	IMC	
Ventura et al. (34)	1	58	F	R capsulo-thalamic	Left	Levitation	
CBD							
Doody and Jankovic (1)	5	57–72	3F,2M	?	2L, 3R	Grasping, IMC, mirror movements	
Rinne et al. (40)	14 (of 36)	NS	NS	?	NS	Wandering, IMC, grasping	
Kompoliti et al. (41)	62 (of 147)	NS	NS		NS	NS	
Callosal tumors							
Brion and Jedynak (2)	3	27,41 56	2M 1F	CC tumor	Left	Callosal disconnection signs	Denial of ownership
Creutzfeldt-Jakob							
MacGowan et al. (43)	2	78	F	?	Left	IMC	Myoclonus
		74	F	?	Left	IMC	Myoclonus
Alzheimer's disease							
Ball et al. (44)	1	68	M		Left	Posturing (dystonia)	Myoclonus
Seizure vs. TIA (paroxysmal)							
Leiguarda et al. (45)	4	34–65	3M,1F	1-L medial frontal atrophy, 1-R medial frontal lymphoma), 1-L parietal AVM, 1-R parietal AVM	Contralateral	Grasping, personification	
Andre et al. (46)	1	62	M	Old strokes-L internal capsule, cerebellum. R occipital lobes. R CA narrowing.	Left	Groping	Probable TIA

F = Female; M = male; R = right; L = left; B = bilateral; IMC = intermanual conflict; CC = corpus callosum; ACA = anterior cerebral artery; PCA = posterior cerebral artery; ICA = internal cerebral artery; AVM = arteriovascular malformation; TIA = transient ischemic attack; NS = not specified.

festations. The alien limb was seen on the side of most prominent rigidity, dystonia, myoclonus, and apraxia. The following alien limb features were elicited most frequently: groping and grasping (21 patients), subtle wandering or searching movements (16), self-restriction (10), a perception of not knowing the limb's location in space (5), intermanual conflict (4), and levitation (2). Pathological confirmation of CBD was made in all four patients who had postmortem evaluations.

Other Etiologies

Alien limb has been associated less frequently with other conditions (Table 2). As discussed previously, Brion and Jedynak described three patients with tumors of the corpus callosum (2). MacGowan described two patients with pathologically proven Creutzfeldt-Jakob disease in whom the only initial manifestation was myoclonic alien hand. In one patient, in addition to myoclonus, the left arm "seemed to have a mind of its own," and would demonstrate spontaneous, seemingly purposeful movements that often "antagonized voluntary movements of her right arm," with prominent intermanual conflict. The patient subsequently developed progressive dementia and the alien limb worsened such that the arm would grab the patient's throat or strike her face (43). Ball et al. described a 68-year-old right-handed man with progressive left alien hand with dystonia of that limb, myoclonus, apraxia, and bilateral parietal dysfunction. The "sensory" component of alien limb was not clearly described, either because it was not present or the patient's cognitive deficits precluded obtaining this information. This patient had severe impairment of visuospatial and perceptual skills as well as global memory impairment, even on initial evaluation, which was considered to be "unusual" for CBD by the authors, and deteriorated cognitively until his death 2 years and 8 months after presentation. Although the clinical diagnosis was CBD, autopsy revealed predominantly Alzheimer histopathology (44). Several authors have described transient or paroxysmal alien hand and have raised the possibility that such a presentation may represent seizure activity or even transient ischemic attacks (45,46).

ANALYTIC ISSUES

Feinberg et al. have proposed two distinct "alien hand syndromes"; (1) the "frontal" variant (secondary to damage to the dominant SMA, anterior cingulate, medial prefrontal cortex, and anterior corpus callosum) typically with reflex grasping, groping, and utilization behavior of the dominant hand; and (2) the "callosal" variant (isolated callosal damage) with prominent intermanual conflict and no frontal features involving the nondominant hand (6). Although intriguing, this categorization may not encompass all cases. First, there is a degree of overlap in the affected areas. For example, for the proposed callosal variant, a number of the reviewed cases demonstrated signs suggestive of more extensive (including frontal) dysfunction in addition to the callosal lesion (1,17,32). In addition, the frontal versus callosal alien limb classification does not fully account for the alien limb syndrome seen in conjunction with etiologies such as CBD, Creutzfeldt-Jakob disease, or possibly Alzheimer's disease, nor is such a classification useful for cases with posterior cerebral pathologies such as that of Levine and Rinn (24), Ay et al. (25), Ventura et al. (capsulothalamic hemorrhage) (34), Dolado et al. (bilateral dorso-parietal-occipital infarctions) (35), and case 6 of one series with nonfrontal lesions of the nondominant hemisphere. Finally, the proposed classification is limited by the fact that the authors did not clearly require the "sensory," primarily subjective, feeling that the limb is foreign or alien, in their definition of alien limb, but only mentioned "uncontrollable movements not due to a movement disorder" (6).

Does the handedness of the patient affect the manifestation of alien limb? All of the reviewed cases were right-handed except for the left-handed patient of Mark et al. (27) and the ambidextrous case 7 of the series reported by Doody and Jankovic (1). Both of these patients demonstrated evidence for bilateral alien hand, with prominent intermanual conflict, in the context of acute right frontal infarct. Although intriguing, a clear pattern cannot be ascertained from such a small sampling of patients, and intermanual conflict clearly occurs in right-handed individuals as well. Yet, these cases suggest the possibility that more disturbed cerebral hemispheric dominance may result in greater interhemispheric disruption from such mesial frontal and callosal lesions.

Is the alien limb a result of single or multiple lesions? The syndrome can clearly be seen in the context of a number of etiologies and locations in the brain, although it is most commonly reported with damage to the medial frontal lobes or corpus callosum. Although the syndrome may be the result of a single process (i.e., ischemic stroke) typically more than one region of the brain is involved (i.e., not isolated callosal or isolated frontal ischemia). In primate studies, unilateral SMA lesions may cause impairment of bimanual coordination, possibly as a result of the remaining SMA producing similar simultaneous movements in both hands (37), although typically without autonomous complex motor activity and this impaired coordination is abolished by callosal sectioning. Thus, unilateral SMA damage is likely not sufficient to account for all the features of alien limb. As cited by Doody and Jankovic, additional callosal lesions or damage to fibers from the SMAs bilaterally are required to produce the full manifestation of the sensation of foreignness and autonomous movements (1). Patients with posterior lesions such as the case of Levine and Rinn (24) illustrate that damage to central sensory tracts in conjunction with parieto-occipital and callosal lesions may result in loss of visual guidance of a limb (optic ataxia) and a loss of sensory information from that limb causing a clinical picture similar to alien limb. Such patients with posterior lesions may be more prone to personification of the affected limb, such as case 6 of one series (1). This multiple area involvement would also be invoked to describe the elements of alien limb seen in rare cases of Alzheimer's disease.

Are there treatment options for patients with alien limb, and what is the expected progression or recovery? Although there is no specific treatment, there have been reports of techniques utilized by patients to suppress or ameliorate the alien limb symptoms. One example is the use of self-restriction, in which patients' unaffected limb will hold or restrain the alien limb. In case 1 of Goldberg et al., the patient would minimize the groping behavior of her right arm by tapping "on her thigh with the right hand as she walked or walk with a cane held in the right hand" (9). The patient reported by Kischka et al. could control the autonomous right-hand movements by use of commands such as "what are you doing?" directed to the affected limb either verbally or nonverbally (30). Patient 1 of Goldberg and Bloom was able to reduce the involuntary movement of her left hand by relaxation or by applying warm water or a shower spray to the left side of her body. Patient 3 in this series could suppress his alien limb (left hand) by visual attention and verbal commands directed to the hand (13). Nicholas et al. reported a 67-year-old man (handedness was not specified) with a right ACA territory infarction with autonomous movements of the left hand, particularly at night. Placing the alien hand in a oven mitt at night successfully controlled this unwanted activity (31).

In terms of progression and duration of alien limb symptomatology, many case reports unfortunately provide limited details as to the patients' course or provide insufficient long-term follow-up to make such determinations. In three cases where the alien limb symptoms persisted for 2 years or longer, the lesions involved cortical and subcortical regions bilaterally (12,15,42). In our experience, the alien symptoms typically resolve over 6 to 12 months following a stroke, and after 1 or 2 years in CBD because the disability progresses and the formerly "alien" limb becomes useless and ceases autonomous activity.

There has been increasing evidence to suggest that, in order for the alien limb to become chronic, there must be mesial frontal cortical dysfunction (5,6,9,10,12,17,29). Della Sala et al. have reported that patients with persistence of alien hand rarely continue to deny ownership of the affected limb and thus they prefer the term "anarchic hand" (47).

CONCLUSIONS AND FUTURE PROSPECTIVES

The alien limb sign combines a subjective sensation that the affected limb is foreign or "alien" to the patient, together with observable autonomous motor activity, most commonly restricted to an upper extremity (1). Core motor features may include grasp reflex, intermanual conflict, impaired bimanual coordination, impulsive grasping and groping, utilization behavior (compulsive manipulation of tools or objects), mirror movements, or autocriticism. Associated motor features are common, such as motor perseveration, cortical reflex myoclonus, apraxia, and motor forms of aphasia. Core sensory features may include impaired recognition of the hand when visual input is removed, personification of the affected limb, and callosal "disconnection" signs (including left hand tactile anomia and impaired intermanual somaesthetic transfer), especially when the alien limb is owing to cerebrovascular lesions.

Etiologies include stroke, ischemic or hemorrhagic, most often affecting the anterior cerebral artery territory distribution or anterior communicating artery aneurysmal rupture, surgical lesions (particularly corpus callosectomy), CBD, Creutzfeldt-Jakob disease, and bifrontal penetrating cerebral injury. Seizures and other neurodegenerative etiologies have been proposed, but are less likely to yield the classic presentation.

Although there are potentially useful maneuvers to control the alien limb manifestations, no adequate therapy is available to date. Many cases of alien limb resolve or improve markedly within 6 months to 1 year after a stroke, and the alien limb may disappear because of progressive disability in degenerative causes such as CBD, but the precise course in neurodegenerative conditions needs to be analyzed more fully. When the anatomy and syndrome clustering of alien limb are better understood, rational surgical interventions might be possible to alleviate symptoms. The primate studies mentioned in which intermanual conflict, induced by SMA lesions, could be abolished by callosal section raise the possibility that limited neurosurgical procedures might be designed to aid certain patients as well. However, clinical studies must demonstrate consistent symptoms secondary to particular etiologies or anatomies, and must assess the relationship between handedness and signs of alien limb before such procedures could be rationally designed.

ACKNOWLEDGMENTS

The authors thank Joseph Jankovic, M.D., and Zeba Vanek, M.D., for their contribution of patient information and helpful insights.

REFERENCES

1. Doody RS, Jankovic J. The alien hand and related signs. *J Neurol Neurosurg Psychiatry* 1992;55:806–810.
2. Brion S, Jedynak CP. Troubles du transfert interhemispherique. A propos de trois observations de tumeurs du corps calleux. Le signe de la main etrangere. *Revue Neurologique* 1972;126:257–266.
3. Wilson DH, Reeves A, Gazzaniga M, Culver C. Cerebral commissurotomy for control of intractable seizures. *Neurology* 1977;27:708–715.
4. Bogen JE. The callosal syndromes. In: Heilman KM, Valenstein E, eds. *Clinical neuropsychology,* 3rd ed. New York: Oxford University Press, 1993:337–407.
5. Tanaka Y, Iwasa H, Yoshida M. Diagonistic dyspraxia: case report and movement-related potentials. *Neurology* 1990;40:657–661.
6. Feinberg TE, Schindler RJ, Flanagan NG, Haber LD. Two alien hand syndromes. *Neurology* 1992;42:19–24.
7. Kety SS. From rationalization to reason. *Am J Psychiatry* 1974;131:957–963.
8. Doody, RS. Alien hand. In: Molgaard CA, ed. *Neuroepidemiology: theory and method.* San Diego: Academic Press, 1993:181–193.
9. Goldberg G, Mayer NH, Toglia JU. Medial frontal cortex infarction and the alien hand sign. *Arch Neurol* 1981;38:683–686.
10. McNabb AW, Carroll WM, Mastaglia FL. "Alien hand" and loss of bimanual coordination after dominant anterior cerebral artery territory infarction. *J Neurol Neurosurg Psychiatry* 1988;51:218–222.
11. Starkstein SE, Berthier ML, Leiguarda R. Disconnection syndrome in a right-handed patient with right hemispheric speech dominance. *Eur Neurol* 1988;28:187–190.
12. Banks G, Short P, Martinez AJ, Latchaw R, Ratcliff G, Boller F. The alien hand syndrome: clinical and postmortem findings. *Arch Neurol* 1989;46:456–459.
13. Goldberg G, Bloom KK. The alien hand sign: localization, lateralization and recovery. *Am J Phys Med Rehabil* 1990;69:228–238.
14. Kuhn MJ, Shekar PC, Schuster J, Buckler RA, Couch SM. CT and MR findings in a patient with alien hand sign. *AJNR* 1990:11;1162–1163.
15. Gasquoine PG. Bilateral alien hand signs following destruction of the medial frontal cortices. *Neuropsychiatry Neuropsycholo Behav Neurol* 1993;6:49–53.
16. Watson RT, Fleet WS, Gonzalez-Rothi L, Heilman KM. Apraxia and the supplementary motor area. *Arch Neurol* 1986;43:787–792.
17. Leiguarda R, Starkstein S, Berthier M. Anterior callosal hemorrhage. A partial interhemispheric disconnection syndrome. *Brain* 1989;1019–1037.
18. Hanakita J, Nishi S. Left alien hand sign and mirror writing after left anterior cerebral artery infarction. *Surg Neurol* 1991;35:290–293.
19. Gottlieb D, Robb K, Day B. Mirror movements in the alien hand syndrome. *Am J Med Rehabil* 1992;71:297–300.
20. Brion S, Jedynak CP. *Les Troubles du Transfert Interhemispherique.* Paris: Masson, 1975.
21. Gasquoine PG. Alien hand sign. *J Clin Exper Neuropsychol* 1993;15(5):654–667.
22. Heilman KM, Gonzalez-Rothi LJ. Apraxia. In: Heilman KM, Valenstein E, eds. *Clinical neuropsychology,* 3rd ed. New York: Oxford University Press, 1993:141–163.
23. Alexander MP, BensonDR, Stuss DT. Frontal lobes and language. *Brain Lang* 1989;37:656–691.

24. Levine DN, Rinn WE. Opticosensory ataxia and alien hand syndrome after posterior cerebral artery territory infarction. *Neurology* 1986;36:1094–1097.
25. Ay H, Buonanno FS, Price BH, Le DA, Koroshetz WJ. Sensory alien hand syndrome:case report and review of the literature. *J Neurol Neurosurg Psychiatry* 1998;65: 366–369.
26. Riley DE, Lang AE, Lewis A, et al. Cortical-basal ganglionic degeneration. *Neurology* 1990;40:1203–1212.
27. Mark VW, McAlaster R, Laser KL. Bilateral alien hand. *Neurology* 1991;41(suppl 1):302. (abstract).
28. Giroud M, Dumas R. Clinical and topographical range of callosal infarction: a clinical and radiological correlation study. *J Neurol Neurosurg Psychiatry* 1995;59:238–242.
29. Trojano L, Crisci C, Lanzillo B, Elefante R, Caruso G. How many alien hand syndromes? follow-up of a case. *Neurology* 1993;43:2710–2712.
30. Kischka U, Ettlin TM, Lichtenstern L, Riedo C. Alien hand syndrome of the dominant hand and ideomotor apraxia of the nondominant hand. *Eur Neurol* 1996;36: 39–42.
31. Nicholas JJ, Wichner MH, Gorelick PB, Ramsey MM. "Naturalization" of the alien hand: case report. *Arch Phys Med Rehabil* 1998;79:113–114.
32. Watson RT, Heilman KM. Callosal apraxia. *Brain* 1983; 106:391–403.
33. Papagno C, Marsile C. Transient left-sided alien hand with callosal and unilateral fronto-mesial damage: a case study. *Neuropsychologia* 1995;33:1703–1709.
34. Ventura MG, Goldman S, Hildebrand J. Alien hand syndrome without a corpus callosum lesion. *J Neurol Neurosurg Psychiatry* 1995;58:735–737.
35. Dolado AM, Castrillo C, Urra DG, Varela de Seijas E. Alien hand sign or alien hand syndrome? *J Neurol Neurosurg Psychiatry* 1995;59:100–101.
36. Akelaitis AI. Studies on the corpus callosum. IV. Diagonistic dyspraxia in epileptics following partial and complete section of the corpus callosum. *Am J Psychiatry* 1944–1945;101:594–599.
37. Brinkman C: Supplementary motor area of the monkey's cortex: short and long term deficits after unilateral ablation and the effects of subsequent callosal section. *J Neurosci* 1984;4:918–924.
38. Walker FO, Hunt VP. Dystonic alien hand. *Neurology* 1991;41(suppl 1);344 (Abstract).
39. Kumar R, Bergeron, Pollanen MS, Lang AE. Cortical-basal ganglionic degeneration. In: Jankovic J, ed. *Parkinson's disease and movement disorders.* Baltimore:Williams & Wilkins, 1998:297–316.
40. Rinne JO, Lee MS, Thompson PD, Marsden CD. Corticobasal degeneration: a clinical study of 36 cases. *Brain* 1994;117:1183–1196.
41. Kompoliti K, Goetz CG, Beoeve BF, et al. Clinical presentation and pharmacological therapy in corticobasal degeneration. *Arch Neurol* 1998:957–961.
42. Gibb WRG, Luther PJ, Marsden CD. Corticobasal degeneration. *Brain* 1989;112:1171–1192.
43. MacGowan DJL, Delanty N, Petito F, Edgar M, Mastrianni J, DeArmond SJ. Isolated myoclonic alien hand as the sole presentation of pathologically established Creutzfeldt-Jakob disease: a report of two patients. *J Neurol Neurosurg Psychiatry* 1997;63:404–407.
44. Ball JA, Lantos PL, Jackson M, Marsden CD, Scadding JW, Rossor MN. Alien hand sign in association with Alzheimer's histopathology. *J Neurol Neurosurg Psychiatry* 1993;56:1020–1023.
45. Leiguarda R, Starkstein S, Nogues M, Berthier M, Arbelaiz R. Paroxysmal alien hand syndrome. *J Neurol Neurosurg Psychiatry* 1993;56:788–792.
46. Andre C, Domingues RC. Transient alien hand syndrome: is this a seizure or a transient ischaemic attack? *J Neurol Neurosurg Psychiatry* 1996;60:232–233 (Letter).
47. Della Sala S, Marchetti C, Spinnler H. Right-sided anarchic (alien) hand. *Neuropsychologia* 1991;29:1113–1127.

Corticobasal Degeneration.
Advances in Neurology, Vol. 82,
edited by I. Litvan, C. G. Goetz, and A. E. Lang.
Lippincott Williams & Wilkins, Philadelphia © 2000.

13

Neuropsychiatric Aspects of Corticobasal Degeneration

Jeffrey L. Cummings* and Irene Litvan†

**Department of Neurology, UCLA School of Medicine, Los Angeles, California 90095-1769; and †Cognitive Neuropharmacology Unit, Defense and Veteran Head Injury Program, Henry M. Jackson Foundation, Bethesda, Maryland 20817-1844*

INTRODUCTION

Corticobasal degeneration (CBD) is a unique clinical and neuropathological entity that has gained increasingly wide attention. CBD has several features unusual in neurological diseases, including prominent involvement of both cortical and subcortical structures and marked asymmetry (1–3). In addition, the presentation of CBD is sometimes behaviorally dramatic, with prominent apraxia and the "alien limb" phenomenon. The neuropathology of CBD also is unique, including achromatic neurons in both cortical and subcortical structures (4,5).

Disease-specific clinical care and research depend on accurate diagnosis. CBD is less common than other middle- and late-life basal ganglia disorders such as Parkinson's disease and progressive supranuclear palsy (PSP), but it is more common than previously appreciated and is underrecognized clinically (Litvan et al., 1997). Clinical diagnosis has depended primarily on recognition of a characteristic motor syndrome—unilateral limb rigidity, bradykinesia, postural imbalance, unilateral limb dystonia, ideomotor apraxia. Characteristic neuropsychological features also have been recognized (6,7). Neuropsychiatric features have received little study in this disorder but preliminary evidence suggests that a distinctive profile of behavioral changes occurs in CBD and may aid in differential diagnosis. In this chapter, we review the available evidence on behavioral changes in CBD, present the results of a recent study of neuropsychiatric features in CBD, contrast the behavioral disturbances of CBD with those of other neurodegenerative diseases, review the neurobiological changes of CBD relevant to behavioral manifestations, and suggest management strategies for the most common behavioral abnormalities reported in CBD patients.

NEUROPSYCHIATRIC SYNDROMES IN CBD

Clinical description or structured assessment of the neuropsychiatric features of CBD rarely have been conducted. In the available literature, three syndromes have been noted: depression, frontal lobe-type behavioral disturbances, and obsessive-compulsive behaviors.

Depression

Depression is common in CBD and may have biologic and reactive determinants. Depression was noted as a prominent phenomenon in a man described by Rey and colleagues (8) with CBD who presented at the age of 67 with a 2-year history of progressive mental and physical fatigue. Assessment with the Beck Depression Inventory revealed moderately severe mood changes (score = 8) at the time of initial assessment. Three years later he was reassessed and continued to exhibit the same level of depressive symptoms (score = 19).

Wenning and coworkers (3) described the natural history of 14 patients with CBD whose diagnosis was confirmed by postmortem examination. Seven of the patients exhibited depression at some point in their illness. One of the 14 had depression as the initial symptom, four had depression at the time of the first clinical assessment, and two had depression at the time of their last visit.

Massman and colleagues (9) used the Geriatric Depression Scale to assess mood changes in their 21 CBD patients. They contrasted the findings in the CBD group to those of 21 patients with Alzheimer's disease displaying no extrapyramidal features and 12 Alzheimer's disease patients with extrapyramidal signs. The mean Geriatric Depression Scale score for the CBD patients was 14.2 (S.D. 8.9), whereas that for the patients with Alzheimer's disease was 5.2 (S.D. 5.0). Geriatric Depression Scale scores of 15 or higher are indicative of a clinically significant depression syndrome, and eight of the 21 CBD patients scored in this range whereas only one of the 21 patients with Alzheimer's disease had a score beyond this cut-off.

Thus, when carefully assessed, depression emerges as a common phenomenon in CBD.

Frontal Lobe-Type Behavioral Alterations

Frontal lobe-type behaviors with disinhibitors, apathy, impulsivity, and tactlessness have been observed frequently in CBD patients, although the exact type of behavioral changes rarely have been described in detail. In an early report of CBD, Gibb and colleagues (4) noted that one of their patients became apathetic as his disease progressed. Rinne and coworkers (4) reported that one of their 36 patients had prominent personality and behavioral changes with impulsiveness. Similarly, Kertesz and Martinez-Lage (10) noted that 22 of their 55 CBD patients had personality and behavioral changes. Wenning and colleagues (3) reported that three of their 14 CBD patients (14%) presented initially with behavioral changes of frontal lobe-type including apathy, irritability, and disinhibition. Four of their patients had these types of behavioral changes at initial visit, three had them at the time of the final visit, and seven manifested them at some time in the clinical course. The presence of these features predicted shorter survival in this patient group.

These reports suggest that frontal lobe-type behavioral changes can occur and be present at anytime in the evolution of CBD.

Obsessive-Compulsive Behavior

Obsessive-compulsive behavior occasionally has been observed in patients with CBD. Rey and colleagues (8), in a case report of a CBD patient, described the individual as displaying stereotyped movements with the right (least involved) hand evidenced by repeated touching of his clothing and reaching for and touching objects in his environment. The movement was interpreted as a compulsive movement although it may also have been a manifestation of forced grasping. The investigators administered the Leyton Obsessional Inventory and found that the patient endorsed a substantial number of obsessive-compulsive-type symptoms, including recurrent thoughts, repetitive acts, indecisiveness, checking behaviors, and preoccupation with perfectionism. This patient was depressed and was receiving L-dopa therapy at the time the obsessive-compulsive behaviors were observed, clinical circumstances that may have contributed to his behavioral syndrome.

Rinne and colleagues (11) noted that one of their series of patients exhibited excessive eating and drinking, possibly consistent with obsessive-compulsive behavior.

These preliminary reports suggest that obsessive-compulsive phenomena may be among the behavioral disturbances of CBD.

NINDS-UCLA STUDY OF NEUROPSYCHIATRIC FEATURES OF CBD

We recently conducted an assessment of 20 CBD patients examined at the National Institute of Neurological Diseases and Stroke (NINDS) (12). The patients had a mean age of 68.1 years (SD 8.8). Ten patients were male. The mean educational level was 15 years (SD 3.2). They had had the illness for a mean of 48.1 months (SD 21.4), and had mean Mini-Mental State Examination scores of 24.9 (SD 5). The study utilized the Neuropsychiatric Inventory (NPI), developed at UCLA by Cummings and colleagues (13), to assess the behavioral symptoms of the CBD patients. The NPI utilizes information from caregivers to rate a variety of behavioral disturbances and has been shown to be valid and reliable. Ten behaviors are routinely assessed, including delusions, hallucinations, agitation, anxiety, apathy, irritability, disinhibition, dysphoria, euphoria, and aberrant motor behavior such as pacing, rummaging and stereotyped motor acts.

Table 1 shows the percent of patients with each of the symptoms assessed by the NPI, along with the mean score for all members of the group and the mean score for patients exhibiting symptoms. The total possible score for each symptom is 12; percentages are calculated by determining the percent of patients with the symptom of any level of severity.

Depression (73%), apathy (40%), irritability (20%), and agitation (20%) were the symptoms most commonly exhibited by CBD patients. Anxiety, disinhibition, delusions and aberrant motor behavior were rare in this population as assessed by the NPI and no patient exhibited euphoria or hallucinations. A factor analysis identified three factors—one including agitation, apathy, disinhibition, and irritability; another including depression, agitation, and aberrant motor behavior; and a third one including depression and anxiety.

Twelve of the CBD patients had primarily left-sided symptoms, and eight had syndromes primarily involving the right limbs. Although the small number of patients prohibited statistical analysis, those with left-sided symptoms (right hemisphere involvement) exhibited greater disinhibition, apathy, and irritability and lower depression scores than those with right-sided (left brain) symptoms.

In the published study (12), the CBD patients were contrasted with NPI assessment results of 34 patients with PSP of similar age and education. A logistic regression identified significantly higher frequencies of depression and irritability in the CBD patients, with fewer patients exhibiting apathy. A discriminant function analysis correctly identified 88% of the CBD patients (sensitivity 67%, specificity 97%).

This study confirms that depression is a common neuropsychiatric disturbance associated with CBD. Moreover, seven of the 14 patients manifesting depressive syndromes had NPI scores in the upper range (eight out of a possible 12, or higher). Several of the patients had suicidal ideation. Apathy, irritability, and agitation are additional behavioral features of CBD.

RELATIONSHIP OF CBD TO OTHER NEURODEGENERATIVE DISORDERS

The profile of neuropsychiatric symptoms found in CBD contrasts with that observed in other neurodegenerative diseases. Patients with Alzheimer's disease more commonly manifest

TABLE 1. *Neuropsychiatric features of 20 patients with corticobasal degeneration*

Neuropsychiatric inventory item	Symptomatic patients (%)	Neuropsychiatric inventory score (mean)	Neuropsychiatric inventory score of patients exhibiting the symptom (mean)
Depression	70	4.4	6.2
Apathy	40	1.7	4.1
Irritability	20	0.95	4.7
Anxiety	15	1.2	8
Disinhibition	15	0.8	8
Delusions	5	0.15	3
Aberrant motor behavior	15	0.7	4.6
Euphoria	0	0	0
Hallucinations	0	0	0
Any NPI symptom	90	10.1	11.2

apathy, agitation, anxiety, aberrant motor behavior, and delusions (14). Patients with frontotemporal degeneration characteristically evidence more disinhibition and euphoria (15). Patients with PSP exhibit higher rates of apathy (16); and patients with Huntington's disease tend to be more irritable, apathetic, and disinhibited. Parkinson's disease patients manifest rates of depression comparable to those of CBD but also manifest high rates of anxiety. Dementia with Lewy bodies, a syndrome sharing many neurologic and neuropsychological features with CBD, has a high rate of visual hallucinations, a phenomenon never observed in the CBD patients included in the NINDS-UCLA study. These different profiles of neuropsychiatric symptoms may aid in differential diagnosis of neurodegenerative diseases. Table 2 lists the frequency of neuropsychiatric symptoms as revealed by the NPI in a variety of neurodegenerative disorders.

POSSIBLE PATHOPHYSIOLOGICAL SUBSTRATE OF BEHAVIORAL CHANGES IN CORTICOBASAL DEGENERATION

Histologic, neurochemical, or neuroimaging correlates of depression in CBD have not been explored. The shared distribution of histologic and biochemical changes of CBD with other neurodegenerative disorders commonly manifesting depression suggest a shared pathophysiology. Examination of the cortex in CBD reveals marked neuronal loss and extensive fibrillary gliosis disproportionately involving layers 3 and 5 in the parietal and posterior frontal cortex. Remaining neurons exhibit cytoplasmic swelling with staining characteristics described as neuronal achromasia. The substantia nigra is involved commonly in CBD and has marked loss of neurons, loss of pigment, and gliosis. Similar changes may be seen in the locus ceruleus and raphe nuclei and there is variable involvement of the lateral thalamic nuclei, globus pallidus, subthalamic nucleus, red nucleus, striatum, and midbrain tegmentum. The cerebral cortical and nigral changes are most severe. The findings are typically bilateral but asymmetric, corresponding to the asymmetric clinical manifestations (5).

There have been few biochemical analyses of CBD brains. One brain examined at postmortem had severe striatal dopamine loss and less marked deficits of dopamine in the substantia nigra. Glutamate content also was markedly reduced in the striatum. Striatal choline acetyltransferase levels were normal (5).

Positron emission tomography (PET) provides additional insight into the pathophysiology of CBD with implications for mood changes in this disorder. Fluorodeoxyglucose-PET typically reveals asymmetric hemispheric involvement with reduced metabolism in the dorsolateral frontal, medial frontal, inferior parietal, sensory-motor and lateral temporal cortex as well as the striatum and thalamus (6,17). Studies of cerebral blood flow using single photon emission computed to-

TABLE 2. *Frequency of endorsement of neuropsychiatric inventory items in CBD and other neurodegenerative diseases*

Neuropsychiatric inventory items	Corticobasal degeneration	Parkinson's disease	Progressive supranuclear palsy	Huntington's disease	Frontotemporal degeneration	Alzheimer's disease
Depression (%)	70	90	18	41	38	38
Apathy (%)	40	41	91	34	95	72
Irritability (%)	20	31	9	38	45	42
Anxiety (%)	15	66	18	34	59	48
Disinhibition (%)	15	12	36	24	68	36
Delusions (%)	5	0	0	10	23	22
Aberrant motor behavior (%)	15	6	9	7	73	38
Euphoria (%)	0	33	0	17	36	8
Hallucinations (%)	0	6	0	0	0	10
Agitation (%)	20	31	5	45	62	60

mography (18) and studies of oxygen utilization with O_{15}-PET (19) revealed similar patterns of abnormalities. F-dopa-PET demonstrates asymmetric reductions of fluorodopa utilization in caudate and putamen (19).

These studies indicate that CBD patients have serotonergic (secondary to involvement of raphe nuclei), noradrenergic (secondary to changes in the locus ceruleus), as well as dopaminergic abnormalities. This biochemic profile is similar to that of Parkinson's disease, a disorder also commonly manifesting depressive symptoms. Striatal abnormalities have been correlated with frontal lobe-type behavioral disturbances and obsessive-compulsive behaviors, presumably secondary to interruption of frontal-subcortical circuits (20).

Refinements in understanding the pathophysiological basis of mood and behavioral disturbances in CBD depend on conducting studies contrasting CBD patients with and patients without these neuropsychiatric symptoms.

TREATMENT OF NEUROPSYCHIATRIC MANIFESTATIONS OF CBD

No studies have been conducted of the response of mood changes in CBD to antidepressant treatment. Depression in Parkinson's disease has been shown to respond to treatment with antidepressant agents (21) and it is reasonable to administer antidepressant agents to CBD patients with mood abnormalities. Depression produces distress, can be life-threatening (through suicide) when severe, increases patient disability and is a source of distress for the caregiver. Treatment should be initiated with a selective serotonin reuptake inhibitor such as citalopram, sertraline, paroxetine, fluoxetine, or fluvoxamine. If patients are unresponsive to or intolerant of these medications, a trial of a tricyclic antidepressant with few cholinergic side effects such as nortriptyline or desipramine is indicated. Electroconvulsive therapy, a treatment successfully applied to depressed patients with Parkinson's disease should be considered in patients who do not respond to pharmacotherapy or where side effects, drug interactions, or the patient's medical condition prohibit use of pharmacologic agents.

SUMMARY

Neuropsychiatric symptoms are present in the majority of patients with CBD. Depression is common in this group of patients and contributes to the morbidity of the disease. Depression is more severe in CBD than in many other neurologic disorders. Neuropsychiatric symptoms should be assessed in all patients with CBD to enhance symptom detection and improve management.

ACKNOWLEDGMENTS

This project was supported by the National Institute of Neurological Diseases and Stroke, a National Institute on Aging Alzheimer's Disease Center grant (AG 10123), an Alzheimer's Disease Research Center of California grant, and the Sidell-Kagan Foundation.

REFERENCES

1. Litvan I, Agid Y, Goetz C, et al. Accuracy of the clinical diagnosis of corticobasal degeneration: a clinicopathologic study. *Neurology* 1997;48:119–125.
2. Schneider JA, Watts RL, Gearing M, Brewer RP, Mirra SS. Corticobasal degeneration: neuropathologic and clinical heterogeneity. *Neurology* 1997;48:959–969.
3. Wenning GK, Litvan I, Jankovic J, et al. Natural history and survival of 14 patients with corticobasal degeneration confirmed at postmortem examination. *J Neurology Neurosurg Psychiatry* 1988;64:184–189.
4. Gibb WRG, Luthert PJ, Marsden CD. Corticobasal degeneration. *Brain* 1989;112:1171–1192.
5. Lang AE, Riley DE, Bergeron C. Cortical-basal ganglionic degeneration. In: Calne DB, ed. *Neurodegenerative diseases.* Philadelphia: WB Saunders, 1994:877–894.
6. Eidelberg D, Dhawan V, Moeller JR, et al. The metabolic landscape of cortico-basal ganglionic degeneration: regional asymmetries studied with positron emission tomography. *J Neurol Neurosurg Psychiatry* 1991;54:856–862.
7. Pillon B, Blin J, Vidailhet M, et al. The neuropsychological pattern of corticobasal degeneration: comparison with progressive supranuclear palsy and Alzheimer's disease. *Neurology* 1995;45:1477–1483.
8. Rey GJ, Tomer R, Levin BE, Sanchez-Ramos J, Bowen B, Bruce JH. Psychiatric symptoms, atypical dementia, and left visual field inattention in corticobasal ganglionic degeneration. *Mov Disord* 1995;10:106–110.
9. Massman PJ, Kreiter KT, Jankovic J, Doody RS. Neuropsychological functioning in cortical-basal ganglionic degeneration: differentiation from Alzheimer's disease. *Neurology* 1996;46:720–726.
10. Kertesz A, Martinez-Lage P. Cognitive changes in corticobasal degeneration. In: Kertesz A, Munoz DG, eds. *Pick's disease and Pick complex.* New York: Wiley-Liss, 1998:121–128.

11. Rinne JO, Lee MS, Thompson PD, Marsden CD. Corticobasal degeneration—A clinical study of 36 cases. *Brain* 1994;117:1183–1196.
12. Litvan I, Cummings JL, Mega M. Neuropsychiatric features of corticobasal degeneration. *J Neurol Neurosurg Psychiatry,* in press.
13. Cummings JL, Mega M, Gray K, Rosenberg-Thompson S, Carusi DA, Gornbein J. The Neuropsychiatric Inventory: comprehensive assessment of psychopathology in dementia. *Neurology* 1994;44:2308–2314.
14. Mega MS, Cummings JL, Fiorello T, Gornbein J. The spectrum of behavioral changes in Alzheimer's disease. *Neurology* 1996;46:130–135.
15. Levy ML, Miller BL, Cummings JL, Fairbanks LA, Craig A. Alzheimer disease and frontotemporal dementias: behavioral distinctions. *Arch Neurol* 1996;53:687–690.
16. Litvan I, Mega M, Cummings JL, Fairbanks LA. Neuropsychiatric aspects of progressive supranuclear palsy. *Neurology* 1996;47:1184–1189.
17. Nagahama Y, Fukuyama H, Turjanski N, et al. Cerebral glucose metabolism in corticobasal degeneration: comparison with progressive supranuclear palsy and normal controls. *Mov Disord* 1997; 12:691–696.
18. Markus HS, Lees AJ, Lennox G, Marsden CD, Costa DC. Patterns of regional cerebral blood flow in corticobasal degeneration studied using HMPAO SPECT; Comparison with Parkinson's disease and normal controls. *Move Disord* 1995:10:179–187.
19. Sawle GV, Brooks DJ, Marsden CD, Frackowiak RSJ. Corticobasal degeneration: a unique pattern of regional cortical oxygen hypometabolism and striatal fluorodopa uptake demonstrated by positron emission tomography. *Brain* 1991;114:541–556.
20. Cummings JL. Frontal-subcortical circuits and human behavior. *Arch Neurol* 1993;50:873–880.
21. Tom T, Cummings JL. Depression in Parkinson's disease: characteristics and treatment. *Drugs Aging* 1998; 12:55–74.

Corticobasal Degeneration.
Advances in Neurology, Vol. 82,
edited by I. Litvan, C. G. Goetz, and A. E. Lang.
Lippincott Williams & Wilkins, Philadelphia © 2000.

14

Speech and Swallowing Disturbances in Corticobasal Degeneration

Carol M. Frattali and Barbara C. Sonies

Speech-Language Pathology Section, Rehabilitation Medicine Department, National Institutes of Health, Bethesda, Maryland 20892

INTRODUCTION

A striking feature of corticobasal degeneration (CBD) is the asymmetry with which the disease presents and pursues its course. Often, a single limb is involved for years before patients experience more generalized deficits. It is this asymmetry and the involvement of both cerebral cortex and basal ganglia that led us to pursue a line of investigation in order to characterize the motoric aspects of CBD that involve speech and swallowing disturbances.

Published studies on the sequelae of CBD document the presence of dysarthria, a collective name for a group of related speech disorders resulting from disturbances in muscular control of the speech mechanism involving respiration, phonation, resonance, articulation, and prosody (1,2). For example, Riley et al. (3) documented the presence of dysarthria in seven of 15 cases. Wenning et al. (4) found dysarthria in 29% of their sample during the first visit (on average 3.0 [SD 1.9] years after onset of symptoms) and 75% of their sample during the last visit (on average 6.1 [SD 2.0] years after onset of symptoms). At last visit, Wenning et al. reported that speech was almost always abnormal (93%). Speech abnormalities were variably described as slurred (n = 9), slow (n = 9), dysphonic (n = 5), mute (n = 5), aphonic (n = 4), unintelligible (n = 4), echolalic (n = 2), or palilalic (n = 1). Speech disorders were reported as initial symptoms in only two (14%) of the Wenning et al. sample.

Similarly, swallowing disorders resulting from CBD have been addressed in only a few clinical studies. Riley et al. (3) reported dysphagia in two of their 15 cases followed. Dysphagia was also reported in four of 13 cases presented in the earlier literature (5–7). The type and severity of dysphagia, as well as specific methods of assessment, however, have not been adequately described.

The purposes of this chapter are threefold:

1. To describe the speech and swallowing characteristics of CBD on the basis of comprehensive and systematic assessment;
2. To differentiate these characteristics from those of other more prevalent neurological disorders; and
3. To speculate on their pathophysiology.

CHARACTERISTIC FEATURES OF CBD

CBD can present with a complex configuration of oral/motor, speech, or swallowing deficits either as initial presenting symptoms or symptoms that arise and worsen as the disease progresses. In order to study the patterns of speech and swallowing disturbances that are characteristic of this neurodegenerative disease, as well as to distinguish patterns of deficits from those of other neurodegenerative diseases, we followed 15 outpatients diagnosed as having CBD at the National Institutes of Health, W.G. Magnuson Clinical Center in Bethesda, MD. All cases met the modified Lang et al. criteria for a diagnosis of

CBD (8), which includes: progressive course of an asymmetric parkinsonism not benefiting from L-dopa therapy; presence of either a dystonic limb or focal myoclonus; presence of either ideomotor apraxia, alien limb syndrome, cortical sensory loss or language disturbances; absence of resting tremor, autonomic disturbance, or laboratory evidence of other disorders.

SUBJECTS

The patients included eight males and seven females ranging in age from 50 to 84 years (mean = 68.1 yrs; SD = 2.6 yrs). All subjects were right-handed, spoke English as their primary language, and had adequate hearing acuity for following instructions and engaging in conversation. Mean education level was 15.7 years (SD = 2.6 yrs). Five patients presented with motor deficits predominating on the right side and 10 patients with motor deficits predominating on the left side. Duration of disease ranged from 12 to 84 months (mean = 54.80 months; SD = 17.98 months) (9–11).

TEST BATTERY

A comprehensive battery of tests, including instrumental procedures, standardized tests, and behavioral/perceptual measures, was compiled to yield reliable and sensitive information on specific oral/motor, speech, and swallowing deficits that could result from CBD (9–13). Table 1 describes this test battery, summarizing each measure's assessment features and purposes. It should be noted that the Swallowing Questionnaire was completed by interviewing both patients and family members to ensure an accurate account of swallowing complaints (11,12).

FINDINGS

Motor Speech Disturbances

Dysarthria

Dysarthria was present in 13 of 14 cases, or 93% of the patient sample; therefore, documenting dysarthria as a prominent feature of CBD, even in the relatively early phases of disease progression (i.e., with mean duration of disease of 3½ years). Differential diagnosis of dysarthria was variable in both type and severity. Of the 13 cases, the majority had mild symptoms, with seven patients presenting with mild dysarthria, five patients with moderate dysarthria, and one case with severe dysarthria.

TABLE 1. *Speech and swallowing assessment battery*

Parameter assessed	Test/measure (with reference)	Description
Oral motor/speech	Oral mechanism examination (9)	Measures strength, symmetry, coordination, and range of motion of speech articulators
	Speech parameters rating (10)	Rates, on a 4-point ordinal scale of severity (1 being normal, 4 being severe), voice quality, resonance, fluency, pitch, intensity, duration, stress, articulation, and facial expression on the basis of a phonetically balanced speech sample
Swallowing	Swallowing questionnaire (11)	Documents specific swallowing complaints related to chewing, swallowing, salivation, regurgitation, and reflux
	Ultrasound imaging of the oropharynx (US) (11,12)	Ultrasonographic study of oropharyngeal functioning during dry, wet, and pudding swallows
	Modified barium swallow study (MBS) (13)	Videofluorographic study of the swallowing mechanism using wet, pudding, and solid bolus textures to evaluate oral, pharyngeal, and esophageal stages of swallowing

Five patients (35.7%) had classic hypokinetic dysarthria, similar to that which characterizes the dysarthria of patients with Parkinson's disease resulting from extrapyramidal damage. This could provide one explanation of the misdiagnosis of CBD for Parkinson's disease. Characteristic features included reduced loudness/monoloudness, monotone stress, fluctuating imprecise speech articulation, slow rate of speech with intermittent rapid-fire bursts, and shallow inhalations. An additional three patients (21.4%) exhibited mixed dysarthria with hypokinetic features predominating (e.g., as in the preceding but with hypernasality and/or strained, strangled vocal quality). Therefore, approximately 57% of the patient sample displayed hypokinetic features of dysarthria. An additional four patients (28.6%) displayed mixed dysarthrias, but with either predominant hyperkinetic or spastic features (e.g., strained, strangled voice, vocal tremor, sudden-forced respiratory patterns). Only one patient had a classic form of spastic dysarthria, as characterized by strained voice, hypernasality, slow-labored and imprecise articulation, excess syllabic stress, and reduced respiratory pressure generation. Table 2 summarizes the types and characteristics of the dysarthrias found in the patient population.

Although type or severity of dysarthria was generally not associated with duration of disease, it should be noted that the patient with shortest disease duration (26 months) did not have dysarthria, and the patient with longest duration of disease (84 months) had severe dysarthria. There was also a trend for mixed rather than specific or "pure" dysarthrias from 3 years of disease duration or longer (seven of nine patients or 78% of sample), likely owing to the involvement of multiple motor systems as the disease progresses.

Apraxia

Oral apraxia (disturbances in purposeful, learned movements of the oral/respiratory structures despite intact strength of the peripheral speech musculature) (1,2,14), or apraxia of speech (an articulatory disorder in which the patient has difficulty programming the positioning of the speech muscles and sequencing the muscle movements for volitional production of phonemes) (1,2), are other types of motor speech disorders that were found to be a characteristic in our patient population. Of 13 patients who were tested for these types of apraxia, six (46%) were found to

TABLE 2. *Dysarthria classifications*

Dysarthria classification	Salient features	Number of patients ($N = 14$)	Percent
Hypokinetic	Reduced loudness, hoarseness, monotone stress, normal resonation, fluctuating and imprecise intelligibility, slow rate with intermittent rapid-fire bursts, and shallow inhalations with reduced exhalatory control	5	35.7
Mixed with predominant hypokinetic features	Features of hypokinetic dysarthria in presence of hypernasality, and/or strained, strangled vocal quality	3	21.4
Mixed with predominant hyperkinetic features	Primarily characterized by strained harsh voice/vocal tremor, variable imprecise articulation, prolongations of sounds, irregular and sudden-forced respiratory patterns, but with hypernasality	2	14.3
Mixed with predominant spastic features	Features of spastic dysarthria in presence of normal resonance and low vocal loudness	2	14.3
Spastic	Strained, strangled voice; hypernasality; slow-labored and imprecise articulation; excess syllabic stress; reduced respiratory pressure generation	1	7.1

have oral apraxia, and five (38%) had combined oral apraxia and apraxia of speech. None of our patients had apraxia of speech in the absence of oral apraxia.

In severe cases of oral apraxia, patients are unable to open their mouths volitionally, pucker their lips, or even take instruction in activities automatic to oral movements (e.g., taking pills, drinking or eating). Two patients demonstrated this deficit during the modified barium swallow study. When instructed to "look straight ahead, hold bolus in mouth momentarily, and swallow," both patients opened their mouths unwittingly, with subsequent loss of bolus. Apologetic comments such as, "I tried as hard as I could" or "my mouth would not cooperate" were made in both cases. Other patients with oral apraxia had more difficulty with respiratory oral gestures (e.g., pretending to blow out a match) than with nonrespiratory oral gestures (e.g., protruding tongue). This finding is consistent with that found in the literature that most patients with oral apraxia have more difficulty producing respiratory oral gestures than producing nonrespiratory oral gestures (14).

Swallowing Disturbances

On the basis of Swallowing Questionnaire findings, which profiled swallowing complaints from the report of patients and their family members, 12 of 14 patients (missing data in one patient) or 86% of our sample reported difficulties in swallowing. Findings are summarized in Table 3. The main complaint was coughing/choking, with 11 patients or 79% of the sample reporting this finding. Seven of 12 patients, or 50% of the patient sample, stated that this problem occurred more frequently with liquids than with solids. In descending order of frequency, other reported difficulties included: slowness of eating (which was also assessed on the basis of slowness of getting food to mouth, as well as bolus transport problems) (64%), difficulty swallowing pills (50%), food spreading over mouth while eating (43%), food getting caught inside cheek and not swallowed (43%), mouth dryness (43%), food falling from mouth (36%), food getting caught lower in throat (29%), a feeling of a lump in the throat (21%), difficulty chewing foods (21%), avoidance of certain foods that are problematic from a swallowing standpoint (21%), food coming out of nose (21%), food getting caught at base of tongue (21%), reflux (14%), and more difficulty with solids than liquids (14%).

On the bases of modified barium swallow (MBS) studies (findings summarized as Table 4), and ultrasound imaging of the oropharynx (US), 12 of 14 (missing data in one patient) or 86%

TABLE 3. *Patient/family reports of swallowing disturbances in CBD as documented on the Swallowing Questionnaire*

Complaint	Number of subjects (*N* = 14)*	Percent
Difficulty swallowing	12	85.7
Coughing/choking	11	78.6
Slow eater	9	64.3
More difficulty with liquids than solids	7	50
Difficulty swallowing pills	7	50
Food spreading over mouth	6	42.9
Food getting caught inside cheek and not swallowed	6	42.9
Dry mouth	6	42.9
Food falling from mouth	5	35.7
Food getting caught lower in throat	4	28.6
Feeling of lump in throat	3	21.4
Difficulty chewing foods	3	21.4
Avoiding foods	3	21.4
Food coming out of nose	3	21.4
Food getting caught at base of tongue	3	21.4
Reflux	2	14.3
More difficulty with solids than liquids	2	14.3

* Missing data for 1 of 15 subjects.

TABLE 4. *Videofluoroscopic findings of swallowing disturbances in CBD**

Symptoms	Number of Subjects	Percent
Oral phase		
Bolus partition (piecemeal deglutition)	10	71.4
Delayed initiation of swallow reflex	9	64.2
Excessive lingual gestures	7	50
Impaired bolus transport	7	50
Nasal reflux	2	14.3
Pharyngeal phase		
Pooling in valleculae	13	92.9
Pooling in pyriform sinus	5	35.7
Bolus falls in pharynx before swallow	4	28.6
Overflow into laryngeal aditus	4	28.6
Aspiration	2†	14.3
Esophageal phase		
Reflux	5	35.7
Esophageal dysmotility	4	28.6

* One of 15 patients had missing data.
† Diet modifications were instituted to prevent further aspiration.

of our sample were found to have swallowing deficits. Predominant oral phase features were excessive lingual gestures (50%), impaired bolus transfer owing to tongue dysmotility (50%), and delayed initiation of swallow reflex (64.2%). Pharyngeal phase findings included bolus pooling in valleculae (92.9%) and, to lesser extent, in the pyriform sinuses (35.7%). Reflux was present in 35.7% of our patient sample in the esophageal phase of swallowing.

During MBS studies, four patients had overflow of bolus into the laryngeal aditus (i.e., the entrance to the laryngeal vestibule including the epiglottis anteriorly, the aryepiglottic folds laterally, and the apexes of the arytenoid cartilages posteriorly); two patients had trace aspiration of liquids. The latter two patients were managed with diet and postural modifications (e.g., thickened liquids, head turn to weaker side during swallowing) to aid in preventing aspiration.

The occurrence of dysphagia as determined by instrumental testing ($n = 12$) coincided with patient and family report on the basis of completion of the Swallowing Questionnaire ($n = 12$). The symptom of reflux, however, was underreported by patients and their families (14%) in comparison with this finding on videofluorographic study (36%). It should be noted, however, that, in all cases, family members assisted in completion of the questionnaire and patients and their family members would sometimes disagree on the presence of specific swallowing disturbances. That is, patients tended to deny certain symptoms when they existed, and family members were found to be more reliable judges when their responses were compared with instrumental test findings. The degree of underreport of swallowing symptoms by patients could be explained, at least in part, by the presence of cognitive deficits and, therefore, reduced awareness of specific deficits. This line of investigation, however, was not systematically conducted and warrants further study.

DIFFERENTIATION WITH CHARACTERISTIC FEATURES OF OTHER NEURODEGENERATIVE DISORDERS

Speech or swallowing deficits found in CBD, considered either singly or together, are not clearly distinguishable from that found in other neurological disorders. Difficulties in differential diagnosis are reported in the literature. For example, when the symptoms of CBD, in general, are determined for purposes of diagnosis, Litvan et al. (15) found that false-negative misdiagnoses occurred frequently, mainly with progressive supranuclear palsy (PSP), vascular parkinsonism, Parkinson's disease (PD), multiple system atrophy, Pick's disease, and Alzheimer's disease.

As described earlier in this chapter, the predominance of hypokinetic features of dysarthria (e.g., soft and monotonal speech) often lead to clinical impressions of PD or Parkinson's plus syndromes, such as PSP. The combination of speech and swallowing deficits can also mimic that found in these diseases. Considered along with other deficits characteristic of CBD (i.e., nonfluent aphasia, motor asymmetry, ideomotor apraxia, and alien limb syndrome), however, a distinctive pattern of deficits emerges that may assist in uniquely characterizing this neurodegenerative disorder. Characteristic speech and swallowing disturbances include:

- *Dysarthria:* Characterized predominantly by hypokinetic features of low vocal intensity, monotonal speech, monoloudness, and imprecise articulation;
- *Oral/verbal apraxia;* and
- *Dysphagia:* Characterized primarily by delay in initiation of swallow reflex, bolus partition, and pooling in valleculae that does not clear adequately with multiple swallows; more difficulty experienced with liquids than solids.

Litvan et al. (15) identified the best predictors for the diagnosis of CBD in their systematic study, primarily from the motor disturbance perspective. At the first visit, the best predictors were absence of gait or balance disturbance, limb dystonia, asymmetric Parkinsonism, and ideomotor apraxia. The best predictors at the last visit were balance or gait disturbance, ideomotor apraxia, cognitive disturbance, focal myoclonus, and limb dystonia.

From our perspective, the motor speech deficit of apraxia assists in ruling out both PD and PSP. Duvoisin (16) supports this position, stating that impaired performance of complex motor acts despite the absence of muscle weakness is common in extrapyramidal syndromes and often begs the question of whether there is an apraxia in PSP. His impression, however, is that true apraxia suggests the possibility of CBD rather than PSP. Albert et al. (17) also described an absence of apraxia in PSP. Thus, apraxia can be a differentiating feature in CBD.

The pathophysiology of Alzheimer's disease, unlike that of PD and PSP, involves cortical damage, and, therefore, may mirror some of the findings characteristic of CBD. What is atypical of Alzheimer's disease, however, is the asymmetry with which the symptoms of CBD present. It should also be noted that Alzheimer's patients have little or no peripheral weakness or incoordination, and have no obvious motor speech deficits until the latest stages of the disease—this being another distinguishing feature from CBD.

SPECULATIONS ON THE PATHOPHYSIOLOGY OF SPEECH AND SWALLOWING DISORDERS

Corpus callosum findings in CBD and correlates with speech, language, and related cognitive deficits have recently been the subject of investigation. For example, Yamauchi et al. (18) investigated whether atrophy of the corpus callosum is associated with cognitive impairment and cerebral cortical hypometabolism in corticobasal degeneration. They found that the atrophy was accompanied by a decreased mean cortical glucose metabolic rate with hemispheric asymmetry and a decrease in the sum of the scaled subtest scores on the Wechsler Adult Intelligence Scale—Revised (19). Therefore, atrophy of the corpus callosum was associated with cognitive impairment and cerebral cortical hypometabolism with hemispheric asymmetry. They suggest that atrophy of the corpus callosum might reflect the severity of the disconnection between cortical regions, which may add to the neuroanatomical explanation of findings of aphasia (described in this volume, Chapter 11). Their report of asymmetrical cerebral atrophy affecting mainly the frontal and parietal lobes can also contribute to the explanation of both motor speech disorders and swallowing disorders. Whereas the presence of motor speech disorders can involve both frontal and parietal lobes, the presence of dysphagia can involve a small portion of the anterolateral cortex immediately in front of the precentral cortex of the frontal lobe.

Motor Speech Disturbances

The various classifications of dysarthria (i.e., hypokinetic and spastic, as well as mixed dysarthrias with hypokinetic, hyperkinetic, or spastic features) suggest lesions in the supratentorial areas involving primarily the frontal and parietal lobes, and the basal ganglia and thalamus, with vascular supply interruption of major cerebral arteries and their branches. Apraxia of speech could also result from cortical damage including premotor and parietal lobe lesions as well as subcortical lesions with involvement of the basal ganglia and anterior limb of the internal capsule, typically with damage to the left hemisphere at this neuroanatomic level (2). This anatomic level would rule out occurrence of flaccid or ataxic dysarthria, which would involve the posterior fossa (pons, medulla, midbrain, or cerebellum), which was not a finding of this current study. It should be noted that hypokinetic dysarthria is associated only with supratentorial (subcortical lesions), which was a predominant finding in our patient population, thus suggesting damage to the extrapyramidal system.

Swallowing Disturbances

Several cortical and subcortical regions mediate the activity of the brainstem pathway to activate and control the oral, pharyngeal, and esophageal phases of swallowing. Although deglutition and ingestion are largely bilateral brainstem activities involving the medulla, pons, and cranial nerves (5,7,9,11,12), a small portion of the anterolateral cortex immediately in front of the precentral cortex of the frontal lobe is involved (20). Although electrical stimulation of the primary motor cortex does not elicit swallowing (21), stimulation of the anterolateral region evokes swallowing that is often associated with mastication (22, 23). Specific cortical sites also play a role in evoking and facilitating the initiation of swallowing. These same cortical regions also modify the duration and intensity of the muscle activity that determines tongue movement, elevation of the hyoid bone, adduction of the vocal cords, and contraction of the upper esophagus during swallowing. The prefrontal region mediates bilateral movements of the face and tongue, repetitive jaw movements, and, in selected regions, pharyngeal and esophageal swallowing. Neural pathways from the anterolateral cortex descend through the internal capsule and subthalamic regions to the level of the upper brainstem. Thus, both cortical and subcortical pathways are involved in swallowing functions, and explain the occurrence of dysphagia in patients with CBD.

CONCLUSIONS

Our investigation found that speech and swallowing disturbances are more prevalent in CBD than that reported in the earlier clinical literature (Table 5). This discrepancy, when compared with the occurrences reported in these published clinical studies, points to the need for thorough and systematic evaluation of oral/motor, speech, and swallowing functions by a speech-language pathologist, using a battery of instrumental and behavioral measures in order to identify these deficits and institute clinical management strategies that can facilitate functional communication and ensure safe swallowing.

TABLE 5. *Occurrence of motor speech and swallowing disturbatices in CBD*

Clinical symptom (Mean duration of disease)	Present findings (*N* = 15) (3. 7 yrs; SD 1.6)	Riley et al. (3) findings (*N* = 15) (5.8 yrs; SD	Wenning et al. (4) findings (at first visit) (*N* = 14) (3.0 yrs; SD 1.9)	Wenning et al. (4) findings (at last visit) (*N* = 14) (6.1 yrs; SD 2.0)
Apraxia (oral and/or verbal)	6 (46%)*	NA	NA	NA
Dysarthria	13 (93%)†	7 (47%)	4 (29%)	9 (75%)
Dysphagia	12 (86%)†	2 (13%)	NA	NA

* Missing data in two patients.
† Missing data in one patient.

The distinguishing features of CBD from other neurodegenerative disorders (specifically, Parkinson's disease, progressive supranuclear palsy [PSP], and Alzheimer's disease) are found in the combination of motor speech and swallowing deficits *when coupled with* findings of asymmetric features, ideomotor apraxia, language disturbances, or the alien limb phenomenon referable to dysfunction of both cerebral cortex and basal ganglia. It is hoped that in-depth clinical investigation can assist in differential diagnosis and bring us closer to a clearer definition of CBD as a distinctive clinical-pathologic entity.

REFERENCES

1. Duffy J. *Motor speech disorders: Substrates, differential diagnosis, and management.* St. Louis: Mosby, 1995.
2. Darley FL, Aronson AE, Brown JR. *Motor speech disorders.* Philadelphia: WB Saunders, 1975.
3. Riley DE, Lang AE, Lewis A, et al. Cortical-basal ganglionic degeneration. *Neurology* 1990;40:1203–1212.
4. Wenning GK, Litvan I, Jankovic J, Granata R, Mangone CA, McKee A. Natural history and survival of 14 patients with autopsy-confirmed corticobasal degeneration. *J Neurol Neurosurg Psychiatry* 1998;64: 184–189.
5. Rebeiz JJ, Kolodny EH, Richardson EP. Corticodentatonigral degeneration with neuronal achromasia. *Arch Neurol* 1968;18:20–33.
6. Watts RL, Williams RS, Growdon JD, Young RR, Haley EC Jr, Beal MF. Corticobasal degeneration (abstract). *Neurology* 1985;35(suppl 1):178.
7. Gibb WR, Luthert PJ, Marsden CD. Corticobasal degeneration. *Brain* 1989;112:1171–1192.
8. Lang AE, Bergeron C, Pollanen MS, Ashby P. Parietal Pick's disease mimicking cortical-basal ganglionic degeneration. *Neurology* 1994;44:1436–440.
9. Sonies B, Weiffenbach J, Atkinson J, Brahim J, Macynski A. Clinical examination of motor and sensory functions of the adult oral cavity. *Dysphagia* 1987a;1:178– 186.
10. National Institutes of Health, W. G. Magnuson Clinical Center, Rehabilitation Medicine Department, Speech-Language Pathology Section. Speech Parameters Ratings. Bethesda, MD: author, 1988.
11. Sonies B, Parent L, Morrish K, Baum B. Durational aspects of the oral-pharyngeal phase of swallowing in normal adults. *Dysphagia* 1987b;3:637–638.
12. Sonies C, Baum B. Evaluation of swallowing pathophysiology. *Otolaryngol Clin North Am* 1988;21:637–648.
13. Logemann JA. *Manual for the videofluorographic study of swallowing.* Austin, TX: Pro-Ed, 1986.
14. Helm-Estabrooks N. *Test of oral and limb apraxia,* normed ed. Chicago, IL: Riverside, 1992.
15. Litvan I, Agid Y, Goetz C, et al. Accuracy of the clinical diagnosis of corticobasal degeneration: A clinicopathologic study. *Neurology* 1997;48:119–125.
16. Duvoisin RC. Clinical diagnosis. In: Litvan I, Agid Y, eds. *Progressive supranuclear palsy.* New York: Oxford University Press, 1992:15–33.
17. Albert ML, Feldman RG, Willis AL. Anatomoclinical and biochemical concepts of subcortical dementia. In: Stahl SM, Iversen SD, Goodman EC, eds. *Cognitive neurochemistry.* New York: Oxford Science Publications, 1974:248–271.
18. Yamauchi H, Jukuyama H, Nagahama Y, Katsumi Y, Dong Y, Hayashi T, Konishi J, Kimura J. Atrophy of the corpus callosum, cortical hypometabolism, and cognitive impairment in corticobasal degeneration, 1998.
19. Wechsler DA. *Wechsler Adult Intelligence Scale—Revised.* New York: Psychological Corporation, 1981.
20. Sonies BC. Swallowing and speech disturbances. In: Litvan I, Agid Y, eds. *Progressive supranuclear palsy.* New York: Oxford University Press, 1992.
21. Murray GM, Sessle BJ. Functional properties of single neurons in the face primary motor cortex of the primate. 1. Input and output features of tongue motor cortex. *J Neurophysiol* 1992;7:747–758.
22. Car A. (1970). La commande corticale du centre deglutiteur bulbaire. *J Physiol (Paris)* 1970;62:361–386.
23. Miller AJ, Bowman, JP. Precentral cortical modulation of mastication and swallowing. *J Dental Res* 1977;56:1154.

Corticobasal Degeneration.
Advances in Neurology, Vol. 82,
edited by I. Litvan, C. G. Goetz, and A. E. Lang.
Lippincott Williams & Wilkins, Philadelphia © 2000.

15

Eye Movement Disorders in Corticobasal Degeneration

Marie Vidailhet* and Sophie Rivaud-Péchoux†

**Department of Neurology, Hôspital Saint Antoine, 75012 Paris, France; and †INSERM U 289, Hôspital de la Salpêtrière, 75651 Paris, Cedex 13 France*

INTRODUCTION

Among the parkinsonian syndromes, corticobasal degeneration (CBD) is remarkable for diversity of neurological features at onset when diagnosis is uncertain. In clinical practice, it is sometimes difficult to differentiate between CBD and progressive supranuclear palsy (PSP) either at an early stage of the disease or when atypical forms of CBD are observed. In the last decade, authors have expanded the description of clinical and pathological features. Initially, little attention was paid to oculomotor abnormalities in CBD; however, subsequently a variety of dysfunctions were clinically described (1–3). In the bedside oculomotor examination, horizontal and vertical saccades and horizontal and vertical smooth pursuit could provide helpful clues for the clinical diagnosis of CBD or PSP. The oculomotor disturbances observed in these two diseases are important to differentiate them from multiple system atrophy and Parkinson's disease where eye movements appear clinically normal (Table 1). In contrast to PSP, in most CBD patients, horizontal eye movements are affected as much as vertical ones (5). At bedside testing, initiation of horizontal saccades can be delayed and some patients seem unable to produce voluntary horizontal saccades, but are improved when something is given to them to look at (1,4). Head movements and eye blinking are used to initiate voluntary saccades (5). Restriction in the range of horizontal or vertical saccadic and pursuit eye movements are observed, often at a late stage of the disease (3). Reflexive visually guided saccades and optokinetic nystagmus can be obtained (5). Additional signs, such as eyelid apraxia and blepharospasm, have also been reported (2,5). In PSP patients, vertical saccades, either in upward or downward directions, are more affected than horizontal ones. From the primary position of gaze to a target, eye movements are slow and hypometric, the eyes reaching the target in multiple steps. Then reduced amplitude is observed in vertical and later in horizontal directions. Eye movement recording is a readily available laboratory test that is very helpful in differentiating between various parkinsonian syndromes (6,7). Moreover, we have shown that the study of horizontal visually guided saccades also distinguishes between CBD and PSP (6). In this chapter, we will review the main disturbances of eye movements found in the early stages of CBD, when the diagnosis is most problematic. We will also confirm that the main discriminative characteristics of CBD are still observed at a later stage of the disease and that repeated eye movement recordings allow the documentation of discriminative parameters that minimize the incorrect diagnosis of CBD, especially in atypical forms of the disease (8).

TABLE 1. *Bedside oculomotor examination*

	Horizontal visually guided saccades	Vertical gaze impairment	Smooth pursuit	Blepharospasm or eyelid apraxia
CBD	Can be impaired at an early stage Eye blinking to initiate voluntary saccades Delay of initiation of saccades	Can appear at a later stage	Normal or slow	Can be present
PSP	Can be impaired at a later stage	Can be impaired at an early stage Slow, hypometric saccades Multiple steps to reach the target Decrease of normal amplitude	Saccadic and slow	Can be present
MSA	Normal	Normal	Normal or saccadic	Rarely present
PD	Normal	Normal	Normal	Very rarely present

EYE MOVEMENT IN CBD AT AN EARLY STAGE OF THE DISEASE

Within parkinsonian syndromes, only CBD and PSP have disorders of ocular motility that could be detected at clinical examination. However, clinicians cannot fully rely on the bedside examination to make the diagnosis. Precise identification of oculomotor dysfunction requires laboratory testing and we showed that simple measurements of eye movements can be used routinely in the examination of these patients, especially at a early stage of the disease (6). Other groups both for vertical and horizontal saccades (7) confirmed these results.

In the following section, we will summarize the main results of a comparative study of eye movements recorded by DC electrooculography (EOG) as described elsewhere (9) in CBD and PSP patients (6). The inclusion criteria for CBD were a parkinsonian syndrome without significant improvement with L-dopa, clear asymmetry of abnormal signs with dystonia and myoclonus, apraxia, and the absence of focal lesions on MRI. In the CBD group, because apraxia is characteristic of the disease, a left and right "apraxia score" was determined for each patient (10). The inclusion criteria (11) for PSP were a parkinsonian syndrome without significant improvement with L-dopa, the presence of at least a slight downward saccade impairment, falls, pseudobulbar palsy or dysarthria, frontal lobe-like signs, a progressive course of the disease, and absence of focal lesions on MRI or CT scan. A global "frontal score" was determined for each patient (12,13).

Vertical Saccades

In the CBD group, downward saccades were slightly impaired in three patients, upward saccades were slightly or moderately impaired in seven patients. In the PSP group, downward saccade paralysis was observed in seven patients, impairment was moderate in two and slight in one.

Horizontal Saccades

The horizontal eye movements observed in CBD patients were relatively homogeneous from one patient to another. Mean results of horizontal eye movements are shown in Table 2. In the CBD group, saccade latency was markedly and significantly increased bilaterally compared with that of the control group and that observed in PSP group ($p < 0.001$). A relationship was observed between the apraxia score and the saccade latency (the longer the saccade latency, the more marked the apraxia). There was a significant correlation for leftward values (Spearman's $r = 0.786$, $p < 0.05$) but not for rightward values.

In the antisaccade task, the percentage of errors in the CBD group did not differ from the control group, whereas in the PSP group, the percentage of errors was markedly and significantly increased compared with that of control group ($p < 0.001$).

TABLE 2. *Mean horizontal saccade values*

	Latency (msec) (mean ± SD)		Antisaccade (mean % of errors, range)	
	Right	Left	Right	Left
Controls ($N = 10$)	203 ± 30	198 ± 20	11 (0–30)	10 (0–30)
CBD ($N = 10$)	355 ± 94	382 ± 97	52 (0–100)	22 (0–60)
PSP ($N = 10$)	183 ± 101	224 ± 72	82 (25–100)	65 (10–100)

This percentage of errors was significantly higher than that existing in the CBD group.

In conclusion, in CBD, horizontal saccade latencies were significantly and markedly increased. Latency of horizontal saccades is increased bilaterally in patients with focal lesions affecting the posterior parietal cortex (14). The relationship between parietal damage and the increase in saccade latency and the correlation found between latency and the "apraxia score" are supported by metabolic studies (15–17) and anatomical studies (1–4,18). In PSP, the decreased velocity of horizontal saccades could be explained by damage to the pontine paramedian reticular formation. The marked percentage of errors in antisaccades that correlated with the frontal score, is in accordance with a prefrontal cortex dysfunction (9). As metabolic studies have shown, there is a bilateral frontal deafferentation from subcortical structures in PSP (11). The main conclusion is that abnormalities of horizontal saccade parameters in the CBD group contrasted with those observed in the PSP group and contribute to an early diagnosis of CBD and PSP.

LONGITUDINAL STUDY OF VISUALLY GUIDED SACCADES IN CBD

Very little is known about the evolution of eye movement disturbances in CBD, in contrast with PSP (9). It has been said that "with further progression of CBD, saccade and pursuit movements may be impaired in a fashion that is more consistent with PSP" (5). We showed (8) that the main discriminative characteristics of CBD described in the preceding are still observed at a later stage of the disease, and that sequential eye movement recordings enhance the documentation of parameters that discriminate between CBD and PSP, especially in atypical forms.

In the following section, we will summarize the main results of a longitudinal study of eye movements in CBD and PSP patients (8). These patients were different from those of the early study (5). Characteristics of the patients are summarized in Table 3. The inclusion criteria (19) for PSP were a gradually progressive disorder, onset at age 40 or later, vertical supranuclear either upward or downward gaze abnormalities, prominent postural instability with falls in the first year of disease

TABLE 3. *Follow up examination*

		Duration of evolution (months)*		
	Age (years) (mean ± SD) (range)	Initial visit (mean ± SD) (range)	Last EOG examination (mean ± SD) (range)	Last clinical visit (mean ± SD) (range)
PSP	69.1 ± 7.7	22.3 ± 7.5	29.4 ± 9.3	33.7 ± 10.3
($N = 7$)	(58–80)	(12–36)	(14–41)	(22–51)
Probable CBD	58 ± 6.5	23.2 ± 5.6	34 ± 4.5	38 ± 7
3 left/3 right	(51–72)	(12–27)	(29–39)	(29–46)
CBD-like	66.3 ± 3.2	26 ± 3.4	43.3 ± 8.4	47.7 ± 10.1
3 left	(64–70)	(24–30)	(38–53)	(40–53)

* Duration of evolution at the first and last EOG examination, and last clinical visit (first EOG examination = initial visit).

onset, absence of other neurological disease, absence of lesion on MRI or CT scan, absence of dementia, hallucinations, autonomic disturbances, or asymmetry of parkinsonian signs. The inclusion criteria (20) for CBD were a chronic progressive course, asymmetric at onset, the presence of higher cortical dysfunction (either ideomotor apraxia, cortical sensory loss or alien limb), a rigid/akinetic syndrome resistant to L-dopa, dystonic posture or focal spontaneous or action-induced myoclonus, absence of cognitive disorders other than apraxia or speech disorders, absence of dementia, absence of dysautonomia or hallucinations. Six patients (Table 3) met all the inclusion criteria and were considered as probable CBD. A subgroup of three patients (Table 3) was identified as "CBD-like" patients. The three patients presented with akineto-rigid parkinsonian syndrome unresponsive to L-dopa, markedly asymmetric, predominating on the left side, with mild to severe hand dystonia. One patient had mild cortical sensory loss. Two patients had left-sided apraxia. One patient had difficulties in fine movements when using objects without apraxia. Because of the lack of apraxia and early postural instability, this patient was included in the CBD-like group. The two other patients classified as CBD-like presented with a severe frontal syndrome and postural instability with frequent traumatic unexpected falls since the early stage of the disease, which were considered to be unusual in CBD.

Vertical Saccades

Vertical saccades were severely impaired in the PSP group, whereas they were only moderately impaired in the probable CBD group. In the CBD-like group, impairment of vertical saccades increased with the disease duration, and reached the level observed in PSP.

Horizontal Saccades

Probable CBD Group

In patients with dystonia present on the left side, significant ($p < 0.05$) increased leftward saccade latency was observed on the first examination, and this was more significant ($p < 0.006$) on the second examination (Table 4). This result was also observed in patients with dystonia observed on the right side but was not significant. Independently, the CBD patients were consistent with the initial diagnosis as shown by the increase in the CBD "score" between the first and last visits (Fig. 1).

CBD-Like Group

In three patients, early square wave jerks (Fig. 2), decreased saccade velocity, and high percentage of errors in the antisaccade test were observed, which are EOG characteristics of PSP. Independently, the initial clinical diagnosis of CBD was questioned and the diagnosis of PSP was subsequently made as more signs of PSP appeared with time, such as marked postural instability and falls and a severe frontal lobe-like syndrome illustrated by an increased "PSP score" (Fig. 3). When compared to the diagnosis obtained from EOG, the clinical diagnosis of PSP was made at the same time as the appearance of oculographic characteristics of PSP in one and only 4 and 6 months later in the two others.

TABLE 4. *Longitudinal study of horizontal saccade values*

	Latency (ms) (mean ± SD)				Velocity (°/s) (mean ± SD)			
	First examination		Last examination		First examination		Last examination	
	Right	Left	Right	Left	Right	Left	Right	Left
Left probable CBD (*N* = 3)	187 ± 4.5	*271 ± 30	199 ± 30	†295 ± 29	298 ± 33	266 ± 41	279 ± 54	273 ± 76
Right probable CBD (*N* = 3)	233 ± 79	195 ± 23	250 ± 25	214 ± 23	296 ± 40	328 ± 55	312 ± 55	307 ± 39
Left CBD-like (*N* = 3)	217 ± 58	247 ± 55	264 ± 79	233 ± 49	182 ± 26	195 ± 23	153 ± 44	147 ± 40
PSP (*N* = 7)	223 ± 79	208 ± 50	226 ± 69	194 ± 32	172 ± 47	161 ± 59	‡147 ± 62	§130 ± 55

Comparison between left and right saccades: *$p < 0.05$; †$p < 0.01$.
Comparison between first and last examination: ‡$p < 0.05$; §$p < 0.01$.

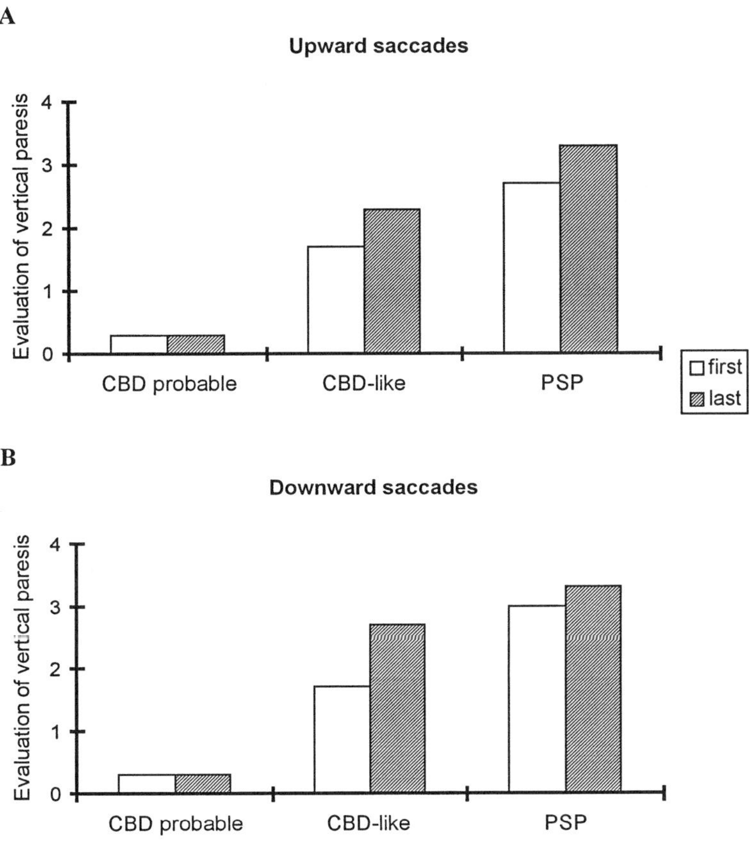

FIG. 1. Longitudinal study of vertical saccade impairment. 0 = normal saccade; 1 = when velocity was decreased but still permits the target to be reached; 2 = both decrease in saccade velocity and reduction in the final amplitude; 3 = when the eyes remain on the medline in one direction; 4 = complete paresis.

PSP Group

In these patients a progressive decrease in saccade velocity throughout the disease was observed (Table 4). During the follow-up clinical study, the diagnosis in the PSP patients remained consistent with the initial diagnosis as shown by the consistency in the "PSP score" between the first and last visits.

Longitudinal study of eye movements in both clinically diagnosed CBD and PSP patients demonstrates that the main characteristic of CBD (i.e., an increase in saccade latency of reflexive visually guided saccades) is consistent during the evolution of the disease and that asymmetry of saccade latency is also a helpful and persistent abnormality, and is characteristic of CBD. In the possible CBD group, early square wave jerks, decreased saccade velocity, and high percentage of errors in the antisaccade test were "red flags" and were more suggestive of the diagnosis of PSP. Independently, in the 4 to 6 months following the EOG recording, the early clinical diagnosis of CBD in our CBD-like group was questioned and the diagnosis of PSP was made.

Two consecutive EOG recordings 6 or more months apart improve the accuracy of diagnosis of CBD versus PSP. In individual patients, EOG abnormalities may precede the clinical diagnosis in accuracy and reliability. This technique may also be helpful in atypical cases of CBD (21–23) or when CBD mimicks Pick's disease (24–26) or PSP. (27,28).

ACKNOWLEDGMENTS

We thank Dr. C. Pierrot-Deseilligny for his help and valuable advice and Drs. Duclos and Vaunaize for kindly allowing us to test their patients.

A

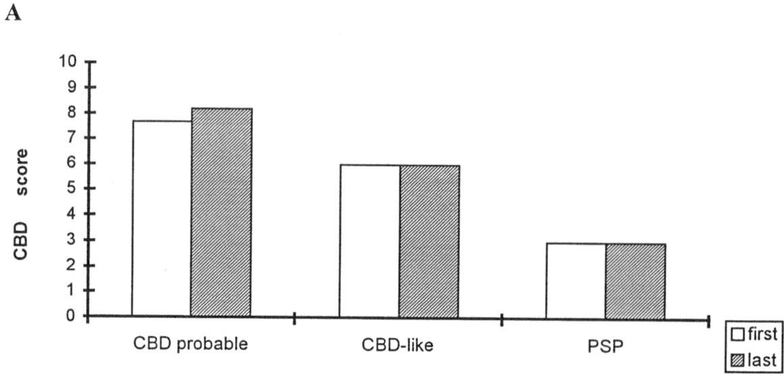

B

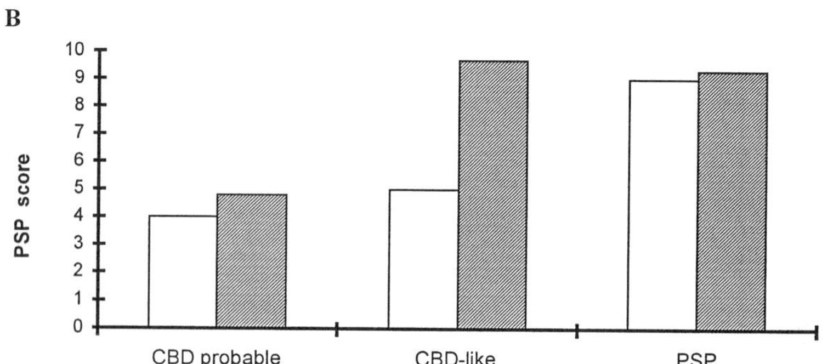

FIG 2. CBD "scores" and PSP "scores" in the probable and possible CBD and in the PSP groups. **A:** CBD "scores" from Litvan et al. (19) (maximum score = 10). Each of the following items = 1: chronic progressive course; parkinsonian syndrome; absence of response to L-dopa; asymmetry at onset; ideomotor apraxia; cortical sensory loss; alien limb syndrome; dystonic limb posture; spontaneous or reflex myoclonus; and absence of cognitive disturbance other than apraxia or speech disorder (at onset). **B:** PSP "scores" from Blin et al. (19) (maximum score = 10). Each of the following items = 1: chronic progressive course; parkinsonian syndrome; absence of response to levodopa; duration < 10 years; postural instability and falls; dysarthria; pseudo-bulbar syndrome; axial rigidity/dystonia; vertical eye movements impairment; and frontal syndrome.

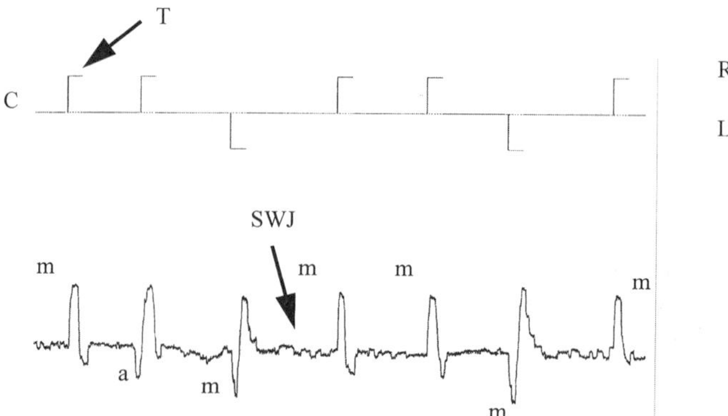

FIG. 3. Eye movement recording of a possible CBD patient in the antisaccade paradigm. C = central fixation; T = target; L = left; R = right; a = antisaccade; m = misdirected saccade; SWJ = square-wave jerks.

REFERENCES

1. Rebeiz JJ, Kolodny EH, Richardson EP. Corticodentatonigral degeneration with neuronal achromasia. *Arch Neurol* 1968;18:20–33.
2. Riley DE, Lang AE, Lewis A, et al. Cortico-basal ganglionic degeneration. *Neurology* 1990;40:1203–1212.
3. Rinne JO, Lee MS, Thompson PD, Marsden CD. Corticobasal degeneration: a clinical study of 36 cases. *Brain* 1994;117:1183–1196.
4. Gibb WRG, Luthert PJ, Marsden CDM. Corticobasal degeneration. *Brain* 1990;53:51–54.
5. Lang AE, Riley DE, Bergeron C. cortical-basal ganglionic degeneration. In: Calne DB, ed. *Neurodegenerative diseases.* Philadelphia: WB Saunders, 1994:877–894.
6. Vidailhet M, Rivaud S, Gouider-Khouja N, et al. Eye movements in parkinsonian syndromes. *Ann Neurol* 1994;35:420–426.
7. Rottach KG, Riley DE, Di Scenna AO, Zivotofosky AZ, Leigh RJ. Dynamic properties of horizontal and vertical eye movements in parkinsonian syndromes. *Ann Neurol* 1996;39:368–377.
8. Rivaud S, Vidailhet M, Gallouedec G, Litvan I, Pierrot-Deseilligny C. Eye movement disorders in corticobasal degeneration. 1999, submitted.
9. Pierrot-Deseilligny C, Rivaud S, Pillon B, Fournier E, Agid Y. Lateral visually-guided saccades in progressive supranuclear palsy. *Brain* 1989;112:471–487.
10. Pillon B, Blin J, Vidailhet M, Deweer B, Sirigu A, Dubois B, Agid Y. The neuropsychological pattern of corticobasal degeneration: comparison with progressive supranuclear palsy and Alzheimer's disease. *Neurology* 1995;45:1477–1483.
11. Blin J, Baron JC, Dubois B, et al. Positron emission tomography study in progressive supranuclear palsy. Brain hypometabolic pattern and clinicometabolic correlations. *Arch Neurol* 1990;47:747–752.
12. Pillon B, Dubois B, Lhermitte F, Agid Y. heterogeneity of cognitive impairment in progressive supranuclear palsy, Parkinson's disease and Alzheimer's disease. *Neurology* 1986;36:1179–1185.
13. Dubois B, Pillon B, Legault F, Agid Y, Lhermitte F. Slowing of cognitive process in progressive supranuclear palsy: comparison with Parkinson's disease. *Arch Neurol* 1988;45:1194–1199.
14. Pierrot-Deseilligny C, Rivaud S, Gaymard B, Agid Y. Cortical control of visually-guided saccades. *Brain* 1991;114:1473–1485.
15. Blin J, Vidailhet M, Pillon B, Dubois B, Feve JR, Agid Y. Corticobasal degeneration: decreased and asymmetrical glucose consumption as studied with PET. *Mov Disord* 1992;7:348–354.
16. Eidelberg D, Dhawan V, Moeller JR, et al. The metabolic landscape of cortico-basal ganglionic degeneration: regional asymmetries studied with positron emission tomography. *J Neurol Neurosurg Psychiatry* 1991; 54:856–862.
17. Brooks DJ. PET studies on corticobasal degeneration. *Mov Disord* 1996;11:349.
18. Wenning GK, Litvan I, Jankovic J, Granata R, Mangone CA, McKee AA, et al. Natural history and survival of 14 patients with corticobasal degeneration confirmed at post mortem examination. *J Neurol Neurosurg Psychiatry* 1998;64:184–189.
19. Litvan I, Agid Y, Calne D, et al. Clinical research criteria for the diagnosis of progressive supranuclear palsy (Steele-Richardson-Olszewski syndrome): report of the NINDS-SPSP international workshop. *Neurology* 1996; 47:1–9.
20. Litvan I, Agid Y, Goetz C, et al. Accuracy of clinical criteria for the diagnosis of corticobasal degeneration. A clinicopathologic study. *Neurology* 1997;48:119–125.
21. Schneider JA, Watts RL, Gearing M, Brewer RP, Mina SS. Corticobasal degeneration: neuropathologic and clinical heterogeneity. *Neurology* 1997;48:959–969.
22. Bergeron C, Pollanen MS, Weyer L, Black SE, Lang AE. Unusual clinical presentations of cortical-basal ganglionic degeneration. *Ann Neurol* 1996;40:893–900.
23. Boeve BF, Maraganore DM, Parisi, JE, et al. Clinical heterogeneity in patients with pathologically diagnosed cortico-basal ganglionic degeneration. *Mov Disord* 1996; 11:351.
24. Cambier J, Masson M, Dairou R, Henin D. Etude anatomo-clinique díune forme pariètale de maladie de Pick. *Rev Neurol* 1981;137:33–38.
25. Lang AE, Bergeron C, Pollanen MS, Ashby P. Parietal Pick's disease mimicking cortico-basal ganglionic degeneration. *Neurology* 1994;44:1436–1440.
26. Jendroska K, Rossor MN, Mathias CJ, Daniel SE. Morphologic overlap between corticobasal degeneration and Pick's disease. A clinicopathological report. *Mov Disord* 1995;10:111–114.
27. Feany MB, Mattiace LA, Dickson DW. Neuropathologic overlap of progressive supranuclear palsy and corticobasal degeneration. *J Neuropathol Exp Neurol* 1996.55: 53–67.
28. Litvan I, Campbell G, Mangone CA, et al. Which clinical features differentiate progressive supranuclear palsy (Steele-Richardson-Olszewski syndrome) from related disorders? *Brain* 1997;120:65–74.

Corticobasal Degeneration.
Advances in Neurology, Vol. 82,
edited by I. Litvan, C. G. Goetz, and A. E. Lang.
Lippincott Williams & Wilkins, Philadelphia © 2000.

16

Corticobasal Degeneration Look-alikes

Kailash P. Bhatia,* Myung S. Lee,* Juha O. Rinne,* Tamas Revesz,† Francesco Scaravilli,† Leo Davies,‡ C. David Marsden* *(d. 09/29/99)*

**University Department of Clinical Neurology and* †*Department of Neuropathology, Institute of Neurology, Queen Square, London WC1N 3BG, United Kingdom; and* ‡*Department of Clinical Neurophysiology, Royal Prince Alfred Hospital, New South Wales, Australia*

INTRODUCTION

Corticobasal degeneration (CBD) is a rare sporadic degeneration neurologic disease that usually begins in the late 50s or 60s. Since the initial description by Rebeiz et al. (1), many more cases with similar clinical features, with or without pathological verification, have been reported under the variable names of corticonigral degeneration with neuronal achromasia (1–3), corticobasal ganglionic degeneration (4–6), corticobasal ganglionic degeneration with neuronal achromasia (CBGD) (7), syndrome of progressive rigidity with apraxia (8), or corticobasal degeneration (CBD) (9–12).

The typical clinical phenotype of CBD (Table 1) is well described (11–15) most recently in three large series of patients (11–13), one of them with postmortem confirmation (12). The characteristic features of CBD are so distinctive that it is often possible to make a confident clinical diagnosis. However, prototypic phenotypes may have atypical (non-CBD) pathology and on the other hand there are also examples of atypical phenotypes who have classic CBD pathology (16). This chapter focuses on specific examples of the first with a review of other cases in the literature.

We describe five cases whose clinical features were suggestive of CBD, but who turned out to have different diseases. Two had extensive periventricular white matter ischemic lesions with multiple cerebral infarctions in the basal ganglia, one had sudanophilic leukodystrophy, one had tau positive inclusion bodies and Pick cells diagnostic of Pick's disease, and one had pathological findings of progressive supranuclear palsy (PSP).

CASE SUMMARIES

Case 1

A 64-year-old right-handed woman slowly developed progressive stiffness and clumsiness of the left hand. She complained that her left arm would not do what she wanted it to do. She had a past history of hypertension and ischemic heart disease. Left hand function deteriorated over the next 4 years, until it became completely useless. Her gait also became unsteady, and she began to fall while walking without obvious reason; the frequency of falls increased to six times a year. She also noted that her movements became slow, although her right arm remained normal. She had a trial of Madopar[R] (L-dopa and benzarazide) without benefit and so it was discontinued. She developed nocturia two to three times a night and urinary urgency, but there was no incontinence.

General physical examination revealed no abnormality other than high blood pressure (170/100 mmHg). She was cooperative and the content of speech was normal. Bedside mental function tests revealed mild short term memory impairment.

TABLE 1. *Symptoms and signs of our five CBD look-alike patients compared to two reported series‡ of patients with typical CBD*

Initial symptoms	Rinne et al. (11)	Wenning et al. (12)	Case 1	Case 2	Case 3	Case 4	Case 5
Clumsiness arm	64%	NA	+	+	+	+	+
Clumsy arm and leg	6%	NA	–	–	+	–	–
Gait	14%	NA	+	+	+	–	–
Speech	3%	NA	–	+	+	+	–
Clinical features		*/†					
Limb rigidity	80%	79/93%	+	+	+	+	+
Unilateral limb dystonia	83%	43/46%	+	+	+	+	+
Focal myoclonus	57%	25/23%	–	–	+	+	+
Bradykinesia	NA	71/92	+	–	+	+	+
Axial rigidity	NA	17/67%	–	–	+	–	–
Ideomotor apraxia	NA	64/75%	+	+	+	+	+
Alien limb phenomenon	50%	29/46%	–	–	+	–	–
Cortical sensory loss	37%	31/40%	–	+	+	–	–
Limited voluntary upgaze	90%	36/62%	+	+	–	+	–
Limited vertical pursuit	90%	31/58%	–	–	–	+	–
Cortical dementia	30%	36/42%	–	–	+	+	+
Frontal lobe release signs	NA	42/73%	–	–	+	+	+
Visual neglect	NA	7/15%	–	H	–	–	–

* The first figure refers to percentage at the first visit, and the second † refers to percentage at the last visit in the study of Wenning et al. (12). H = hemianopia; NA = not available.
‡ (From refs. 11 and 12, with permission.)

Psychometry revealed a verbal IQ of 115 and a performance IQ of 97. Her posture was stooped, and her gait was slow and cautious, wide-based, with some difficulty in heel-to-toe walking, but no definite gait ataxia. Romberg test was negative. Postural reflexes were impaired. There was slight limitation of upgaze, but otherwise the range of eye movement was full. Smooth pursuit eye movements were broken, and saccadic eye movements were hypometric bilaterally. Tongue movements were slow. Muscle tone was increased by rigidity in her left arm and leg, but axial tone was normal. The left arm showed dystonic posturing with flexion of the elbow, wrist, and little and ring fingers. There was no resting tremor or myoclonic jerks. She could not perform simple movements to verbal commands with her left arm and hand. She also failed to imitate complex postures with either hand. Right hand movements were slow. She had no ideational apraxia. Muscle power and cerebellar function in the right limbs were normal. Deep tendon reflexes were hyperactive in all four limbs, but more exaggerated in her left upper extremity. The plantar responses were flexor. Sensory function tests were normal.

Laboratory examinations, including full blood cell counts, serum biochemistry, VDRL (venereal disease reference laboratory), and TPHA (treponema pallidum haemagglutination assay), were all normal. There was a delay in cortical evoked potentials, especially on the left side, suggesting abnormal conduction of central sensory pathways. Brain MRI scan showed diffuse high signal intensities in the centrum semiovale and periventricular white matter bilaterally, with multiple small lesions in both the basal ganglia and the right insula, compatible with bilateral ischemic changes owing to small vessel disease. There was some asymmetry with a dilated lateral ventricle and sylvian fissure on the right side, suggesting a mild degree of cerebral atrophy.

Summary

This patient exhibited a progressive asymmetric syndrome of apraxia with rigidity and dystonia associated with abnormal eye movements and dysequilibrium. Although the clinical diagnosis was that of CBD, investigation showed extensive ischemic cerebrovascular diseases in the setting of hypertension.

Case 2

A 69-year-old right-handed man slowly developed clumsiness in his right hand. His first symptom was difficulty in tying a bow tie. He noticed increasing unsteadiness on walking and general slowness of movements from 1 year after the onset, but there were no falls. The right hand became increasingly clumsy, and 3 years after the onset, it developed jerky irregular tremor on movement. He described his right hand as not belonging to him; "Often I am unaware of my right hand and it won't do what I want it to do." He thought his left hand was normal. His right hand became useless. For example, he could not feed himself or pour a cup of tea. He had difficulty in reading because of problems scanning to the right. His speech became less fluent, and sometimes he noted a difficulty in finding the right word. He could not concentrate, and noticed some deterioration of ability to calculate. Initially, he had been treated with Sinemet^{R} 110 mg (L-dopa 100/carbidopa 10) four times a day and Madopar^{R} 250 mg (L-dopa 200/benserazide 50) six times a day, but there was no benefit and the drugs were discontinued. He complained of urinary frequency and occasional nocturia associated with hesitancy and poor stream, but no episodes of urinary incontinence.

He had a past history of occasional attacks of migraine. Nine years before the onset of the illness he suddenly became febrile, dysphasic, and subsequently stuporous. He recovered after 5 days, but was amnesic for the illness. The cerebrospinal fluid contained 15 white blood cells/mm^3 and 127 mg/dL of protein, but no further information was available.

There was no abnormality on general physical examination, except a raised blood pressure of 170/100 mmHg. He was unable to recall the present date, month, or name of the Prime Minister. His speech was slightly dysarthric, but with good volume. There were occasional hesitations in finding words, but his naming ability was good. Neuropsychological tests revealed a superior range verbal IQ of 123 and an average range performance IQ of 107. He had an impassive face. There was a right homonymous hemianopia with preservation of the fields along the horizontal meridian bilaterally. There was a slight bilateral optic atrophy. Upgaze was limited, and pursuit eye movements were jerky. Saccadic eye movements were hypometric with slow onset in all directions. The other cranial nerves were normal. His gait was unsteady and slow, and he carried his right arm flexed in front of him while walking. There was dystonic flexion at his right elbow and wrist, and he did not use this limb spontaneously. There was a jerky action tremor of the right arm, involving the proximal parts of the limb, but no rest tremor or stimulus sensitive myoclonus. Tone was increased by rigidity in the right arm and leg. Power was normal in all four limbs. There was no cerebellar dysfunction. Deep tendon reflexes were normal and symmetric. The plantar responses were flexor. Cutaneous sensation was normal, but joint position sense and stereognosis were defective in his right hand. He failed to imitate complex postures with either hand. There was no ideational apraxia.

Routine laboratory examinations including chest x-ray, full blood cell count, thyroid function tests, serum electrolytes, random blood sugar, liver function tests, cholesterol, and triglycerides were all normal. Serum B_{12} and folate were normal. Treponemal serology tests were negative. Protein C, protein S, antithrombin III, and lupus anticoagulant were normal. Cerebrospinal fluid examination was normal apart from a slightly increased protein of 62 mg/dL; there were no oligoclonal bands.

Nerve conduction studies were normal. Electroencephalogram revealed minor nonspecific abnormalities in the temporal region. Visual evoked potentials revealed abnormal asymmetrical delay in his right visual fields of both eyes, suggesting a right hemifield defect. T2-weighted MRI images of the brain (Fig. 1) revealed bilateral diffuse high signal intensities in the central

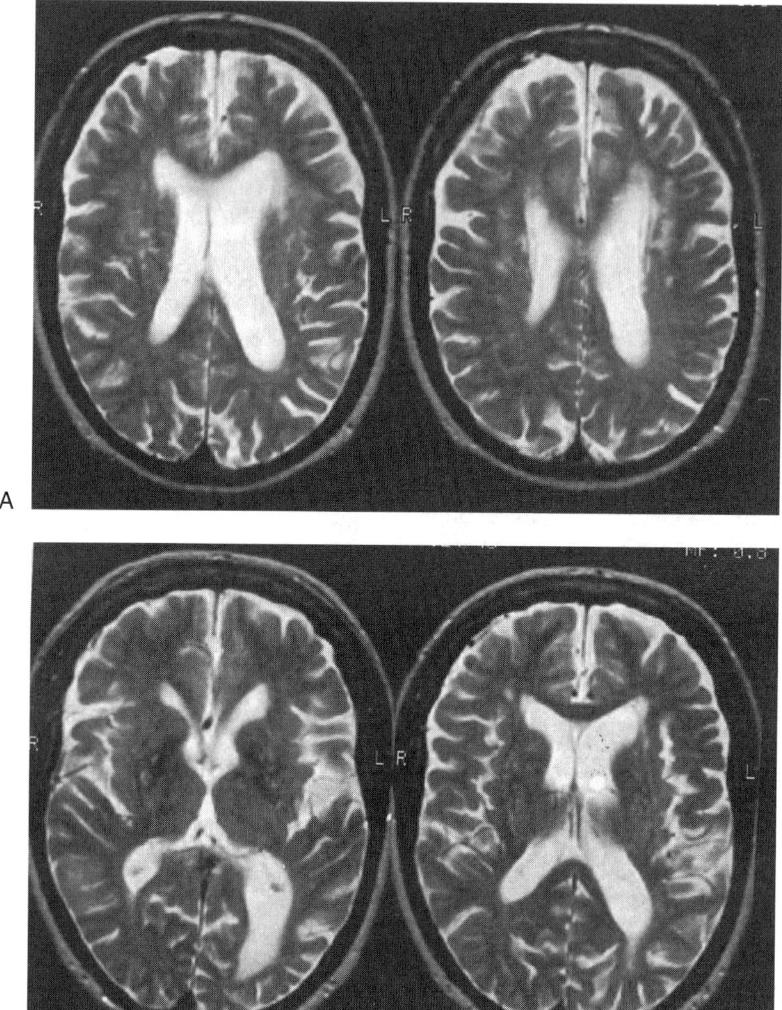

FIG. 1. A: T2 weighted axial MRI brain image of the Case 2 shows multiple scattered high signals lesions in the bilateral periventricular region, and **B:** multiple bilateral small high-signal intensity lesions involving basal ganglia and internal capsule.

and periventricular white matter, and multiple small lesions in the bilateral basal ganglia and pons (Fig. 1B), suggesting infarction owing to small vessel disease. T1-weighted coronal image showed asymmetrical ventricular dilatation.

Summary

Again, this patient exhibited a progressive asymmetric akinetic apraxic dystonic rigidity, with abnormal eye movements. However, atypically for CBD, he had a hemianopia, the character of which indicated a lesion of the lateral geniculate body, and brain imaging revealed widespread cerebrovascular disease.

Case 3

A 40-year-old right-handed motor mechanic developed the gradual onset of progressive difficulty in using his right hand. He dated his illness to a fall while playing football 6 months previously, although there was no head injury or alteration of consciousness. The next day he developed a pain in his right elbow, which disappeared over the course of a few days.

About 6 months later he gradually developed a tightness of his right hand and arm, causing difficulty in using the limb. About another 6 months later, he noticed jerky involuntary movements of the right hand. He also had pain in the right ankle while walking, which gradually worsened. He had a tendency to lose his balance while standing on his right leg, but no falls. The right leg became increasingly stiff, and he had to give up driving because of difficulty in operating the pedals with the right foot. An L-dopa challenge was negative, and oral treatment with Madopar^{R} (L-dopa 200/bensarazide 50) 750 mg and trihexyphenidyl 4 mg daily was of no benefit, so was stopped. After a year he began to notice that his right arm behaved as if it had a mind of its own. Involuntary, but apparently purposive, movements of that arm appeared. For example, while getting dressed his right hand gripped the clothes, and he needed to use his left hand to uncurl his right fingers. The shaking and jerking of his right arm worsened, and he became unable to write. His speech became slurred and he had difficulty in turning in bed. Two years after the onset, he was unable to stand because of dystonic contractures of his right foot, and he was confined to a wheelchair. He denied any changes in memory or sphincter control.

His 73-year-old mother and his two siblings were well. His father died at the age of 66 from a severe dementing illness. This began with headache, intermittent confusion, and an unsteady gait at the age of 65 years. Examination of his medical records showed that he had severe cognitive impairment with dysphasia, broad-based gait with a positive Romberg's test, and terminal intention tremor of both hands. The knee jerks were hyperactive bilaterally, and the right plantar reflex was equivocal, although his left was flexor. An air encephalogram was reported to show communicating hydrocephalus. An electroencephalogram revealed asymmetrical suppression of the background activity over the left hemisphere. Cerebrospinal fluid contained no cells, but a slightly increased protein of 60 mg/dL. VDRL was negative. No further information was available. There was no other family history.

Neurological examination 2 years after onset revealed a odd gait with circumduction of his right leg, and decreased right arm swing. There was axial rigidity and mild retropulsion, but postural reflexes were preserved. The visual fields were full and optic discs, retinae, and visual acuities were normal but he had red and green color blindness. He had a slow hypometric voluntary saccadic eye movements bilaterally. He had a reduced blink rate with a mask-like face. There was a grasp reflex of the right hand, but no snout or palmomental reflexes. There were hemidystonic postures on the right limbs with adduction of the shoulder, flexion of the elbow and wrist, and inversion of the foot. There were irregular spontaneous jerks of his right arm, but no stimulus sensitivity could be demonstrated. There was no utilization behavior or intermanual conflict, but his right hand closed involuntarily and followed the examiner's fingers. He was unable to mimic hand postures with either hand. He also failed to copy simple movements. He had ideomotor and ideational apraxia. His performance on visual perceptual tests remained normal. There was a slight increase in tone, mild pyramidal weakness and slow initiation of movements of the right limbs. Vibration, pain, and touch sensations were all normal, but joint position sense was slightly reduced in the right fingers and toes. Two point discrimination was mildly impaired on the fingers and there was a mild dysgraphesthesia. Romberg's sign was negative. His tandem gait was normal. Deep tendon reflexes were brisker on the right side. Left plantar reflex was flexor, but was equivocal on the right side. There were no abnormal cerebellar signs of his left extremities. Repeated psychometric tests over an interval of 14 months revealed no significant deterioration, and the last test revealed that he had a dull, average range verbal IQ of 89 and borderline defective range performance IQ of 74.

Routine investigations and serum ceruloplasmin and copper were all normal. Antithrombin III was within normal range, but protein C and protein S were increased to 150% (normal range: 70% to 140%) and 178% (normal range: 60% to

140%), respectively. Cerebrospinal fluid contained two white blood cells/mm^3, protein 38 mg/dL, and negative oligoclonal bands. Twenty-four-hour urinary vanyl mandelic acid was raised to 58 μmole/L. Screening for anticardiolipin antibodies and lupus anticoagulant were negative. White cell enzymes including β-hexosaminidase, total β-hexosaminidase, β-galactosidase, galactocerebrosidase, α-fructosidase, and arylsulfatase A were normal. Serologic tests for antibodies, including influenza A, influenza B, mycoplasma pneumoniae, adenovirus, psittacosis, coxiella, herpes simplex, herpes zoster, and measles were all negative. Poliovirus serology revealed BK virus titer of 1/10 and JC virus of 1/320. Long chain fatty acids ($C^{22,24,26}$) were normal. A jejunal biopsy looking for Whipple's disease was normal. Electroencephalography and motor evoked potentials were normal, as were cortical sensory evoked potentials to stimulation of the right median nerve. Electromyography revealed a small amplitude rapid action tremor of the right arm. Nerve conduction studies were normal. A left carotid angiogram only revealed mild irregularity of the internal carotid artery proximal to the siphon. T2-weighted MRI brain scan showed areas of high signal intensity in the corona radiata bilaterally (Fig. 2), suggesting a diffuse white matter disorder. T1-weighted coronal images showed asymmetric cerebral atrophy, more severe on the left side.

MRI stereotactic brain biopsy of the cerebral white matter lesions was performed. Peripheral parts of the sample contained well or relatively well preserved myelin, whereas central portions showed severe myelin loss. There was a gradual transition between the two areas. The lesion contained numerous astrocytes and occasional binucleated macrophages. The macrophages contained coarse granular material in their cytoplasm, which was yellowish in color in H&E staining, and dark-blue in the luxol fast blue and cresyl violet preparations. The granules were negative on the Perl's, but positive on the Schiff and Masson-Fontana staining for melamin preparation (Fig. 3A). There was loss of axons, but this was less severe than the demyelinating process. Axonal spheroids were also found (Fig. 3B). No evidence of an inflammatory process was found. Electron microscopic study showed some macrophages containing indistinct linear and circular profiles.

Summary

This man developed an asymmetric jerky dystonic apraxic rigid syndrome, with abnormal eye movements, and a suggestion of pyramidal signs and cortical sensory loss in the most affected

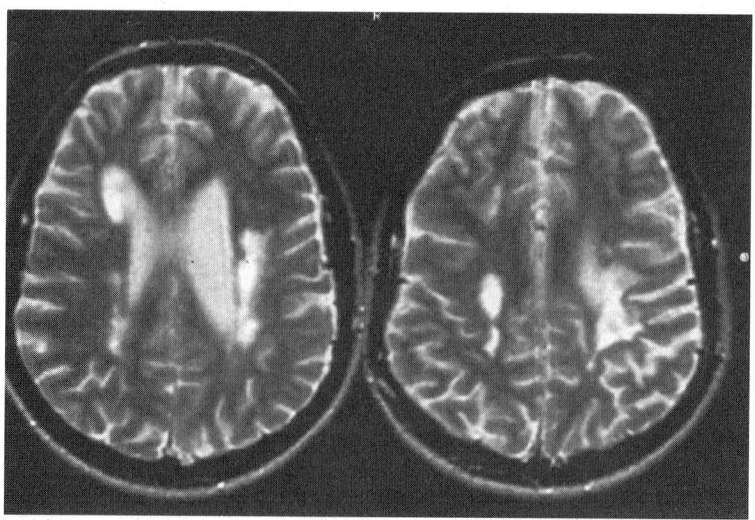

FIG. 2. T2-weighted saggital brain MRI image of Case 3 shows confluent patchy high-signal intensity lesions in the bilateral periventricular regions.

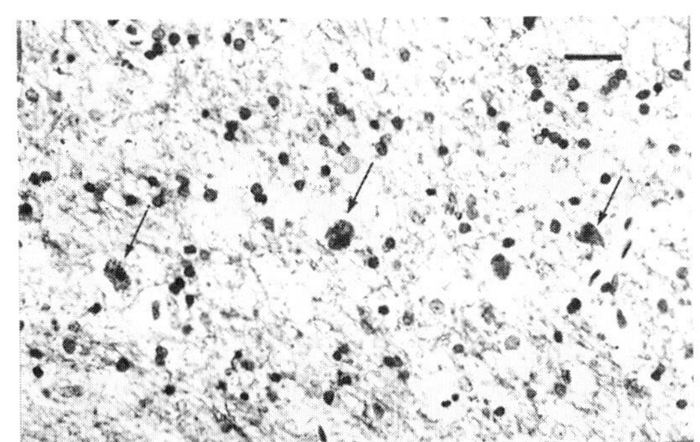

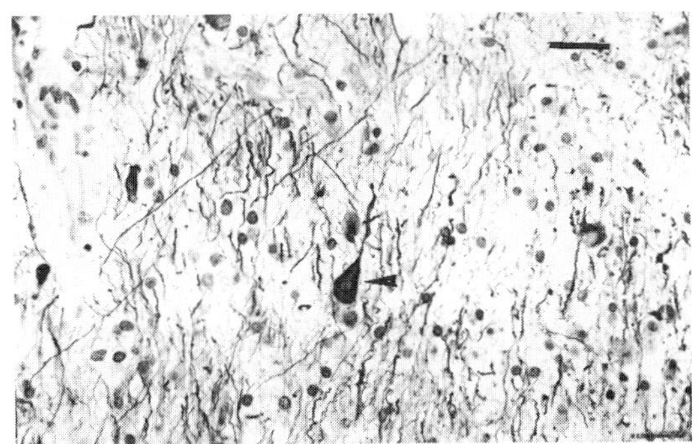

FIG. 3. A: A photomicrograph of cerebral white matter showing severe myelin loss and increased cellularity. Scattered macrophages with intracytoplasmic pigment are present (*arrows*). Luxol fast blue with cresyl violet ×150 (1 cm bar = 60 μm). **B:** Silver impregnation for axons demonstrating relative preservation of axons and occasional swelling (*arrowhead*). Glees and Marsland preparation ×150 (1 cm bar = 60 μm).

limbs. The clinical diagnosis was of CBD until the brain MRI revealed extensive white matter change. Brain biopsy revealed the pathology of a sudanophilic leukodystrophy.

Case 4

A 55-year-old right-handed woman developed gradual onset of clumsiness of her right hand. Initially, the difficulty was confined to fastening buttons and using a fork and knife, but it slowly progressed to affect other tasks such as writing. She was aware that her hand was not weak, but stated that "It just won't do what I want it to do." Her right arm became progressively stiff and would jerk whenever she attempted to use it. Along with the deterioration of right arm function, she developed language problems over a period of 2 years from the onset. Her speech became slurred and she noted difficulty in finding the right words. She also had difficulty in reading, and was intermittently unable to comprehend words that she had previously been able to understand. She had increasing problems with arithmetic, and was no longer able to calculate money when she shopped. She denied memory deterioration, and her husband reported that her personality was not changed. There were no symptoms referable to her legs and left arm. She developed urinary frequency. There was no significant family history of a dementing illness or of other neurologic diseases. Her past history was unremarkable.

On neurologic examination 2 years after the onset of the illness she was still alert and oriented. Spontaneous speech was reduced, slow and poorly articulated, and there was a nominal dysphasia. Posture and gait were normal. The initiation of voluntary saccades was impaired in both vertical and horizontal directions. She used head thrusts to break fixation and initiate eye movements. She was able to follow a moving target through a full range and optokinetic nystagmus was normal. She was unable to mimic movements with her face or either hand. She also failed to use simple objects with her hands. Tendon reflexes were normal and the plantar responses were flexor. There were bilateral grasp reflexes. Sensory examination was normal. CT brain scan showed mild cerebral atrophy.

The condition progressed so that 4 years after the onset she became totally dependent on her husband for daily living. Examination at this time showed that she required assistance to stand from a chair. Her posture was stooped, and gait was wide-based with normal-sized steps. There was no arm swing when she walked. Speech was barely intelligible with dysphasic errors. Visual fields were normal, and fundoscopic findings were unremarkable. There was a supranuclear vertical and horizontal saccadic gaze abnormality. Pursuit eye movements were jerky. She was able to close her eyes on command but they immediately reopened. Rooting reflex was prominent. Tone was increased in the right arm more than the left arm.

The right hand was held in a fist with flexion of the fingers and adduction of the thumb, which protruded between the middle and ring fingers. The right arm was flexed at the elbow and adducted at the shoulder. Voluntary movement of the right arm was limited to elevation of the shoulder and slight flexion of the shoulder. Action and stimulus sensitive myoclonus was present in the right arm. There was plastic rigidity in all four limbs and the power appeared to be normal. Tendon reflexes were brisk, particularly on the right with finger jerks. The plantar reflexes were extensor on both sides. Sensory tests were normal. Routine investigations were normal. Cerebrospinal fluid examination was normal, and there was no oligoclonal bands. Electroencephalogram was of low amplitude, but exhibited no specific abnormalities. Psychometry revealed a verbal IQ of 78 and a performance IQ of 96, which were not significantly different from her performance 4 years previously. Verbal memory was intact, but there was a significant deterioration in visual memory.

A right frontal cortical biopsy performed 4 years after the onset showed a normal arrangement of cortical architecture and subcortical myelin, but there was an increase in the number of astrocytes. In the deeper cortical layers there were achromatic swollen cells with eccentric nuclei and complete loss of Nissl's substance.

Immunohistochemical staining for phospholated neurofilaments (RT 97), tau protein, and ubiquitin was carried out. The cytoplasm of some of the ballooned cells was positive on all three preparations (Fig. 4A). Intracytoplasmic inclusions with morphological features of Pick bodies showed an immunoreaction with anti-tau and anti-ubiquitin antibodies. Some inclusions had a sharply demarcated outer margin, but the majority had a fibrillary pattern with a blurred outer margin. Tau immunohistochemistry showed the presence of cortical neuropil threads and tau positive oligodendroglial cells in the white matter underlying cortex.

Summary

This patient developed a progressive jerky dystonic right hand, with buccofacial and limb apraxia and abnormal eye movements. She also exhibited early and slowly progressive dyscalculia dysphasia. However, psychometric tests in the first 4 years of the illness revealed no definite deterioration. Progressive dystonia and generalized parkinsonian features were prominent subsequent findings. Although early cognitive impairment was thought to be unusual, the most possible clinical diagnosis was CBD. However, the frontal cortical biopsy revealed tau-positive inclusions with morphological features of Pick bodies and tau-positive oligodendroglial cells suggestive of Pick's disease.

Case 5

The patient presented at the age of 57 when he noticed difficulty in performing routine tasks with his right hand. He worked as a collator in a printing works and the earliest difficulties were with handling multiple sheets of paper. Over the 6 months preceding his initial consul-

A
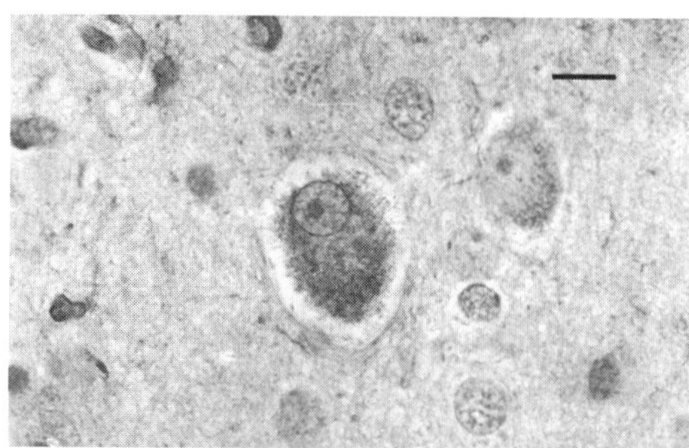
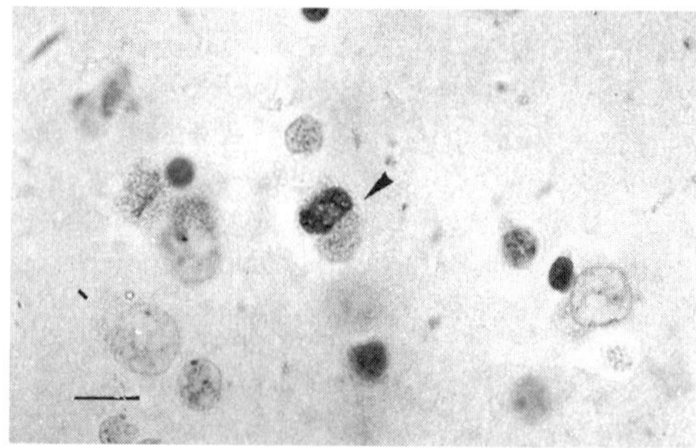
B

FIG. 4. Both the cytoplasm of Pick's cells (**A**) and the Pick bodies in small neurons (**B**) are positive on anti-tau immunostain (×750) (1 cm bar = 12 μm).

tation he had developed difficulty with writing, using his knife, and combing his hair with his right hand. He had also noticed that his hand tended to grasp things spontaneously if his palm brushed against them and that his hand would tend to make slow rhythmic involuntary squeezing movements. The patient was divorced and lived on his own. He drank to excess, averaging 150 grams of alcohol per day taken as beer. He took no medication and had no significant family history.

On examination he was found to be a man of normal intellect who gave a good account of his history and habits. He walked without swinging his right arm but with good stride length and turned freely. His facial expression was normal and dynamic. His visual acuity, fundi, eye movements, and lower cranial nerves were normal. There was rigidity in the right arm of plastic type but the tone in the other limbs was normal tone. The reflexes were normal and symmetrical and there were no Babinski signs. There was no tremor. The right arm was clumsy and he needed a mental effort to make movements with it. Proximal movements were made slowly but with near normal strength but he was unable to make rapid tapping movements with the fingers of the right hand. Although the patient could hold a pen, this was done in an awkward manner with exaggerated wrist flexion and a mass grasping movement with the fingers. No recognizable letters could be produced. Hand writing samples from a year previous showed a fair hand. The patient had a prominent grasp reflex to any palmar stimulation. Once the object was grasped the hand then tended to rhythmically grasp and release the object at about 1 Hz. The patient was aware of this but was unable to prevent it. The same rhythmic movements could be provoked by stroking the volar surface of the right forearm. Fine tapping movements of the left hand were very mildly impaired. There was no postural hypotension. A trial of Madopar (L-dopa and benserazide) to a maximum dose of 1.5 grams of L-dopa per day produced no effect on any of the symptoms or signs and the treatment was withdrawn. An MRI scan of the brain was reported to show mild generalized cerebral atrophy and moderate cerebellar atrophy. An FDG PET study of the brain showed marked hypometabolism of the left striatum and thalamus with relative hypometabolism of the left orbito-frontal cortex.

The patient was followed at 6-month intervals over the next 4 ½ years. Over this period the difficulties in the right arm slowly progressed. The arm became fixed in a flexed posture across the chest and the rhythmic movements became almost imperceptible because of the development of flexion contractures in the arm and hand. The fingers were held flexed with the thumb opposed against the first interphalangeal joint of the index finger. The left hand began to be noticeably involved with the development of rigidity in the left arm and clumsiness of the hand for fine tasks. The gait remained narrow-based with a reasonable stride length but the patient had several falls. In one of these he fractured his right olecranon process as he fell onto the useless right arm. He had some difficulty maintaining his stance against a push or pull, but no festination or retropulsion was evident. He retained an erect upright posture and the eye movements remained normal for both saccadic and pursuit movements in all directions of gaze.

At the age of 62 the patient was assaulted by an unknown assailant and died some days later. The general autopsy showed multiple bruises and contusions and bilateral hypostatic pneumonia. The brain weighed 1349 grams. On macroscopic examination there was moderate atrophy of the medial third of the left precentral gyrus. There was moderate ventricular dilatation and some darkening of the inner segment of the globus pallidus. There was mild atrophy of the cerebellar vermis and mild pallor of the substantia nigra.

On microscopic examination there was quite marked widespread vascular pathology affecting vessels in the white matter and the gray–white junction. This took the form of widened perivascular spaces with tortuous vessels and perivascular gliosis. Hemosiderin laden macrophages were evident in the perivascular spaces. Sections from the left motor cortex showed a focal area of damage with loss of lamination and thinning of the cortex. This area had few surviving neurons and a spongy state. There were neurofibrillary tangles in some of the remaining neurons. Ubiquitin stains were negative. The comparable area from the opposite side was normal. The hippocampus and inferior temporal cortex did not show any Alzheimer changes. Neurofibrillary tangles were present in the subthalamic nucleus, substantia nigra (pars compacta and reticulata), A10 dopaminergic nuclei, dorsal raphe, periaqueductal gray, and the locus ceruleus. The substantia nigra showed mild cell loss and gliosis but no Lewy bodies were seen. Sections through the cerebellum showed loss of Purkinje cells and vermian atrophy with corresponding cell loss in the inferior olives of the medulla. Tau stains showed the presence of tufted astrocytes that were tau-positive. There were no astrocytic tau plaques.

Summary

This patient developed an asymmetric rigid clumsy and increasingly dystonic arm followed by gait instability and falls without eye movement or bulbar problems, suggesting a clinical diagnosis of CBD. However, the distribution of the neurofibrillary changes on neuropathology and the presence of tufted astrocytes (and no astrocytic plaques) on tau stains were consistent with a diagnosis of PSP rather than CBD. In addition, there were changes of cerebral atheroma with focal cortical involvement and alcohol-related cerebellar degeneration.

DISCUSSION

All five cases had symptoms and signs compatible with the protype of typical CBD on clinical grounds (Table 1). The most prominent and early clinical features of these patients was a clumsy asymmetric rigid dystonia of an arm. They had other features characteristic of CBD, including ideomotor apraxia, difficulty in imitating finger postures, and alien limb behavior. They also had abnormal eye movements, gait disturbance, and impaired postural reflexes. All these deficits led us to suspect that they had CBD. However, atypical features were recognized in some of them. For example, Case 2 had a history of transient encephalitic illness. He had difficulty in reading owing to a right homonymous hemianopia, and had optic atrophy owing to a lateral geniculate body infarction. Case 4 gave a history of a father with a dementing illness. Cases 1 and 2 had an evidence of widespread cerebrovascular disease, and Case 3 had diffuse white matter lesions on brain MRI scans. In Cases 4 and 5 brain imaging studies showed only nonspecific degenerative changes; however, Case 4 had prominent early, but relatively stable, language problems and dyscalculia.

Cases 1 and 2 had extensive white matter lesions and multiple basal ganglia infarctions compatible with Binswanger's disease (17,18). About two-thirds of patients with Binswanger's disease present with slowly progressive deterioration of cognitive function, an abnormal gait, or postural impairment (19). They also may present with unexplained falls without warning or loss of consciousness, as in those with CBD (11). In such cases, there may be no apparent neurologic abnormalities between the falls. However, as the disease progresses, persistent abnormalities of gait become evident (20,21). Many also develop asymmetrical pyramidal, cerebellar, or extrapyramidal deficits (19). Rarely, apraxia has been reported (22). However, the clinical phenotype of CBD has not been widely reported with diffuse cerebrovascular disease.

Pigmentary sudanophilic leukodystrophy is a rare familial or sporadic adult onset neurologic disease usually characterized by a progressive frontal lobe syndrome and spastic tetraparesis (23–25). The demyelination mainly affects the centrum semiovale, internal capsule, and corpus callosum. Sometimes there is atrophy of the superior frontal and inferior temporal cortex (24,26), and of the thalamus, cerebellar dentate nucleus, and basal ganglia including caudate, globus pallidus, and subthalamic nucleus (24,27–29). Behavior changes with progressive cognitive impairment are the most frequent initial symptoms. Stimulus sensitive asymmetric myoclonus (24,25), and mild parkinsonian features including cogwheel rigidity, a mask-like face, and a short-stepped gait have been described (24,28,29). There have been rare reports of other leukoencephalopathies presenting with an akinetic rigid syndrome (30). However, no cases with sudanophilic leukodystrophy have been reported with the clinical features of CBD.

Classic Pick's disease associated with well demarcated frontotemporal atrophy often starts with behavioral and personality changes before the age of 65 years (31–33). Litvan et al. (34) recently suggested that the best predictors for an accurate diagnosis of Picks disease apart from frontal dementia were absence of apraxia and of a gait disturbance at onset. Patients with Pick's disease usually develop symmetrical mild extrapyramidal symptoms in the late stage of the illness, but additional movement disorders are rare (35–38). The majority have clinical features quite different from those of typical CBD.

However, the pathological and clinical boundaries between atypical cases of Pick's disease and CBD are not so clear. Pick bodies are found only in about one-third of the cases who were pathologically diagnosed as having Pick's disease (32,39). Many of those without Pick bodies share common pathologic features with CBD, with cerebral atrophy affecting the frontal lobes but extending posteriorly to the precentral cortex, and with relative preservation of the white matter and temporal cortex; degeneration of the basal ganglia and thalamus are common (32,37,38). The ultrastructural and histochemical characteristics of the inclusion bodies in such cases of generalized Pick's disease may be different from those seen in classical Pick's disease, raising the possibility that they may have a different pathogenesis (36). Patients with generalized Pick's disease have additional extrapyramidal deficits more frequently than those with classical Pick's disease, although some cases with severe degeneration of the frontal cortex and basal ganglia may have no parkinsonian features during life (35–38).

Atypical cases of Pick's disease showing clinical features suggestive of CBD have been described. Cambier et al. (40) reported a 66-year-old woman who initially presented with difficulty in using her right hand. Later, she developed dystonia, myoclonus, and athetosis of that arm. The other limbs were progressively affected, but there was no cognitive deterioration. Pathological study revealed bilateral asymmetrical parietal lobe atrophy with Pick's bodies, but the basal ganglia were preserved. Another report mentions a patient who initially developed speech and memory impairment at the age of 67 years (41). Subsequently increased tone and cogwheel rigidity appeared in all four limbs. Eight years after the onset, she developed an asymmetric dystonic posture of the left arm. Postmortem pathological study revealed asymmetric superior frontal lobe atrophy with swollen achromatic neurons. There was marked degeneration in the basal ganglia and thalamus.

Although no Pick bodies were found, the authors preferred the diagnosis of Pick's disease to CBD because of the preservation of parietal lobe and the presence of neuronal fiber loss in the white matter (41). More recently, Lang et al. (42) described a patient with pathologically proven asymmetric Pick's disease involving the parietal lobe who displayed a combination of parkinsonism, dyspraxia, and myoclonus mimicking CBD.

On the other hand, atypical cases of pathologically diagnosed CBD with prominent cognitive impairment from the onset or early in the course of the illness also have been reported (2,3,11, 16,43). Lippa et al. (3) reported two cases with pathology compatible with "corticonigral degeneration with neuronal achromasia." Their first case initially developed word finding difficulty, 1 year later symmetrical parkinsonian features, and 4 years after the onset, a dystonic posture of the right hand. Their second case initially developed memory deficit, and 1 year later, symmetrical parkinsonian features, but there were no dystonic postures. In both cases gross examination of the brain revealed moderate frontal atrophy with pale swollen cells, but no Pick bodies or neurofibrillary tangles were found. In subcortical nuclei only the substantia nigra was affected exclusively. Rinne et al. (11) reported a case (Case 9) who initially presented with gait difficulty and falls, and subsequently developed profound behavioral and personality changes. Pathological study revealed swollen ballooned cells in the deep layer of the frontal, parietal, temporal, and insular cortex and basophilic inclusions in the subcortical nuclei, but no Pick bodies were found.

Recently, Bergeron et al. (16) described three patients with the distinctive pathology of CBD who presented with cognitive change and only mild or delayed motor symptoms. In two of these patients who had severe dementia the pathological changes of CBD were extensive in the anterior frontal lobe, amygdala, and hippocampus, suggesting that the clinical presentation depended on the topographic distribution of the lesions (16).

Litvan et al., using the neuropsychiatric inventory (NPI) tool, found that patients with CBD commonly exhibit depression, apathy, irritability, and agitation (43). Clearly, there is an appreciable overlap between the clinical features and pathologic findings in atypical cases of Pick's disease and CBD. Whether CBD is a variant of Pick's disease, defined by its unusual topography of degeneration, which may itself determine the absence of clinical Pick bodies, remains to be established. Alternatively, Pick's disease or CBD may have different causes, but share common clinical and pathological features. A significant breakthrough in the pathological definition of these conditions has been the use of tau immunohistochemistry to differentiate the isoforms of tau in these conditions (44). Tau accumulates in the CBD brain as two polypeptides of 68 and 64 kDa, which are not recognized by antibodies specific to the adult tau sequences encoded by exons 3 and 10 of the tau gene in contrast to the tau doublet of Pick's disease (or of PSP) (44,45). CBD tau also has a unique ultrastructural appearance (45).

Apart from Pick's disease, mild to moderate symmetrical extrapyramidal deficits are common in patients with advanced Alzheimer's disease (46,47). However, rarely cases with clinical feature similar to those of CBD have been reported (8,48,49). For example, postmortem pathological study of a patient who had a progressive rigidity, apraxia, dysphasia, and synkinetic limb movements showed findings compatible with Alzheimer's disease (8).

PSP usually presents with unexpected falls as well as symmetric axial and proximal rigidity in contrast to unilateral predominant limb rigidity and dystonia in CBD. Apraxia, myoclonus, and cortical sensory loss seen in CBD are generally absent in PSP. Unilateral limb dystonia has been rarely described in pathologically confirmed cases of PSP (50). There is also a report of PSP proven on pathology in a patient who had an asymmetric akinetic-rigid syndrome with dystonia of the affected arm, abnormal eye movements (but normal downgaze), an alien limb, dyarthria and dysphagia, and an impaired gait (51). Clues pointing to PSP were normal sensation, absence of apraxia, and disproportionate atrophy of the midbrain in the brain MRI. Spontaneous arm levitation (without full-blown alien limb syndrome) can be seen in PSP (52). Marganore et al. (53) in an abstract also mention a case with the clinical features of CBD with the pathology of PSP.

Pathologically, there appears to be some overlap between PSP and CBD. However, there are also differences. Swollen neurons, which are abundant in CBD, are rare in the neocortex in PSP. Although neuronal and glial tau can be seen in both disorders, CBD cases exhibit a higher density of lesions in both cortex and subcortical white matter. Tau accumulates in PSP brains as a doublet repeat of polypeptides that differs from the tau triplet observed in Alzheimer's disease and the tau doublet of CBD or Pick's disease (44). Also, some suggest that tufted astrocytes occur in PSP and astrocytic plaques in CBD (54).

In conclusion, the cases reported here along with others in the literature indicate that the clinical phenotype of CBD forms a syndrome and may be owing to a number of different pathologies. Widespread cerebrovascular disease, sudanophilic leukodystrophy, Alzheimer's disease, and Pick's disease proper all must be considered in the differential diagnosis. Other causes include hemiatrophy-hemiparkinson syndrome (55), leukodystrophies (29), motor neuron disease (56), antiphospholipid syndrome (Huw Morris and Andrew Lees, personal communication) and some others may well be identified in the future. The clinical features CBD should prompt a review of such a differential diagnosis, and the presence of features atypical for classical CBD should increase the suspicion that some other pathology may be responsible.

REFERENCES

1. Rebeiz JJ, Kolondy EH, Richardson EP. Corticodentatonigral degeneration with neuronal achromasia: a progressive disorder of late adult life. *Trans Am Neurol Assoc* 1967;92:23–26.
2. Case Records of the Massachusetts General Hospital. Case 38-1985. *N Engl J Med* 1985;313:739–748.
3. Lippa CF, Smith TW, Fontneau N. Corticonigral degeneration with neuronal achromasia. A clinicopathological study of two cases. *J Neurol Sci* 1990;98:301–310.
4. Watts RL, Williams RS, Young RR, Haley EC. Corticobasal ganglionic degeneration. *Neurology* 1985;35 (suppl 1):178.
5. Riley DE, Lang AE. Corticobasal ganglionic degeneration (CBGD): further observations in six additional cases. *Neurology* 1988;38(suppl 1):360.

6. Greene PE, Fahn S, Lang AE, Watts RL, Eidelberg D, Powers JM. Case 1, 1990: progressive unilateral rigidity, bradykinesia, tremulousness, and apraxia, leading to fixed postural deformity of the involved limb. *Mov Disord* 1990;5:341–351.
7. Watts RL, Mirra SS, Young RR, Burger PC, Villier JA, Heyman A. Cortico-basal ganglionic degeneration (CBGD) with neuronal achromasia: Clinical-pathological study of two cases. *Neurology* 1989;39 (suppl 1):140.
8. LeWitt P, Friedman J, Nutt J, Korczyn A, Brogna C, Truong D. Progressive rigidity with apraxia: The variety of clinical and pathological features. *Neurology* 1989;39 (suppl 1):140.
9. Gibb WRG, Luthert PJ, Marsden CD. Corticobasal degeneration. *Brain* 1989;112:1171–1192.
10. Thompson PD, Marsden CD. Corticobasal degeneration. In: Rossor MN, ed. *Clinical neurology,* Vol. 1 (no 3). *Unusual dementia.* London: Baillière Tindall. 1992: 677–686.
11. Rinne JO, Lee MS, Thompson PD, Marsden CD. Corticobasal degeneration: a clinical study of 36 cases. *Brain* 1994;117:1183–1196.
12. Wenning GK, Litvan I, Jankovic J, et al. Natural history and survival of 14 patients with corticobasal degeneration confirmed at postmortem examination. *J Neurol Neurosurg Psychiatry* 1998;64:184–189.
13. Kompoliti K, Goetz CG, Boeve BF, et al. Clinical presentation and pharmacological therapy in corticobasal degeneration. *Arch Neurol* 1998;55:957–961.
14. Rebeiz JJ, Kolondy EH, Richardson EP. Corticodentatonigral degeneration with neuronal achromasia. *Arch Neurol* 1968;18:20–33.
15. Watts RL, Mirra SS, Richardson EP, Jr. Corticobasal ganglionic degeneration. In: Marsden CD, Fahn S, eds. *Movement Disorders 3.* Stoneham, UK: Butterworth-Heineman, 1994:282–289.
16. Bergeron C, Pollanen MS, Weyer L, Black SE, Lang AE. Unusual clinical presentations of cortico-basal ganglionic degeneration. *Ann Neurol* 1996;40:893–900.
17. Huang K, Wu L, Luo Y. Bingswanger's disease: Progressive subcortical encephalopathy of multi-infarct dementia. *Can J Neurol Sci* 1985;12:88–94.
18. Zimmerman RD, Fleming CA, Lee BCP, Saint-Louis L, Deck MDF. Periventricular hyperintensity as seen by magnetic resonance: prevalence and significance. *AJNR* 1986;7:13–20.
19. Babikan V, Ropper AH. Binswanger's disease: a review. *Stroke* 1987;18:2–12.
20. Thompson PD, Marsden CD. Gait disorder of subcortical arteriosclerotic encephalopathy: Binswanger's disease. *Mov Disord* 1987;2:1–8.
21. Nutt JG, Marsden CD, Thompson PD. Human walking and higher-level gait disorders, particularly in the elderly. *Neurology* 1993;43:268–279.
22. Dubas F, Gray F, Roullet E, Escourolle R. Leucoencephalopathies arteriopathiques. *Rev Neurol* 1985; 141:93–108.
23. Oepen H. Klinische, pathologisch-anatomische und genealogische Untersuchung einer spätadulten Leukodystrophie. *Arch Psychiat Nervenkr* 1964;206:115–130.
24. Tuñón T, Ferrer I, Gállego J, Degado G, Villaneuva JA, Martinez-Peñuela JM. Leukodystrophy with pigmented glial and scavenger cells (pigmentary type orthochromatic leukodystrophy). *Neuropathol Appl Neurobiol* 1988;14:337–344.
25. Okeda R, Matsuo T, Kawahara Y, et al. Adult pigment type (Peiffer) of sudanophilic leukodystrophy. Pathological and morphological studies on two autopsy cases of siblings. *Acta Neuropathol* 1989;78:533–542.
26. Gray F, Destee A, Bourre J-M, et al. Pigmentary type of orthochromatic leukodystrophy (OLD): a new case with ultrastructural and biochemical study. *J Neurop Exp Neurol* 1987;46:585–596.
27. Poser CM, Dewulf A, Bogaert LV. Atypical cerebellar degeneration associated with leukodystrophy. *J Neuropathol Exp Neurol* 1957;16:209–237.
28. Tsuchiya Y, Numabe T, Yokoi S. Neuropathological and neurochemical studies of three cases of sudanophilic leudodystrophy. *Acta Neuropathol (Berl)* 1970;16:353–366.
29. Pietrini V, Tagliavini F, Pilleri G, Trabattoni CR, Lechi A. Orthochromatic leukodystrophy with pigmented cells. *Acta Neurol Scand* 1979;59:140–147.
30. Bhatia KP, Morris JH, Frackowiak RSJ. Primary progressive multifocal leukoencephalopathy presenting as an extrapyramidal syndrome. *J Neurol* 1996;243:91–95.
31. Constantinidis J, Richard J, Tissot R. Pick's disease. Histological and clinical correlation. *Eur Neurol* 1974;11: 208–217.
32. Tissot R, Constantinidis J, Richard J. Pick's disease. In: Vinken PJ, Bruyn GW, Klawans HL, Frederiks JAM, eds. *Handbook of Clinical Neurology,* Vol 46, Amsterdam: Elsevier Science Publishers, 1985.233–246.
33. Mendez MF, Selwood A, Mastri AR, Frey WH. Pick's disease versus Alzheimer's disease. A comparison of clinical characteristics. *Neurology* 1993;43:289–292.
34. Litvan I, Agid Y, Sastrj BS, et al. What are the obstacles for an accurate clinical diagnosis of Pick's disease? A clinicopathological study. *Neurology* 1997;49:62–69.
35. Winkelman NW, Book MH. Asymptomatic extrapyramidal involvement in Pick's disease. *J Neuropathol Exp Neurol* 1994;8:30–42.
36. Munoz-Garcia D, Ludwin SK. Classic and generalized variants of Pick's disease: a clinicopathological, ultrastructural, and immunocytochemical comparative study. *Ann Neurol* 1984;16:467–480.
37. Uchihara T, Tsuchiya K, Kosaka K. Selective loss of nigral neurons in Pick's disease: a morpholometric study. *Acta Neuropathol* 1990;81:155–161.
38. Kosaka K, Ikeda K, Mehraein P. Striatopallidonigral degeneration in Pick's disease: a clinicopathological study of 41 cases. *J Neurol* 1991;238:151–160.
39. Escourolle R. *La maladie de Pick. Etude critique d'ensemble et synthèse anatomo-clinique,* MD thesis. Paris: Foulton, 1956.
40. Cambier J, Masson M, Dairou R, Henin D. Étude anatomo-clinique d'une forme pariétale de maladie de Pick. *Rev Neurol* 1981;137:33–38.
41. Case Records of the Massachusetts General Hospital. Case 16-1986. *N Engl J Med* 1986;314:1101–1111.
42. Lang AE, Bergeron C, Pollanen MS, Ashby P. Parietal Pick's disease mimicking cortico-basal ganglionic degeneration. *Neurology* 1994;44;1436–1440.
43. Litvan I, Cummings JL, Mega M. Neuropsychiatric features of corticobasal degeneration. *J Neurol Neurosurg Psychiatry* 1998;65:717–721.
44. Feany MB, Dickson DW. Neurodegenerative disorders with extensive tau pathology: a comparative study and review. *Ann Neurol* 1996;40:139–148.
45. Ksiezak- Reding H, Morgan K, Mattice LA, Davies P, Liu W-K, Yen S-H, Weidenheim K, Dickson D. Ultra-

structure and biochemical comparison of paired helical filaments in cortico-basal degeneration. *Am J Pathol* 1994; 145:1496–1508.

46. Mölsä PK, Marttila RJ, Rinne UK. Extrapyramidal signs in Alzheimer's disease. *Neurology* 1984;34:1114–1116.
47. Chui HC, Teng EL, Henderson VW, Moy AC. Clinical subtypes of dementia of Alzheimer type. *Neurology.* 1985;35:1544–1550.
48. Crystal HA, Horoupian DS, Katzman R, Jotkowitz S. Biopsy-proved Alzheimer disease presenting as a right parietal lobe syndrome. *Ann Neurol* 1982;12:186–188.
49. Ball JA, Lantos PL, Jackson M, Marsden CD, Scadding JW, Rossor MN. Alien hand sign in association with Alzheimer's histopathology. *J Neurol Neurosurg Psychiatry* 1993;56:1020–1023.
50. Rafal RD, Friedman JH, Limb dystonia in progressive supranuclear palsy. *Neurology* 1987;37:1546–1549.
51. Annonymous Case Records of the Massachusetts General Hospital Weekly clinicopathological exercises. Case 46-1993. A 75-year-old man with right sided rigidity, dysarthria, and abnormal gait. *N Engl J Med* 1994; 330:448.
52. Barclay CL, Bergeron C, Lang AE. Arm levitation in progressive supranuclear palsy. *Neurology,* in press.
53. Maraganore DM, Boeve B, Parisi J. Disorders mimicking the "classical" clinical syndrome of cortico-basal ganglionic degeneration. *Mov Disord* 1996:11:347 (abstract).
54. Bergeron C, Davis A, Lang AE. Corticobasal ganglionic degeneration and progressive supranuclear palsy presenting with cognitive decline. *Brain Pathol* 1998;8: 355–365.
55. Giladi N, Fahn S. Hemiparkinsonism-hemiatrophy syndrome may mimic early-stage cortico-basal ganglionic degeneration. *Mov Disord* 1992;7:384–385.
56. Grimes DA, Bergeron CB, Lang AE. Motor neuron disease-inclusion dementia presenting as cortico-basal degeneration. *Mov Disord* 1999;14:674–680.

Corticobasal Degeneration.
Advances in Neurology, Vol. 82,
edited by I. Litvan, C. G. Goetz, and A. E. Lang.
Lippincott Williams & Wilkins, Philadelphia © 2000.

17

Phenotypes and Prognosis: Clinicopathologic Studies of Corticobasal Degeneration

Irene Litvan,* David A. Grimes,† and Anthony E. Lang‡

**Cognitive Neuropharmacology Unit, Defense and Veteran Head Injury Program, Henry M. Jackson Foundation, Bethesda, Maryland 20817-1844; †Department of Medicine, The Ottawa Hospital, Ottawa, Ontario K1Y 4E9, Canada; and ‡Division of Neurology, Toronto Western Hospital, Toronto, Ontario M5T 2S8, Canada*

INTRODUCTION

The first clinicopathologic description of corticobasal degeneration (CBD) was made by Rebeiz et al. (1), who described three patients with asymmetric akinetic-rigid parkinsonism with involuntary movements and signs of cognitive disturbance. Typically, CBD presents with unilateral L-dopa-unresponsive akinesia and rigidity, dystonia or myoclonus, as well as focal cortical signs such as limb apraxia, aphasia, and cortical sensory loss (1–6). Most initial reports focused on the motor features, but more recently pathologically confirmed CBD cases of patients presenting with primary aphasia, dementia, visual inattention, or rapidly progressive mutism reveal that this disorder exhibits a striking clinical heterogeneity (6–13).

Because clinical studies may include disorders that can simulate features of CBD such as progressive supranuclear palsy (PSP), Pick's disease, Alzheimer's disease (AD), hemiatrophy-parkinsonism (9,14–17), pathologic confirmation still remains the absolute diagnostic gold standard.

To better delineate the spectrum of clinical features of CBD, we compared two pathologically confirmed data sets consisting of 27 cases: 14 from the files of seven medical centers located in Austria, the United Kingdom, and the United States (the National Institutes of Health [NIH] series) (6), and 13 collected through the Canadian Brain Tissue Bank and the Toronto Hospital Movement Disorders Centre (the Toronto series) (13). The cases from the NIH series have been previously reported (6). We evaluated the characteristics of each data set, estimated the frequency of features in the combined data set, and then compared the findings of these cases to those in the largest clinical series from one center reported up-to-date (5). In addition, we analyzed the clinical predictors of survival in the combined data set.

Study Sample and Methods

In both series, all patients were evaluated at least once by a neurologist; the majority were assessed in movement disorder clinics, less frequently in dementia clinics. These two case series were generated from different sources: the NIH series came mostly (but not exclusively) from movement disorder clinics, whereas the Toronto series was derived from a brain bank used by both movement disorder and dementia specialists. Because the clinical data were retrospectively collected in most patients, a feature that was not specifically recorded was coded as absent if the neurological examination was stated as being normal. However, this may imply that all patients were examined to rule out each feature, resulting in a possible underestimation of certain symptoms and signs. Only seven of the 13 patients in the Toronto series had a follow-up visit. However, when we estimated percentages, we included in the denominator the subjects evaluated and those who exhibited the particular analyzed feature at earlier stages of the disease, assuming that features present once would remain present later because CBD is a progressive disorder. Thus, the data at the last visit should be interpreted as features present in the course of the disease since in our clinical experience patients may at later stages no longer exhibit signs they presented earlier, such as alien limb syndrome.

The NIH cases met the National Institute of Neurological Disorders and Stroke (NINDS) (18) neuropathologic criteria for CBD which included fronto-parietal atrophy with severe cortical neuronal loss and intense astrogliosis as well as swollen and achromatic neurons (without Pick bodies) in the affected cortex. Several cytoskeletal abnormalities were present including neuropil threads, neurofibrillary tangles, basophilic inclusions (the latter in basal ganglia areas), and tau-positive astrocytic inclusions forming cortical "astrocytic plaques." There were no other pathologic associated nosologic disorders. The Toronto series was characterized by cortical neuronal loss, gliosis, swollen achromatic neurons with substantia nigra degeneration, corticobasal inclusions, and widespread cortical and subcortical tau-positive neuronal and glial inclusions with associated astrocytic plaques (13,14).

Statistical analyses included analysis of variance (ANOVA), logistic regression and discriminant function analyses. To explore the relationships among the main disease features (e.g., motor, cognitive, and behavioral disturbances) at early stages, Spearman correlation coefficients were calculated for all CBD patients using data from the first visit. This exploratory analysis was not meant to establish strict significance, and thus a type 1 error was considered preferable to missing a possible correlation (type 2 error). For this reason, no Bonferroni adjustment was made and significance was considered at $p < 0.05$. Note, however, that several correlations achieved an alpha level of 0.005, required for significance if the Bonferroni adjustment was used. Survival was estimated with the Kaplan-Meier analysis.

Demographics and survival

There were no between-data set differences in demographics (Table 1). The combined data set consisted of 27 patients (14 women, 13 men); mean age (±SD) at onset 63.5 ± 6.7 years; mean symptom duration to death 7 ± 2 years; and mean age at death 70.5 ± 7 years. Only one patient from the Toronto series had a familial parkinsonian disorder.

Patients from the Toronto series tended to have a shorter survival (6.0 ± 0.6 years) than those from the NIH series (7.8 ± 0.6; $p < 0.06$, Kaplan-Meier method) (Fig. 1). Between-center differences in survival were statistically significant ($p < 0.04$) when parametric survival statistics (Weibull) were used. Mean (± SEM) survival from onset for the combined data set was 7.0 ± 0.5 years (range, 2.5 to 12.5). Mean survival of patients with attentional disturbances (e.g., impaired immediate memory in tasks such as digit span) at the first visit was shorter (5.8 ± 0.9 years) than those with normal attention (7.6 ± 0.5 years, $p < 0.05$). Similarly, those with short-term memory disturbances (e.g., learning a word list) and those with dementia (memory and at least another cognitive disturbance) had a shorter survival (6 ± 0.6 years and 6.2 ± 0.6 years, respec-

TABLE 1. *Demographics**

Characteristics	NIH (*N* = 14)	Toronto (*N* = 13)	Rinne[†] (*N* = 36)
Sex	8F/6M	6F/7M	20F/16M
Age at onset (yrs)	63 ± 7.7 (45–75)	64 ± 5.8 (52–73)	60.9 ± 9.7 (40–76)
Disease duration (yrs)	7.9 ± 2.6 (2.5–12.5)	6.1 ± 2.0 (3–10)	5.9 ± 1.2 (4–8)[‡]

* Data are mean ± SD and range.
[†] Only six patients had pathologically confirmed CBD.
[‡] Disease duration is included for 10 patients who died.

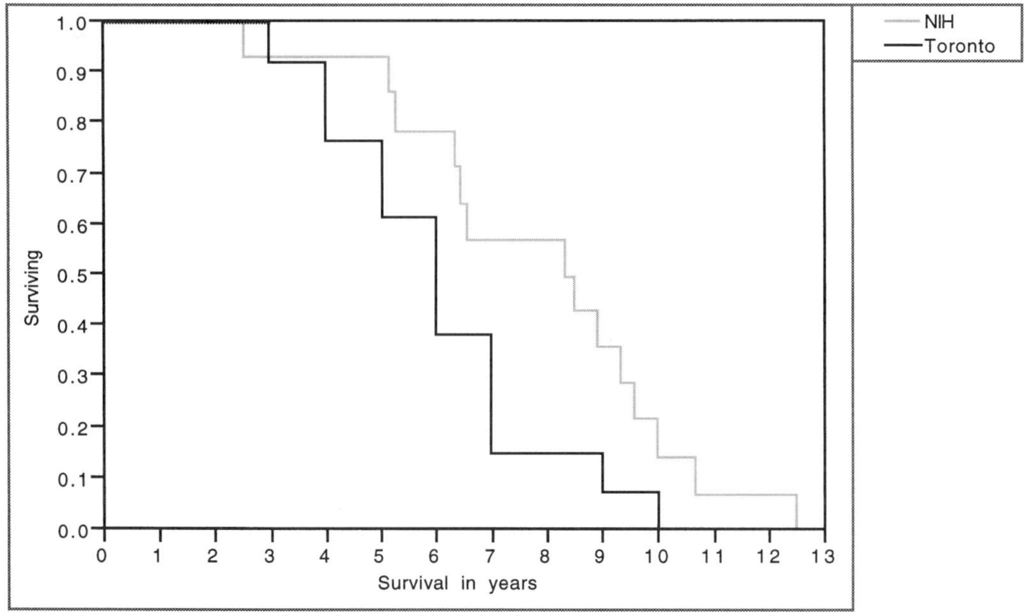

Fig. 1. Kaplan-Meier survival analysis of patients with CBD grouped by center (Toronto and NIH series). The Y axis refers to the proportion of patients who are alive (surviving) at a given time point.

tively) than those with normal memory (8.2 ± 0.5, $p < 0.01$) and without dementia (7.7 ± 0.6 years, $p < 0.03$). Mean survival of patients with bilateral bradykinesia at the first visit tended to be shorter (6 ± 0.8 years) than those without (8.2 ± 0.6 years; $p < 0.06$). Moreover, the presence of bilateral bradykinesia, and immediate or short-term memory impairment at the first visit predicted shorter survival ($p < 0.01$). Neither age at onset nor early onset of dysphagia, incontinence, falls, gait disturbances, aphasia, pyramidal signs, dystonia, or oculomotor disturbances, had an effect on survival.

The Onset

The information analyzed in this section was obtained from the patients' medical histories and does not include their examinations. Limb clumsiness was present at onset in 50% of the patients in the NIH series but in only 23% in the Toronto series ($p < 0.05$). Sensory disturbances in one limb (e.g., paresthesias, pain) were recorded in 29% of the patients from the NIH series (none in the Toronto series, $p < 0.05$) and led to (ineffective) surgical decompression of peripheral nerves in some of them. On the other hand, cognitive disturbances as a first symptom occurred more frequently in the Toronto series, although these between-data set differences were not significant.

When considering the combined series, one-third of the patients experienced as their first symptom cognitive problems, particularly, memory disturbances (Table 2). Behavioral changes, mostly suggestive of frontal dysfunction (e.g., apathy), occurred in one-third of the patients. During the first year of symptom onset, gait disturbances occurred in 26% of the patients (7 of 27), but falls were infrequent; two patients, 15%. Speech disturbances at onset occurred in 22% of the patients. Rinne et al. (5) clinical series reported a similar frequency of unilateral motor symptoms (limb clumsiness) to those found in the NIH series and similar gait disturbances than in the Toronto series. In contrast to these two pathologically confirmed series, cognitive or behavioral symptoms were not described at onset in the Rinne et al. clinical series (5).

TABLE 2. *Initial symptoms in patients with autopsy confirmed CBD*

Primary symptom	NIH (*N* = 14)	Toronto (*N* = 13)	Combined (*N* = 27)	Rinne* (*N* = 36)
Limb clumsiness	7 (50%)	3 (23%)	10 (37%)	19 (53%)
Jerking	3 (21%)	1 (8%)	4 (15%)	7 (19%)
Speech disorder	2 (14%)	4 (31%)	6 (22%)	1 (3%)
Cognitive problems (memory loss)	3 (21%)	6 (46%)	9 (33%)	0
Behavioral changes	3 (21%)	6 (46%)	9 (33%)	0
Gait disorder	5 (36%)	2 (15%)	7 (26%)	5 (14%)
Sensory problems	4 (29%)	0†	4 (15%)	3 (9%)
Depression	1 (7%)	0	1 (4%)	0

* Only six patients had pathologically confirmed CBD. Patients may have more than one feature.
† $p < 0.05$.

Early Motor, Pseudobulbar, and Oculomotor Features

At the first visit in the NIH series (3.0 ± 1.9 years since symptom-onset), 64% (nine of 14) of the patients had unilateral or grossly asymmetrical akinesia, dystonia or myoclonus or history of unilateral onset of "tremor." In contrast, in the Toronto series (similar duration since symptom-onset, 2.9 ± 1.4 years), motor asymmetry was present in only 31% of the patients and bilateral parkinsonism was more frequent, although not statistically different ($p < 0.06$). Bladder incontinence was significantly more frequent in the Toronto series (Table 3).

When considering the combined series, unilateral limb dystonia was present in eight (30%) patients at the first visit. Irregular tremor present at rest was documented in four (15%) patients; transient pill-rolling tremor was reported by a general neurologist in one (4%) patient. Four (15%) patients had focal myoclonus. Gait disorders were present on first neurological examination in 15 (56%) patients [small-stepped (n = 5), bradykinetic (n = 8), unstable (n = 6), broad-based (n = 4)] and associated with falls in nine (33%), three patients required assistance when walking, and three were wheelchair-bound. Patients who were wheelchair-bound at the first visit had similar symptom duration (3 ± 0.9 years) than those who were not (2.9 ± 0.4 years). Four of six L-dopa-treated patients did not benefit from treatment, whereas two had a moderate (30 to 50%) unsustained response of unknown duration.

Pyramidal signs were present in 26% of the patients (unilateral in three, and bilateral in four) (Table 3). Speech was affected in 14 patients (52%), dysarthria in six (22%), aphonia or anarthria in four (15%), and unintelligibility in four (15%). Dysphagia was only reported in one patient.

Voluntary and pursuit vertical gaze suggestive of supranuclear gaze palsy was found in a few patients (n = 4) in the NIH series, one of whom also exhibited an abnormal horizontal supranuclear gaze palsy.

When we compared the frequency of features in each of these pathologically confirmed series to the large Rinne et al. (5) clinical series, only certain motor features, particularly unilateral dystonia, gait and speech disturbances, occurred in similar proportion. On the other hand, in the Rinne et al. (5) series, early oculomotor disturbances were very frequent (75%) and could be characterized in some patients as an "oculomotor apraxia" (difficulty to initiate voluntary saccades, voluntary or pursuit gaze with preservation of optokinetic nystagmus), whereas only supranuclear gaze palsy (also affecting vertical gaze) was described in the NIH series, and only saccadic pursuit was noted in a few patients in the Toronto series.

Early Cognitive and Behavioral Features

In the Toronto series, attention, disorientation, memory dysfunction, and cortical dementia were significantly more frequent than in the NIH series. These features, in addition to aphasia, were also the most frequent cognitive disturbances in this particular series. In contrast, in the NIH series limb apraxia (impaired ability to mimic ges-

TABLE 3. *Early motor features of patients with pathologically confirmed CBD*

Features	NIH ($N = 14$)	Toronto ($N = 13$)	Combined ($N = 27$)	Rinne* ($N = 36$)
Motor				
Gait disorder	7 (50%)	8 (62%)	15 (56%)	19 (53%)
Postural instability	5 (36%)	3 (23%)	8 (30%)	19 (53%)
Falls	6 (43%)	3 (23%)	9 (33%)	19 (53%)
Unilateral bradykinesia	5 (36%)†	1 (8%)	6 (22%)	19 (53%)
Bilateral bradykinesia	5 (36%)	5 (38%)	10 (37%)	8 (22%)
Axial rigidity	2 (17%)	4 (31%)	6 (22%)	NA
Unilateral limb rigidity	3 (25%)	0	3 (11%)	19 (53%)
Bilateral limb rigidity	8 (57%)	10 (77%)	18 (67%)	8 (22%)
Tremor				
Rest	3 (21%)	1 (8%)	4 (15%)	NA
Action	1 (7%)	3 (23%)	4 (15%)	NA
Unilateral limb dystonia	6 (43%)	2 (15%)	8 (30%)	12 (33%)
Neck dystonia	1 (7%)	0	1 (4%)	NA
Focal myoclonus	3 (21%)	1 (8%)	4 (15%)	16 (50%)
Cerebellar signs	4 (29%)	1 (8%)	5 (19%)	NA
Pyramidal signs	3 (21%)	4 (31%)	7 (26%)	14 (39%)
Pseudobulbar				
Speech disturbances	6 (43%)	8 (62%)	14 (52%)	15 (42%)
Dysarthria (slurred)	4 (29%)	2 (15%)	6 (22%)	15 (42%)
Aphonia/anarthia	1 (7%)	3 (23%)	4 (15%)	NA
Dysphagia	1 (7%)	0	1 (4%)	NA
Bladder incontinence	1 (7%)	6 (46%)†	7 (26%)	NA
Emotional lability	1 (7%)	0	1 (4%)	NA
Oculomotor				
Limited vertical voluntary	5 (36%)	0	5 (19%)	‡
Limited vertical pursuit	4 (29%)	0	4 (15%)	‡
Limited horizontal voluntary	1 (7%)	0	1 (4%)	‡
Limited horizontal pursuit	1 (7%)	0	1 (4%)	‡
Eyelid apraxia	2 (14%)	1 (8%)	3 (11%)	2 (6%)

* Only six patients had pathologically confirmed CBD.
† $p < 0.05$.
‡ Oculomotor disturbances including difficulty to initiate saccades were described in 75% of the patients of this series. Because percent is based on the total number of patients of each series, rather than on those with detailed information, some features may be underrepresented.
NA = not available.

tures and hand postures usually associated with complaints of disability) was significantly more frequent (seven patients, 50%) than in the Toronto series (15%).

When considering the combined series, cognitive disturbances were present in 48% of the patients during the first year after symptom onset and in 55% at the first visit. Moreover, 44% of the patients were thought to meet dementia criteria (Diagnostic Statistical Manual, DSM III-R). Overall six (22%) patients developed an early alien limb phenomenon (complex unintentional movements of one limb interfering with normal motor tasks) which affected most frequently the upper extremity (Table 4). Patients with alien limb syndrome had concomitant limb apraxia or dystonia, and one also had cortical sensory loss. Visual neglect was reported in only one patient.

Inappropriate social behavior and frontal release signs as early features, were significantly more frequent in the Toronto series. Other frontal lobe-type of behaviors such as apathy, irritability, and disinhibition, had similar frequency in both series. Depression was only documented in the NIH series. None of the patients exhibited hallucinations unrelated to medications; one patient had drug-induced hallucinations.

Cognitive disturbances, in particular language and praxis disturbances, were again less frequent in the Rinne et al. (5) series. In this latter series, the alien limb phenomenon was more frequently reported than limb apraxia (5), although the alien

TABLE 4. *Early cognitive and behavioral features of patients with pathologically confirmed CBD*

Features	NIH (*N* = 14)	Toronto (*N* = 13)	Combined (*N* = 27)	Rinne* (*N* = 36)
Cognitive				
Cognitive disturbances 1st yr	5 (36%)	8 (62%)	13 (48%)	NA
Cognitive disturbances 3rd yr	6 (43%)	9 (69%)	15 (55%)	7 (19%)
Cortical dementia	3 (21%)	9 (69%)†	12 (44%)	7 (19%)
Attention disorder	3 (21%)	9 (69%)†	12 (44%)	NA
Disorientation				
Time	1 (7%)	8 (62%)†	9 (33%)	NA
Place	1 (7%)	8 (62%)†	9 (33%)	NA
Memory disturbance				
Immediate	2 (14%)	7 (54%)†	9 (33%)	NA
Short-term	5 (36%)	10 (77%)	15 (55%)	NA
Remote	4 (29%)	9 (69%)	13 (48%)	NA
Limb apraxia	7 (50%)†	2 (15%)	9 (33%)	2 (6%)
Alien limb phenomenon	4 (29%)	2 (15%)	6 (22%)	14 (39%)
Aphasia	4 (29%)	7 (54%)	11 (41%)	2 (6%)
Dysexecutive syndrome	5 (36%)	3 (23%)	8 (30%)	2 (6%)
Constructive apraxia	7 (50%)	2 (15%)	9 (33%)	NA
Visual neglect	1 (7%)	NA	NA	NA
Visual agnosia	0	4 (31%)	4 (15%)	NA
Sensory cortical signs	4 (31%)	NA	NA	9 (25%)
Behavioral				
Apathy	4 (29%)	2 (15%)	6 (22%)	NA
Inappropriate social behavior	3 (21%)	9 (69%)†	12 (44%)	1 (3%)
Irritability	4 (29%)	3 (23%)	7 (26%)	NA
Disinhibition	3 (21%)	3 (23%)	6 (22%)	1 (3%)
Outburst	1 (7%)	2 (15%)	3 (11%)	1 (3%)
Depression	5 (36%)	0	5 (19%)	NA
Frontal lobe release signs	5 (42%)	11 (85%)†	16 (59%)	13 (36%)

* Only six patients had pathologically confirmed CBD. Because percent is based on the total number of patients of each series, rather than on those with detailed information, some features may be underrepresented.
NA = not available.
† $p < 0.05$.

limb phenomenon is usually present in an apraxic limb (19).

Motor and Cognitive Associations

Using nonparametric correlations, we identified different patterns of presentations. At early stages (Table 5), asymmetric parkinsonism was significantly associated with unilateral dystonia ($r = 0.62$) and limb apraxia (0.59). However, asymmetric parkinsonism was inversely associated with cognitive features at onset (–0.55) or development at the first visit of attention disturbances (–0.48) or dementia (–0.48). Unilateral dystonia at the first visit was also inversely associated with history of cognitive features at onset (–0.62). These associations suggest that patients with an asymmetric parkinsonism or unilateral dystonia at the first visit did not, exhibit at onset, cognitive disturbances. In addition, patients with an asymmetric parkinsonism did not usually exhibit dementia at the first visit.

When patients had bilateral bradykinesia at the first visit they were also likely to exhibit pyramidal signs (0.69) or incontinence (0.47). Pyramidal signs at the first visit were associated with incontinence (0.57) and cognitive features at onset (0.44), although not associated with dementia. Incontinence at the first visit was associated with history of cognitive features at symptom onset (0.66), and at the first visit, of attention disturbances (0.57), aphasia (0.41), and dementia (0.48). Moreover, incontinence was inversely associated with limb apraxia (–0.51). Cognitive features at onset were associated with the development at the first visit of aphasia (0.56), attention disturbances (0.57), and dementia (0.48), but inversely related to the presence of limb apraxia

TABLE 5. *Correlation (Spearman) between relevant early motor and cognitive features*

	Asymmetric parkinsonism	Unilateral dystonia	Bilateral bradykinesia	Pyramidal	Incontinence	Cognitive 1st Sx	Personality changes	Limb apraxia	Alien limb syndrome	Attention disturbance	Aphasia
Unilateral dystonia	0.62*										
Bilateral bradykinesia	–0.06	–0.06									
Pyramidal	–0.24	–0.31	**0.69**†								
Incontinence	–0.31	–0.23	0.47‡	0.57*							
Cognitive 1st Sx	**–0.55**†	–0.62*	0.06	0.44‡	**0.66**†						
Personality changes	–0.37	–0.19	0.19	0.37	0.27	0.46‡					
Limb apraxia	**0.59**†	0.29	–0.11	–0.40	–0.51*	–0.48‡	–0.22				
Alien limb syndrome	0.44	0.48	0.16	–0.14	–0.18	–0.44	0.25	0.56‡			
Attention disturbance	–0.48‡	–0.04	0.30	0.39	0.57*	0.57*	0.45	–0.60*	0.09		
Aphasia	–0.41†	–0.31	0.03	0.20	0.41‡	**0.56**†	0.29	–0.23	–0.09	0.49*	
Dementia	–0.48†	0.15	0.03	0.09	0.48*	0.48*	**0.57**§	–0.41	0.32	**0.65**§	**0.62**§

* $p < 0.01$; † $p < 0.005$; ‡ $p < 0.05$; § $p < 0.001$.
The variables that meet an adjusted alpha level of significance are indicated in bold.

(−0.48). The presence of limb apraxia at the first visit was associated with alien limb syndrome (0.56), but not with an attention disorder (−0.60). Thus, there are at least two alternative patterns of presentations. One includes the presence of cognitive disturbances at onset and later development (usually within 3 years of symptom onset) of aphasia, attention disturbances, dementia, and incontinence. An additional pattern includes patients with bilateral bradykinesia who had associated pyramidal signs and incontinence but did not exhibit dementia at the first visit. Incontinence at the first visit was present in the context of dementia or of bilateral motor (pyramidal or extrapyramidal) disturbances.

Late Motor, Pseudobulbar, and Oculomotor Features

In the NIH series all the patients had a late follow-up visit (criteria for inclusion into the study) but in the Toronto series only seven patients were followed. In general, symptoms and signs apparent early in the course of the disease steadily progressed up to the last visit. The last clinical visit occurred a mean of 6.1 ± 2.0 years after symptom onset in the NIH series.

All patients eventually developed an unstable and bradykinetic gait, 62% had falls, and 57% were wheelchair-bound (Table 6). In most cases, bilateral bradykinesia and rigidity dominated the extrapyramidal syndrome, although the par-

TABLE 6. *Late motor features of patients with pathologically confirmed CBD**

Features	NIH† (*N* = 14)	Toronto (*N* = 7)‡	Combined (*N* = 21)‡	Rinne§ (*N* = 30)
Motor				
Gait disorder	14 (100%)	12/12 (100%)	26/26 (100%)	29 (97%)
Postural instability	12 (86%)	6 (86%)	18 (86%)	NA
Falls	9 (64%)	4 (57%)	13 (62%)	NA
Bradykinesia	11 (79%)	8/8 (100%)	19/22 (86%)	NA
Axial rigidity	6 (43%)	9/9 (100%)	15/23 (65%)	NA
Limb rigidity	13 (93%)	13/13 (100%)	26 (96%)	24 (80%)
Tremor				
Rest	3 (21%)	0	3 (14%)	NA
Action	1 (7%)	2 (29%)	3 (14%)	NA
Unilateral limb dystonia	6 (43%)	2/8 (25%)	8/22 (36%)	25 (83%)
Bilateral limb dystonia	1 (7%)	2 (29%)	3 (14%)	25 (83%)
Neck dystonia	1 (8%)	NA	NA	NA
Focal myoclonus	3 (21%)	4 (57%)	7 (33%)	17 (57%)
Cerebellar signs	2 (15%)	0	2 (10%)	NA
Pyramidal signs	5 (36%)	6/8 (75%)	11/22 (50%)	22 (73%)
Pseudobulbar				
Speech disturbances	13 (93%)	8/10 (80%)	21/24 (88%)	NA
Dysarthria (slurred)	10 (71%)	5 (71%)	15 (71%	21 (70%)
Aphonia/anarthia	5 (33%)	5/10 (50%)	10/24 (42%)	NA
Dysphagia	5 (36%)	2 (29%)	7 (33%)	NA
Bladder incontinence	8 (57%)	8/12 (67%)	16/26 (62%)	NA
Emotional incontinence	3 (21%)	1 (14%)	4 (19%)	NA
Oculomotor				
Limited voluntary vertical gaze	8 (57%)	3 (43%)	11 (52%)	27 (90%)**
Limited vertical pursuit	7 (50%)	2 (29%)	9 (43%)	27 (90%)**
Limited voluntary horizontal gaze	4 (29%)	2 (29%)	6 (29%)	27 (90%)**
Limited horizontal pursuit	5 (36%)	2 (29%)	7 (33%)	27 (90%)**
Eyelid apraxia	4 (29%)	3 (43%)	7 (33%)	4 (13%)

* $p < 0.05$.
† Because percent is based on the total number of patients of each series, rather than on those with detailed information, some features may be underrepresented.
‡ Unless specified, the percentages were calculated based on the seven patients examined at the last visit. However, when a feature was present at the first examination, it was considered present at a later evaluation, and percentages were calculated accordingly.
§ Only six patients had pathologically proven CBD. NA = not available.
** Not clarified if voluntary or pursuit movements or if vertical and horizontal gaze palsy.

kinsonism remained asymmetric in the NIH series. Axial and limb rigidity were present in most of the patients in the Toronto series; however, limb more than axial rigidity was more often reported in the NIH series. Dystonia was present in 11 patients in the combined series, mostly unilateral in the NIH series. Six patients with dystonia had superimposed myoclonus. Three (21%) patients had "irregular tremor present at rest," and one also had focal myoclonus. Overall, 40% of the patients presented pyramidal signs such as Babinski (n = 11), although one-half of the patients had hyperreflexia. Cerebellar signs were infrequent.

Speech was almost always abnormal in the combined series (88%). In the NIH series, it was variably described as dysarthric (n = 10), slow (n = 9), aphonic/anarthric (n = 5), unintelligible (n = 4), echolalic (n = 2), or palilalic (n = 1). Dysphagia was reported in only one-third of the patients in the combined series. Bladder incontinence occurred in more than one-half of the patients.

In the Rinne et al. (5) series, the most frequent characteristics were gait disturbance, limb dystonia, myoclonus, and pyramidal features.

Late Cognitive and Behavioral Features

Cortical dementia was very frequent in the Toronto series (85% of the patients) but also occurred in almost one-half of the NIH patients. Memory disturbances were described in more than one-half of the patients of each series (Table 7). Aphasia was described in five (36%) patients in the NIH series, and in nine (75%, considering seven who had it at the first visit

TABLE 7. *Late cognitive and behavioral features of patients with pathologically confirmed CBD**

Features	NIH† (N = 14)	Toronto (N = 7)‡	Combined (N = 21)‡	Rinne§ (N = 30)
Cognitive				
Cortical dementia	6 (43%)	11/13 (85%)	17/27 (63%)	9 (30%)
Attention	6 (43%)	11/12 (92%)	17/26 (65%)	NA
Acute disorientation	2 (15%)	3 (43%)	5 (24%)	NA
Disorientation				
Time	6 (43%)	11/13 (85%)	17/27 (63%)	NA
Place	3 (21%)	9/13 (69%)	12/27 (44%)	NA
Memory				
Immediate	8 (57%)	10/13 (77%)	18/27 (67%)	NA
Short-term	8 (57%)	12/13 (92%)	18/27 (67%)	NA
Remote	7 (50%)	9/13 (69%)	16/27 (59%)	NA
Anomia	8 (57%)	8/11 (73%)	18/25 (72%)	NA
Aphasia	5 (36%)	9/12 (75%)	14/26 (54%)	NA
Executive dysfunction	8 (57%)	3/9 (33%)	11/23 (48%)	NA
Constructive apraxia	9 (64%)	3/3	12	NA
Limb apraxia	9 (64%)	4 (57%)	13 (62%)	30 (100%)
Alien limb phenomenon	6 (43%)	4 (57%)	10 (48%)	15 (50%)
Sensory cortical signs	4 (29%)	NA	NA	11 (37%)
Visual neglect	2 (15%)	NA	NA	NA**
Behavioral				
Personality changes	10 (71%)	12/12 (100%)	22/26 (85%)	NA
Apathy	6 (43%)	3 (43%)	9 (43%)	NA
Inappropriate social behavior	5 (36%)	9/13 (69%)	14/27 (52%)	NA
Irritability	5 (36%)	5 (71%)	10 (48%)	NA
Disinhibition	4 (29%)	3 (43%)	7 (33%)	NA
Depression	4 (29%)	NA	NA	NA
Frontal lobe release signs	8 (57%)	12/12 (100%)	20/26 (77%)	NA

* $p < 0.05$.
† Because percent is based on the total number of patients of each series, rather than on those with detailed information, some features may be underrepresented.
‡ Unless specified, the percentages were calculated based on the seven patients examined at the last visit. However, when a feature was present at the first examination, it was considered present at a later evaluation, and the percent was calculated accordingly.
§ Only six patients had pathologically proven CBD. NA = not available.
** Defects in visuospatial vision, the nature of which was unspecified, were reported in 10 patients.

and two who developed it) in the Toronto series. Interestingly, the patients who developed aphasia had the onset of their motor symptoms on the right (four of eight with symptom onset on the right) or both extremities (although in nine of these 12 patients motor disturbances predominated on the right). In the NIH series, executive dysfunction was present in eight patients who also manifested frontal lobe behavioral disturbances (apathy, irritability, or disinhibition) and had evidence of frontal lobe release signs. Visual neglect was only described in the NIH series. Limb apraxia occurred in more than 50% of the patients in the combined series and alien limb phenomenon in approximately 50% (Table 7). In contrast, at the last visit in the Rinne et al. series (5), limb apraxia was present in all patients, but alien limb phenomenon was less frequently observed. Personality changes were only reported in the pathologically confirmed series.

Clinical Diagnosis and Cause of Death

Misdiagnosis was very frequent in both series, but more so in the Toronto series. Because patients in the Toronto series usually presented with cognitive disturbances, they were often misdiagnosed as having AD. Overall, CBD was only diagnosed in six of the 27 patients (22%) at the first visit (Table 8). At the follow-up visit when more classical motor signs developed, an additional three patients in the Toronto series were accurately diagnosed as having CBD.

TABLE 8. *Initial clinical diagnosis of pathologically confirmed CBD cases*

Clinical diagnosis	NIH ($N = 14$)	Toronto ($N = 13$)
Corticobasal degeneration	5	1
Alzheimer's disease	1	6
Frontotemporal dementia	1	1
Atypical progressive supranuclear palsy	1	0
Atypical Parkinson's disease	0	1
Bulbar amyotrophic lateral sclerosis	0	1
Multiple system atrophy	1	0
Unknown or symptomatic diagnosis	5	3

Neuropathologic Findings

From a neuropathologic point of view, the cases in the NIH series were considered "typical." They showed neuronal loss and gliosis, neurofibrillary tangles, neuropil threads, and astrocytic plaques in the frontoparietal areas. However, 11 of the 13 cases in the Toronto series had predominantly frontal involvement. Only six cases in the Toronto series had a neuropathologic diagnosis of CBD previous to using immunohistochemistry. Most cases were diagnosed before immunostaining as having "atypical Pick's disease" because of frontal involvement with cell loss and gliosis, swollen neurons, and neuronal inclusions. However, in all the Toronto cases there were typical tau immunodeposits in the frontal cortex consisting of neurofibrillary tangles, neuropil threads and astrocytic plaques, characteristic of CBD, not present in Pick's disease (20) (see Chapter 2). In both series, there was severe neurodegeneration in the substantia nigra but varied neuronal loss and gliosis in the striatum and globus pallidum.

COMMENTS

This is the largest combined series of pathologically confirmed CBD cases reported to date. Although pathologically confirmed studies may include more atypical clinical patients, the demographics in both series is similar to that of clinical series (5). Because this combined series includes patients recruited in movement disorder and dementia clinics, the study may allow the evaluation of the full spectrum of features in CBD. On the other hand, because this is a retrospective study, the way neurologists examined or recorded the evaluation of their patients was not standardized. Only well-designed, prospective studies will avoid bias in recruitment, lack of uniformity in data collection, and missing data.

The CBD patients in this pathologically confirmed series usually presented in the seventh decade and never before age 45. The current analysis confirms that CBD has an heterogeneous clinical presentation reflecting its diverse anatomic involvement. Some CBD patients presented with what have been considered "typical" signs, unilateral, L-dopa-unresponsive parkinsonism, and limb apraxia. The parkinsonism in CBD usually does not benefit from L-dopa because in addition to a severe involvement of the substantia nigra (with consequent dysfunction of subcortical projections to premotor-motor and supplementary motor subcortical circuits), several output nuclei, in particular pallidum and putamen, are affected (21). Early involvement of cortical parietal areas contribute to the distinctive parietal syndrome usually manifesting as limb apraxia but also as paresthesias, agraphesthesia, constructive apraxia, sensory and visual neglect, and eventually alien limb syndrome.

In addition to this distinctive presentation, CBD patients presented with cognitive disturbances at onset and were found to develop aphasia, attention disorder, incontinence, and dementia at early stages. Moreover, cognitive disturbances at onset, particularly in the Toronto series, tended to occur in the absence of motor signs. In fact, some patients presented with bilateral motor disturbances, parkinsonism, pyramidal signs, and developed early incontinence. These different phenotypes have different prognosis and survival. Cognitive features at onset predicted an early development of dementia and incontinence, features usually associated with an early placement in nursing home facilities. Additionally, patients in the Toronto series tended to have shorter survival. In fact, early presence of dementia, severe or bilateral parkinsonian features, and memory or attention disturbances predicted a poor survival in this combined series of CBD patients. These features were unrelated to symptom duration until the first visit. Whether an early bilateral frontal rather than an asymmetric frontoparietal involvement represents a more aggressive form of the disease, different genotypes or is a statistical artifact, needs further investigation.

Only six patients were accurately diagnosed as having CBD at early stages. This poor diagnostic accuracy may be, in part, related to the lack of awareness of the clinical spectrum of this disorder. Patients in the NIH series were diagnosed more accurately probably because in this series the most common initial manifestation was limb clumsiness, reported by one-half of the patients. In contrast, in the Toronto series, the most common feature presentations were memory, behavioral, and speech disturbances, features usually not associated with CBD. Poor diagnostic accuracy suggests that the frequency of this disorder has been underestimated, and therefore, CBD may be more frequent than has been previously reported.

In the early stages, the presence of unilateral parkinsonism overlapping with distinctive features of CBD such as unilateral limb apraxia, focal myoclonus, dystonia, or alien limb phenomenon occurred in only 40% of patients ($n = 11$). Left visual neglect and left-sided parkinsonism occurred infrequently, and were previously reported in CBD (11). Thus, in the absence of vascular events, the presentation of limb apraxia, left visual or sensory neglect, in addition to unilateral motor signs, should raise the suspicion of CBD (6). It is conceivable that diagnostic accuracy may improve if neurologists develop an early index of suspicion and search for focal cognitive features such as neglect, aphasia, limb apraxia, and the alien hand phenomenon, when they examine patients with L-dopa-unresponsive asymmetric parkinsonism, myoclonus, or dystonia. Despite this, in the NIH series (6), at least two-thirds of the patients eventually developed limb apraxia; this figure is probably an underestimate since neurologists do not always search for it. On the other hand, it is possible that because of restrictive diagnostic inclusion criteria, in some of the clinical series, such as that of Rinne et al. (5), limb apraxia may be overestimated.

The dementia (44%) in CBD was usually characterized by attention and memory disturbances and aphasia. Nine patients who experienced memory problems at the onset of their illness presented at the first neurological visit, features suggestive of cortical dementia that in addition to memory and attention disturbances included aphasia ($n = 7$) and frontal lobe behavioral ($n = 9$) disturbances, but none had limb apraxia. Thus, CBD should be considered in the differential diagnosis of patients presenting with cortical dementia, particularly when attention, frontal behavioral symptomatology (e.g., apathy, irritability, inappropriate social behavior), or language disturbances predominate. In addition, CBD should be strongly suspected when the frontal dementia is accompanied by early speech disturbances, incontinence, pyramidal signs or parkinsonism, features usually not recognized as being associated with CBD. The presentation of CBD with memory, attention, and frontal disturbances as well as with aphasia has been insufficiently stressed in the literature (3,5,22,23). Differentiation from Pick's disease may be difficult in this situation (8,10,24). Not surprisingly, patients with this type of presentation showed cortical neuronal degeneration predominantly in the frontal lobes. Lesions in the dorsolateral frontal and premotor cortices and dorsolateral caudate found in CBD, contribute to the executive dysfunction CBD patients exhibit (22). These disturbances were associated with the presence of executive dysfunction, slowness of thought, attention disturbances, and aphasia. The memory disturbances observed in these patients are thought to be related to an impaired ability to organize their retrieval strategies as well as attention disturbances owing to their frontal lobe involvement. Involvement of both medial and orbitofrontal circuits may explain the neuropsychiatric disturbances described in these series as well as in clinical series (25). Although inappropriate social behavior, disinhibition, apathy, and depression were the dominant behavioral changes in these two pathologically confirmed series, in the clinical series depression is much more pervasive (see Chapter 14). In addition to mood disturbances, the orbitofrontal syndrome is associated with enforced utilization of objects in the environment (26).

Other early common motor features included gait disturbances (56%) and speech disturbances (52%), but in contrast to what occurs in PSP (27), less frequently associated with falls (33%) and swallowing disturbances. These symptoms in addition to the presence of supranuclear gaze palsy and frontal lobe disturbances, may frequently lead to an erroneous diagnosis of PSP (28). The gross asymmetry of parkinsonism and the presence of limb apraxia should, however, caution against this misdiagnosis, although patients with PSP may develop mild ideomotor apraxia (e.g., use of body parts) and infrequently asymmetric motor features (29,30). In contrast, the limb apraxia in CBD is usually moderate-to-severe and could be better characterized as a limb kinetic apraxia: In addition to a grotesque or unrecognizable gesture imitation, patients complain of difficulty in performing activities of daily living such as folding (upper extremity) or walking (lower extremity). Moreover, it may be associated with ideational apraxia (19). Furthermore, before the development of supranuclear gaze palsy, CBD patients usually present oculomotor apraxia (5,31). In addition, in CBD there is usually an equally severe vertical and horizontal gaze palsy, unlike the disproportionate involvement of vertical gaze in PSP as well as absence of oculomotor apraxia. Degeneration of the caudate, frontal, and parietal eye fields may explain the oculomotor abnormalities observed. The frontal eye field, principally involved in controlling intentional saccades to visible or predicted targets; the supplementary eye field, contributing to trigger saccades concerned with motor complex programming; and the prefrontal cortex controlling the inhibition of unwanted reflexive saccades are all involved. In addition to these difficulties, CBD patients have severe saccade and smooth pursuit paresis secondary in part to bilateral lesions affecting both the frontal and parietal eye fields.

Interestingly, most patients eventually developed motor features (bradykinesia, rigidity, gait disorder, and dysarthria). Although cortical dementia was present in most of the patients from the Toronto series, it was present in less than one-half of the patients in the NIH (6) and Rinne et al. (5) series. Furthermore, supposedly characteristic features such as asymmetric fixed dystonia, alien limb syndrome, or myoclonus were also absent in one-third to one-half of the patients in these series.

Average disease duration (7 years) was slightly longer than previously reported (5,32), but similar to what has been reported for other atypical parkinsonian syndromes such as PSP and multiple system atrophy (33,34). Most of our CBD patients died from pneumonia as a result of dysphagia and immobility. However, in contrast to what has been suggested in PSP, early dysphagia did not predict shorter survival (34). Whether dysphagia has a later onset in CBD or this finding is the result of the retrospective method of information collection, needs further investigation.

The present series suggests that in addition to the fixed dystonic jerky and apraxic arm, neurologists should suspect CBD when patients present with less distinctive features such as unilateral limb bradykinesia in conjunction with focal cognitive disturbances (e.g., limb apraxia or hemineglect) even in the absence of superimposed dystonia or myoclonus. Moreover, CBD should be also suspected when patients present with cortical dementia characterized by attentional, memory, language, and behavioral disturbances, particularly when associated with early motor signs. Clinicians should also suspect CBD in patients with bilateral parkinsonism, pyramidal signs, and incontinence, when associated with cognitive disturbances.

Because the analyzed series may include more atypical cases, the frequency of these various clinical presentations of this disorder needs to be evaluated in prospective clinicopathological studies focusing not only in motor, but also in cognitive and behavioral features. Differentiating these phenotypes seems important for prognosis, but it needs to be investigated if the various presentations also carry different genotypes.

ACKNOWLEDGMENTS

We thank Drs. S. Daniel, D. Dickson, D. S. Horoupian, J. Jankovic, K. Jellinger, P. L. Lantos, and A. McKee for providing cases for the NINDS database and Dr. C. Bergeron for providing the Toronto cases. We also thank Drs. K. Ray Chaudhuri, L. D'Olhaberriague, and R. K. B. Pearce for collecting the clinical data and D. G. Schoenberg, M. S. for skillful editing.

REFERENCES

1. Rebeiz JJ, Kolodny EH, Richardson EP. Corticodentatonigral degeneration with neuronal achromasia. *Arch Neurol* 1968;18:20–33.
2. Gibb WRC, Luthert PJ, Marsden CD. Clinical and pathological features of corticobasal degeneration. *Adv Neurol* 1990;53:51–54.
3. Riley DE, Lang AE, Lewis A, et al. Cortical-basal ganglionic degeneration. *Neurology* 1990;40:1203–1212.
4. Greene PE, Fahn S, Lang AE, Watts RL, Eidelberg D, Powers JM. Case 1, 1990: progressive unilateral rigidity, bradykinesia, tremoulousness, and apraxia, leading to fixed postural deformity of the involved limb. *Mov Disord* 1990;5:341–351.
5. Rinne JO, Lee MS, Thompson PD, Marsden CD. Corticobasal degeneration. A clinical study of 36 cases. *Brain* 1994;117:1183–1196.
6. Wenning GK, Litvan I, Jankovic J, et al. Natural history and survival of 14 corticobasal degeneration patients confirmed at autopsy. *J Neurol Neurosurg Psychiatry* 1998;64:184–189.
7. Lippa CF, Cohen R, Smith TW, Drachman DA. Primary progressive aphasia with focal neuronal achromasia. *Neurology* 1991;441:882–886.
8. Lennox G, Jackson M, Lowe J. Corticobasal degeneration manifesting as a frontal lobe dementia. *Ann Neurol* 1994;36:273–274.
9. Lang AE, Bergeron C, Pollanen MS, Ashby P. Parietal Pick's disease mimicking cortical-basal ganglionic degeneration. *Neurology* 1994;44:1436–1440.
10. Oda T, Ikeda K, Akamatsu W, et al. An autopsy case of corticobasal degeneration clinically misdiagnosed as Pick's disease. *Seishin Shinkeigaku Zasshi* 1995;97: 757–769.
11. Rey GJ, Tomer R, Levin BE, Sanchez-Ramos J, Bowen B, Bruce JH. Psychiatric symptoms, atypical dementia, and left visual field inattention in corticobasal ganglionic degeneration. *Mov Disord* 1995;10:106–110.
12. Bergeron C, Pollanen MS, Weyer L, Black SE, Lang AE. Unusual clinical presentations of cortical-basal ganglionic degeneration. *Ann Neurol* 1996;40:893–900.
13. Grimes DA, Lang AE, Bergeron C. Dementia is the most common presentation of cortical-basal ganglionic degeneration. *Neurology* 1998;50:96 (abstract).
14. Bergeron C, Davis A, Lang AE. Corticobasal ganglionic degeneration and progressive supranuclear paly presenting with cognitive decline. *Brain Pahol* 1998;8:355–365.
15. Ball JA, Lantos PL, Jackson M, Marsden CD, Scadding JW, Rossor MN. Alien hand sign in association with Alzheimer's disease histopathology. *J Neurol Neurosurg Psychiatry* 1993;56:1020–1023.
16. Maraganore DM, Boeve BF, Parisi J. Disorders mimicking the "classical" clinical syndrome of cortical-basal ganglionic degeneration. In: Lang A, ed. *Cortical-basal ganglionic degeneration and its relationship to other asymmetrical cortical degeneration syndromes.* Movement Disorder Society Satellite Symposia. Washington, D.C.: Mov Disord 1995:354 (abstract).
17. SantaCruz P, Torner L, Cruz-Sanchez F, Lomena F, Catafau A, Blesa R. Corticobasal degeneration syndrome: a case of Lewy body variant of Alzheimer's disease. *Int J Geriatric Psychiatry* 1996;11:559–565.
18. Litvan I, Agid Y, Goetz C, et al. Accuracy of the clinical diagnosis of corticobasal degeneration: a clinicopathological study. *Neurology* 1997;48:119–125.
19. Hauw JJ, Daniel SE, Dickson D, et al. Preliminary NINDS neuropathologic criteria for Steele-Richardson-Olszewski syndrome (progressive supranuclear palsy). *Neurology* 1994; 44:2015–2019.
20. Leiguarda R, Lees AJ, Merello M, Starkstein S, Marsden CD. The nature of apraxia in corticobasal degeneration. *J Neurol Neurosurg Psychiatry* 1994; 57:455–459.
21. Feany MB, Dickson DW. Widespread cytoskeletal pathology characterizes corticobasal degeneration. *Am J Pathol* 1995;146:1388–1396.
22. Tsuchiya K, Uchihara T, Oda T, Arima K, Ikeda K, Shimada H. Basal ganglia lesions in corticobasal degeneration differ from those in Pick's disease and progressive

supranuclear palsy: a topographic neuropathological study of six autopsy cases. *Neuropathology* 1997;17:208–216.
23. Pillon B, Blin J, Vidailhet M, Deweer B, Sirign A, Dubois B, Agid Y. The neuropsychological pattern of corticobasal degeneration: comparison with progressive supranuclear palsy and Alzheimer's disease. *Neurology* 1995;45:1477–1483.
24. Kertesz A, Hudson L, Mackenzie IR, Munoz DG. The pathology and nosology of primary progressive aphasia. *Neurology* 1994;44:2065–2072.
25. Litvan I, Agid Y, Sastri N, et al. What are the obstacles for an accurate diagnosis of Pick's disease? A clinicopathologic study. *Neurology* 1997;49:62–69.
26. Litvan I, Cummings JL, Mega M. Neuropsychiatric features of corticobasal degeneration. *J Neurol Neurosurg Psychiatry* 1998;65: in press.
27. Jacobs DH, Adair JC, Heilman KM. Visual grasp in corticobasal degeneration [letter]. *Ann Neurol* 1994;36: 679–680.
28. Litvan I, Sastry N, Sonies BC. Characterizing swallowing abnormalities in progressive supranuclear palsy. *Neurology* 1997;48:1654–1662.
29. Litvan I, Agid Y, Jankovic J, et al. Accuracy of clinical criteria for the diagnosis of progressive supranuclear palsy (Steele-Richardson-Olszewski syndrome). *Neurology* 1996;46:922–930.
30. Leiguarda RC, Pramstaller PP, Merello M, Starkstein S, Lees AJ, Marsden CD. Apraxia in Parkinson's disease, progressive supranuclear palsy, multiple system atrophy and neuroleptic-induced parkinsonism. *Brain* 1997;120: 75–90.
31. Pharr V, Litvan I, Brad DG, Troncoso J, Reich S, Stark M. Ideomotor apraxia in progressive supranuclear palsy: a case study. *Mov Disord* in press.
32. Vidailhet M, Rivaud S, Gouider-Khouja N, et al. Eye movements in parkinsonian syndromes. *Ann Neurol* 1994;35:420–26.
33. Gibb WR, Luthert PJ, Marsden CD. Corticobasal degeneration. *Brain* 1989;112:1171–1192.
34. Ben-Shlomo Y, Wenning GK, Tison F, Quinn NP. Survival of patients with pathologically proven multiple system atrophy: a meta-analysis. *Neurology* 1997;48: 384–393.
35. Litvan I, Mangone CA, McKee A, et al. Natural history of progressive supranuclear palsy (Steele-Richardson-Olszewski syndrome) and clinical predictors of survival: a clinicopathological study. *J Neurol Neurosurg Psychiatry* 1996;60:615–620.

Corticobasal Degeneration.
Advances in Neurology, Vol. 82,
edited by I. Litvan, C. G. Goetz, and A. E. Lang.
Lippincott Williams & Wilkins, Philadelphia © 2000.

18

Magnetic Resonance Imaging in CBD, Related Atypical Parkinsonian Disorders, and Dementias

Mario Savoiardo, Marina Grisoli, and Floriano Girotti

Department of Neuroradiology,
Istituto Nazionale Neurologico "C. Besta," 20133 Milano, Italy

INTRODUCTION

Neuroradiological reports on the computed tomographic (CT) or magnetic resonance imaging (MRI) features of corticobasal degeneration (CBD) are still scanty (1–3). This is owing to two problems: first, the clinical diagnosis of CBD has been made only in the past 10 years and only in specialized centers experienced in studies on movement disorders; second, the MRI findings that were described in the first reports are rather inconspicuous, since they are mainly represented by asymmetrical frontoparietal atrophy and by minimal, and perhaps not constant, signal abnormalities in the atrophic cortex (3,4).

As the diagnosis of CBD is not yet the diagnosis of the standard clinical neurologist, MRI diagnosis of CBD generally is not even considered by the neuroradiologist. In order to make or suggest this diagnosis, the neuroradiologist must first be aware of the importance of observing the atrophic brain for asymmetries.

In fact, when we became aware of the existence of CBD and of the demonstration of asymmetrical frontoparietal atrophy at postmortem examination of CBD cases, we reexamined the MRI studies of the patients clinically diagnosed as CBD at our Institute, that we had simply labeled as "atrophic." In all the cases reviewed, we were able to recognize very easily the asymmetry, and, without knowledge of the clinically affected side, were able to correctly identify the most atrophic frontoparietal region, which was contralateral to the clinically affected side (3,4).

In this chapter, we will review the literature and describe our MRI observations in CBD, comparing them with the findings observed in progressive supranuclear palsy (PSP), and frontotemporal dementia (FTD). We will also briefly describe the MRI findings in other extrapyramidal disorders and dementia, such as multiple system atrophy (MSA) of the striatonigral degeneration (SND) type, and Alzheimer's disease (AD).

The neuroradiological discussion will be focused on MRI, with brief mention of CT findings, since CT has very little importance in the diagnosis of these disorders in comparison with MRI.

CORTICOBASAL DEGENERATION

Clinical diagnosis of probable CBD was made on the basis of the presence of slowly progressive, asymmetric, akinetic-rigid syndrome with one or more of the following signs: ideomotor apraxia, myoclonus, sensory deficit of cortical origin, and alien limb syndrome associated with late-onset disorders of walking and stability. Lack of response to L-dopa and absence of other diseases that could explain the symptoms and signs ware essential for the diagnosis (5).

A total of 25 patients (9 males, 16 females; mean age: 67.1 years, range: 53 to 76 years) met these criteria. All the patients had some degree of cerebral cortical atrophy with widening of cisterns and sulci, seven slight, 18 marked. Asymmetrical atrophy with focal distribution involving the posterior frontal and parietal regions contralateral to the clinically most involved side was observed in 24 patients (96%) (Fig. 1).

Extension of the involved area was judged according to the combined observation of sagittal, coronal, and axial images. The asymmetry was mild in 11 cases (44%), marked in 13 (52%). Particularly in cases with marked asymmetry, dilata-

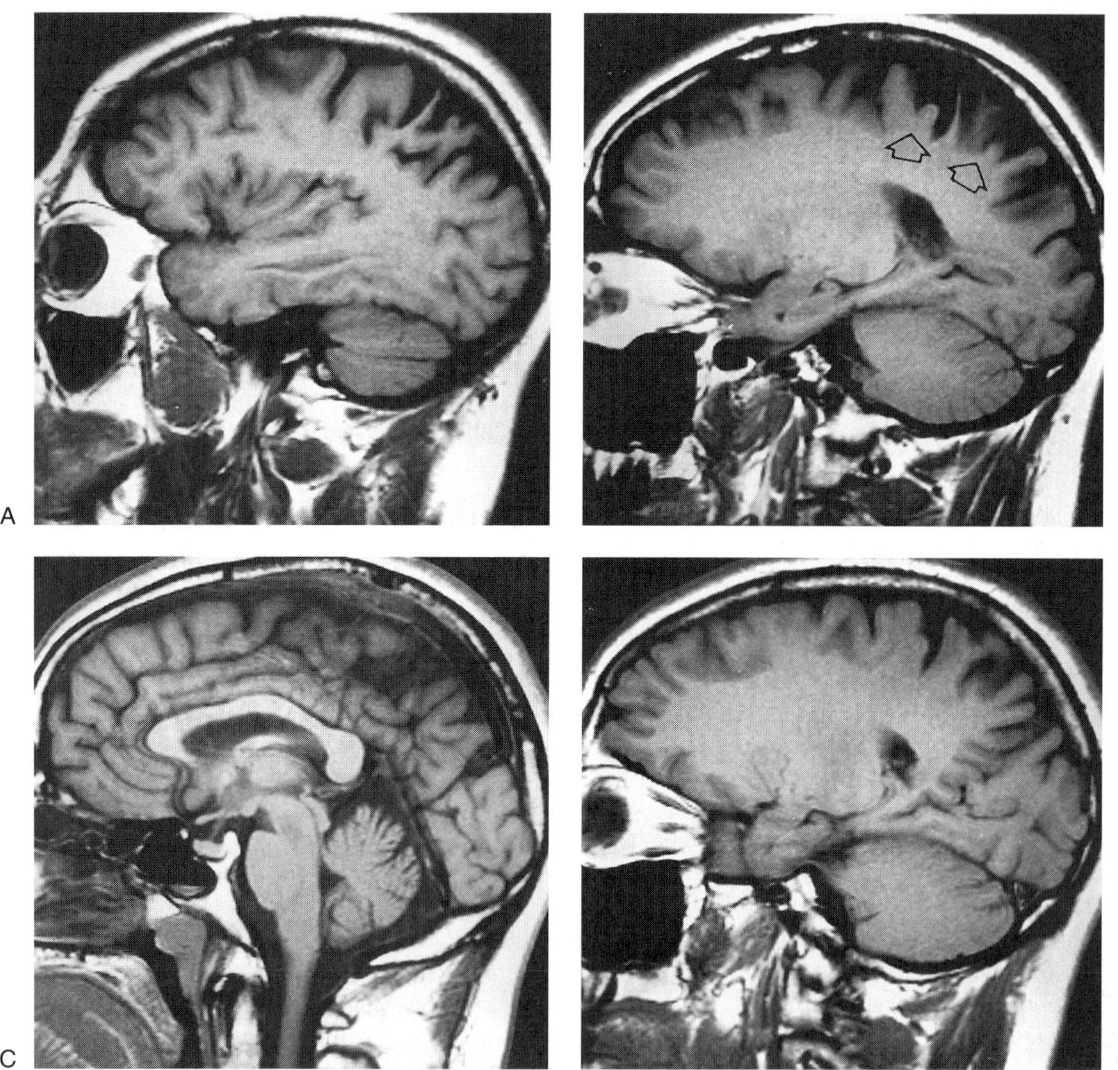

FIG. 1. CBD. 1.5 T MRI. Sagittal T1-weighted images, **A** to **D** from left to right. Atrophy of the left posterior frontal and parietal region is marked on the superior part of the convexity (**B,** *arrows*) and extends inferiorly to the middle parietal area (**A**). The midline section shows a normal midbrain (**C**). Parietal atrophy on the right hemisphere is mild (**D**). Coronal proton density (**E**) and T2-weighted (**F,** adjacent section) images confirm the asymmetry of parietal atrophy; the atrophic left parietal cortex is hyperintense in proton density (**E,** *arrowhead*). Axial proton density images (**G** and **H**) of follow-up 0.5 T MRI 1 year later demonstrate thin, hyperintense left frontoparietal cortex (*arrowheads*).

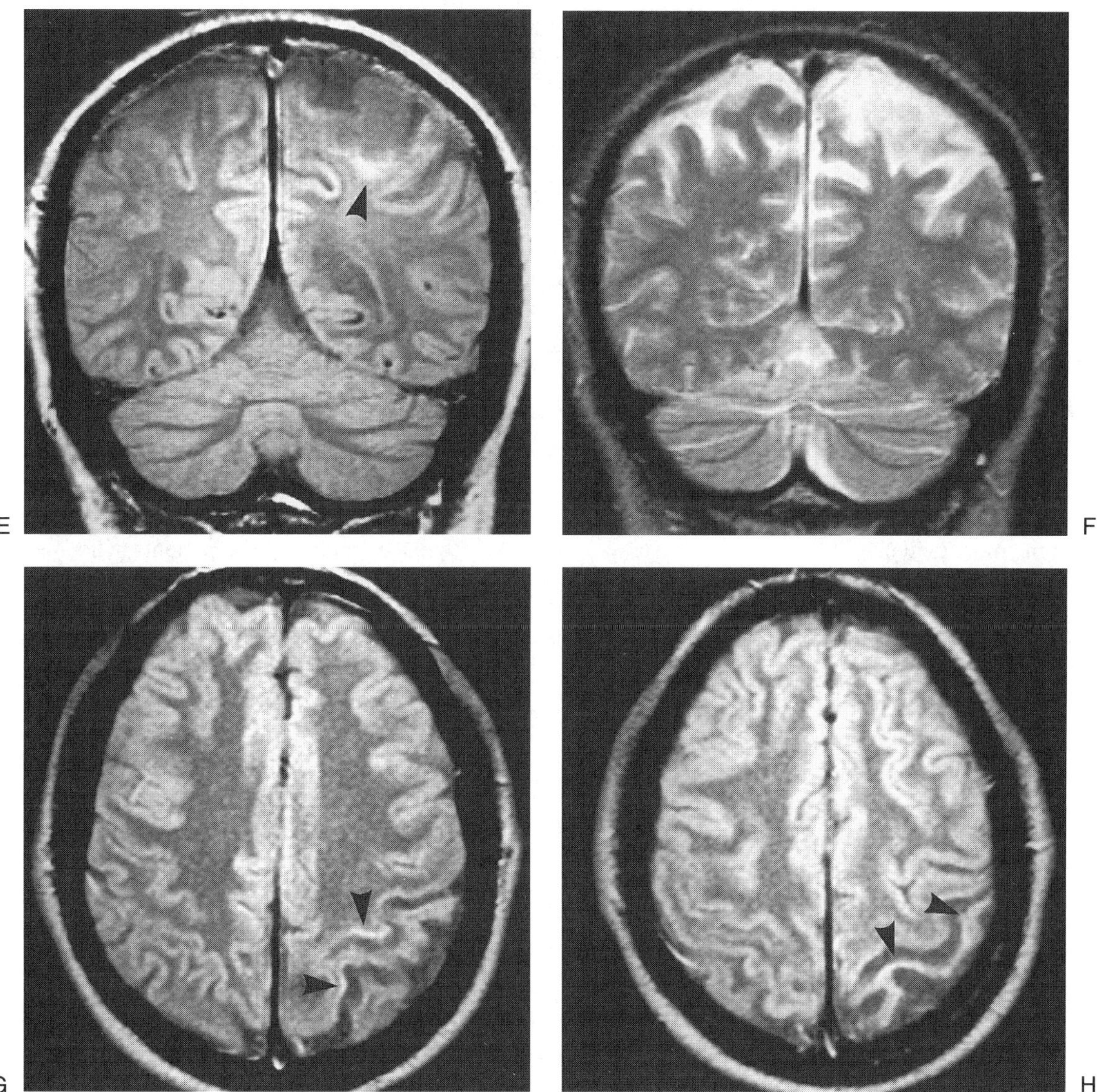

FIG. 1. (*Continued*)

tion of the ipsilateral ventricle was obvious. The white matter underlying the atrophic cortex had a decreased bulk, particularly evident in coronal sections by comparison with the opposite side, but had normal signal intensity. The cortex, on the contrary, appeared thin and often exhibited a slight increase in signal intensity in proton density images (Fig. 1 E, G, H). In standard spin echo (SE) T2-weighted images, the signal abnormality of the atrophic cortex was not detected, probably because of overshadowing by the high signal intensity of the adjacent cerebrospinal fluid (CSF) (Fig. 1 F); in fact, the abnormality of the cortex became more easily detectable when we started to use FLAIR sequences, which are T2-weighted, but with suppression of the signal of the CSF.

In spite of the pathological changes in the basal ganglia found in postmortem studies, at MRI basal ganglia abnormalities were not found in most of the patients. In four of the seven cases studied at 1.5 T, some hypointensity was seen in T2-weighted images in the putamina, almost equal to that seen in the pallida; this finding was similar to the one we often see in MSA-SND type, but the hypointensity was not more marked than that present in the pallida and was not accompanied by a thin lateral rim of hyperintensity. No signal abnormalities were present in the basal ganglia in the 18 patients studied with 0.5 T MRI.

In two other CBD patients, the midbrain was mildly atrophic, a feature usually seen in PSP patients; in both cases slight hyperintensity was also seen in proton density images in the periaqueductal region, another feature pointing to PSP. The charts of these patients were reviewed but failed to indicate clinical features clearly suggesting PSP. It will be interesting to follow up these patients both clinically and with MRI to see whether a mixed aspect of CBD and PSP will become more evident.

No other significant findings were present in our series of CBD patients. Occasional small areas of increased signal intensity in T2-weighted images in the periventricular white matter were seen; these areas were similar or less prominent than those usually found in patients of the same age, and attributed to chronic ischemic changes.

In conclusion, our series of CBD patients presented almost constantly asymmetric posterior frontal and parietal atrophy, more marked on the side contralateral to the more affected limbs. Mild signal changes in the atrophic cortex were seen particularly in proton density and FLAIR sequences. Basal ganglia abnormalities were generally absent; in a few cases, findings suggesting iron deposition in the putamina were observed, similar to (but not as marked as) those observed in SND patients. Two cases presented midbrain abnormalities as observed in PSP.

A final observation regards a difference between our initial series of 10 patients with diagnosis of CBD (3), of whom eight had marked asymmetrical atrophy, and the additional recent 15 cases in which only five had marked asymmetry, whereas nine had mild asymmetric atrophy, and one had no definite asymmetry. This probably reflects the evolution in the diagnostic criteria or in the ability in making a clinical diagnosis; the first patients had an advanced and well-defined clinical syndrome, while the subsequent patients had more subtle signs, reflecting the increased ability and confidence of the neurologist in making an early diagnosis. A longer follow-up and postmortem confirmation will be necessary to avoid possible misdiagnoses.

PROGRESSIVE SUPRANUCLEAR PALSY

CBD and PSP are at times difficult to differentiate clinically (5). Using Litvan et al. criteria (6), probable PSP was diagnosed on the basis of parkinsonism with age at onset over 40 years, supranuclear vertical gaze palsy, postural instability in the first years of illness, late mild dementia, and poor or absent response to L-dopa, in the absence of other diseases that could explain the symptoms and signs.

We recently reviewed 24 patients who met these criteria. Sixteen were male, eight female; mean age was 64.9 years (range: 52 to 75 years).

MRI studies demonstrated cerebral atrophy in 19 patients (79.2%), marked in 8 (33.3%), and slight in 11 (45.8%). Asymmetrical cortical atrophy was never found in PSP patients. Midbrain atrophy was found in 22 cases (91.7%), severe in 13 (54.2%), slight in 9 (37.5%). No definite midbrain atrophy was detected in the remaining two cases (8.3%).

Atrophy of the midbrain—that could be detected also in CT scans (7)—was more recognizable on MRI studies, because it was very easy to see in the sagittal T1-weighted images. In these images the midbrain appeared reduced in all its dimensions, sometimes very short in its caudocranial extension, with a superiorly concave aspect of the profile delineating the floor of the third ventricle (normally convex) (Fig. 2 A, B). The tectum was usually thin, particularly in its cranial part (2,4,8,9).

A peculiar feature was sometimes observed: in spite of attempting to correctly position the patients, they tended to keep their head hyperextended and this position suggested, at first glance, the possibility of PSP.

As a result of midbrain atrophy, the third ventricle enlarged, with the consequent deformity of the profile in the midline sagittal section already mentioned; the atrophy, however, extended cranialward to involve diencephalic structures and

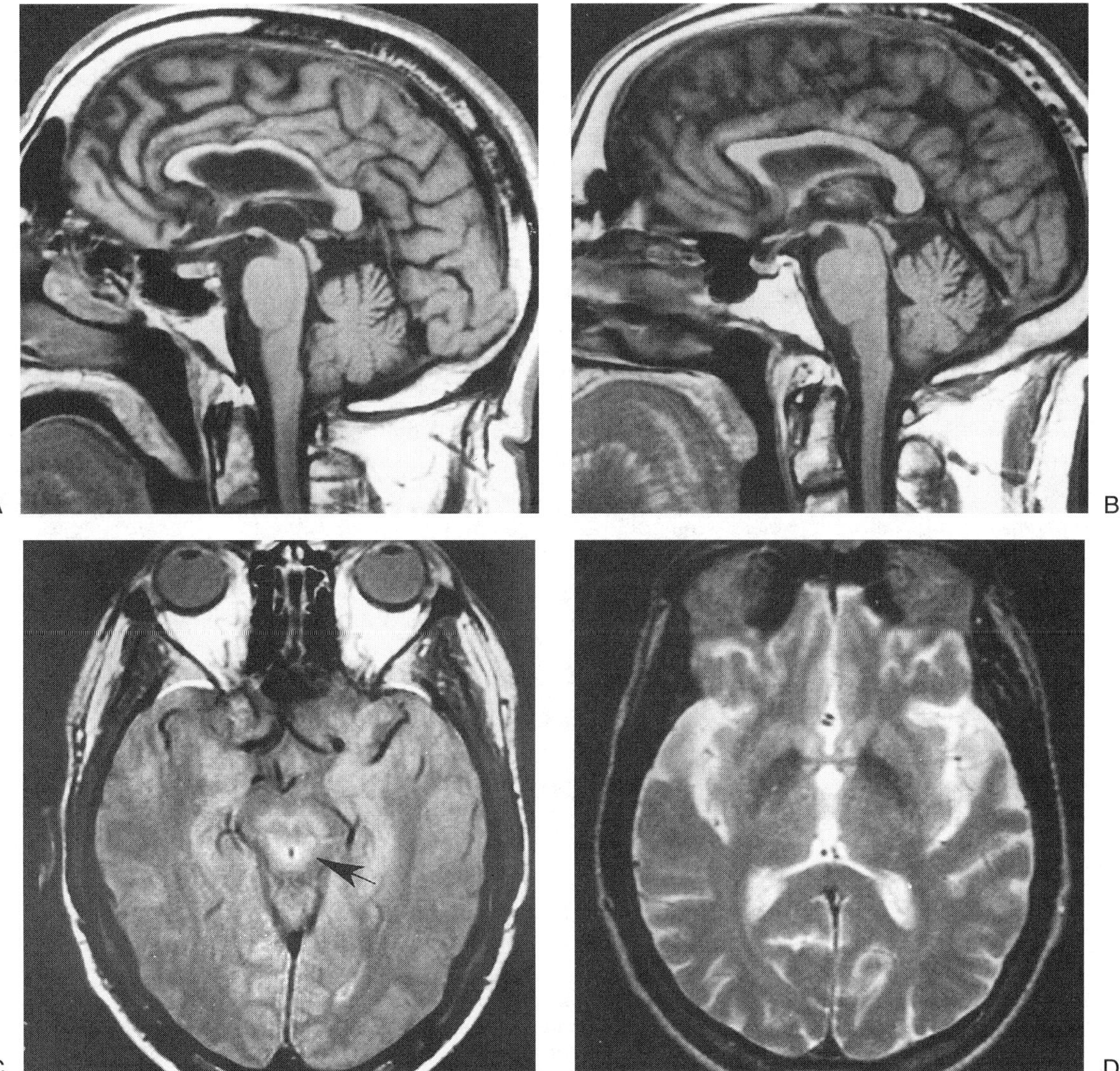

FIG. 2. PSP. 1.5 T MRI. In a severely affected patient (**A**) the sagittal midline T1-weighted image shows marked midbrain atrophy. In a less severely affected patient (**B** to **D**), the midbrain is mildly but definitely atrophic (**B**); compare the size and shape of the midbrain with the normal midbrain of Fig. 1, **C.** Axial proton density image through the midbrain shows periaqueductal hyperintensity (**C,** *arrow*). Axial T2-weighted image through the basal ganglia (**D**) shows normal pallidal hypointensity with normal signal in the putamina; the third ventricle is slightly enlarged.

this resulted in an enlargement of the third ventricle also visible in coronal and axial sections (Fig. 2 D). About one-fourth of the patients had, in fact, a disproportionate enlargement of the third ventricle compared to the size of the lateral ventricles.

The most common signal abnormality, present in 16 patients (66.7%), was a slight increase of signal intensity in proton density and FLAIR images in the periaqueductal region, consistent with cell loss and gliosis that are known to occur in this region (10) (Fig. 2 C).

Abnormalities in the basal ganglia were conspicuously absent. No signal abnormalities were seen at 0.5 T; in 1.5 T studies (eight cases), occasional slight hypointensity in T2-weighted images was seen in the putamina, consistent with iron deposition, never approaching the level of hypointensity normally present in the pallida. The putaminal hypointensity was judged consistent with the patient's age, as in a 79-year-old man with marked hypointensity, previously reported (4). The only patient in the present series who presented marked putaminal hypointensity was a 73-year-old man.

In the only case of PSP in which postmortem examination was carried out with Perls' stain and with 1.5 T MRI on a 1-cm thick coronal slice on the basal ganglia, no abnormal iron deposition was found (8).

Occasional hyperintensities of the white matter in T2-weighted images consistent with chronic ischemic changes did not exceed what could be expected in a normal population of the same age. In conclusion, our neuroradiological diagnosis of PSP has improved over time. At the beginning of our experience (8), we found that obvious atrophy of the midbrain was present in only about half of the patients with clinical diagnosis of PSP. This is still true; however, we are now confident in recognizing on the MR images milder degrees of midbrain atrophy that remarkably increase the percentage of MRI positive cases, reaching a level higher than 90%.

These findings should be validated by objective measurements in a prospective study. Measurements could not be obtained in this retrospective review, but we are convinced that, in a clinical setting, measurements are not necessary and experience of the neuroradiologist on the specific neurologic disorder under study is more important.

MRI differentiation of PSP from CBD is usually straightforward, although atypical presentations probably due to variations in the distribution of pathological changes may occur. The most characteristic MRI features of CBD, PSP, and the other disorders discussed in this chapter are summarized in Table 1.

FRONTOTEMPORAL DEMENTIA

Frontotemporal dementia (FTD) is caused by degeneration of the anterior frontal and temporal lobes and is characterized by severe modifications of the personality and social behavior. In our patients, FTD was diagnosed according to the criteria proposed by the Lund and Manches-

TABLE 1. *Distribution of characteristic MRI abnormalities in CBD and related atypical parkinsonian disorders and dementias*

	CBD	PSP	FTD	SND	AD
Atrophy	Fronto-parietal, asymmetrical	Midbrain, with diencephalic extension	Anterior frontal and temporal, basal ganglia, mainly caudate nucleus	(May be associated with pontine and cerebellar atrophy of OPCA)	Temporal, hippocampal, and diffuse
Signal abnormalities	Rare, slight hyperintensity in PD and T2-w.i. of atrophic cortex	Slight hyperintensity in PD-w.i. in periaqueductal area	Hyperintensity in PD and T2-w.i. of cortex and white matter in atrophic areas	1.5T: Hypointensity in T2-w.i. in posterior lateral putamen with lateral rim of hyperintensity 0.5T: Usually only hyperintensity in PD and T2-w.i. in posterior lateral putamen (may be associated with signal changes of OPCA)	No constant, specific signal abnormalities

PD = proton density; PD-w.i. = proton-density-weighted images; T2-w.i. = T2-weighted images.

ter groups (11); under this denomination different histopathological entities are included, mainly frontotemporal lobar degeneration and Pick's disease (12).

Our first MRI observation of Pick's disease regards a case of a woman 53 years of age, clinically affected by a frontotemporal dementia, whose sister had died after a progressive dementia with identical clinical features and course: her brain presented the histopathological features of Pick's disease.

Following this case, we observed nine other patients clinically characterized by a similar progressive course of frontotemporal dementia, without pathological proof but with identical MRI features. Therefore, without trying to distinguish Pick's disease from other forms of frontotemporal dementia by MRI, we will describe the highly characteristic MRI features observed in these patients, similar to those reported in other series (13–15).

The brain appears very markedly atrophic in the frontal and temporal regions, in a symmetrical or slightly asymmetrical way (Fig. 3 A, B). In the most advanced cases, the atrophy extends posteriorly to involve to a lesser degree the parietal regions, with the pre- and postcentral gyri remaining relatively unaffected (Fig. 3 A, B). In the most severely affected patients, only the occipital lobes were spared. The distribution of atrophy is particularly well demonstrated in the sagittal sections that show the "knife edge" aspect of the anterior frontal and temporo-polar gyri. The bulk of the white matter is greatly diminished in the axis of the convolutions and in the whole anterior part of the brain. The supratentorial ventricles enlarge, mainly anteriorly (Fig. 3 D). To the enlargement of the ventricles the atrophy of the basal ganglia contributes; the caudate nucleus is particularly atrophic, with its head almost vanishing in the most severely affected cases, causing a ballooning of the frontal horns. The atrophy of the head of the caudate nucleus was in some patients more marked than the severest atrophy ever observed by us in Huntington's chorea. In proton density and T2-weighted images, the signal abnormalities are remarkable; the extremely thin cortex and, even more, the subjacent white matter present an increased signal intensity that is marked in the anterior frontal and temporal regions and progressively diminishes backward (Fig. 3 C, D). In coronal sections through the chiasm, the normal T2 hypointensity of the chiasm stands out against the abnormal signal intensity of the cerebral hemispheres. As we go backward with the sections, we sometimes observe a preserved signal hypointensity of the optic radiations against the fading abnormal background of the white matter, which, in severely affected cases, becomes normal only in the occipital regions.

Another peculiar feature, always recognizable in axial sections in the advanced cases of our series, is the widening of the interpeduncular fossa. This is likely owing to atrophy of the frontopontine fibers which run in the medial part of the cerebral peduncles (Fig. 3C).

The distribution of all the findings and the signal changes described correspond to the distribution of the pathologic changes described in Pick's disease (16), but also in other types of frontotemporal dementia. What is important, in our opinion, is that we can demonstrate the distribution and the extention of the MRI abnormalities, thus giving unquestionable support to the diagnosis of FTD.

MULTIPLE SYSTEM ATROPHY: STRIATONIGRAL DEGENERATION

We shall not discuss here all the neuroradiological aspects of MSA. As the clinical and pathological studies demonstrate, MSA is a degenerative disorder that involves the basal ganglia, infratentorial structures, and the autonomic system. The involvement of the latter, however, is in the intermediolateral cell columns of the spinal cord and escapes demonstration by MRI. The involvement of infratentorial structures regards the olivopontocerebellar system; sporadic olivopontocerebellar atrophy (OPCA) is beautifully demonstrated by MRI (4,9,17). A recent review by Schrag et al. (18) of a Queen Square series demonstrates that all 16 cases with clinical diagnosis of OPCA type of MSA had the characteristic abnormalities in the brainstem and cerebellum, thus indicating 100% of sensitivity; specificity was higher than 90% both versus controls and idiopathic Parkinson's disease patients.

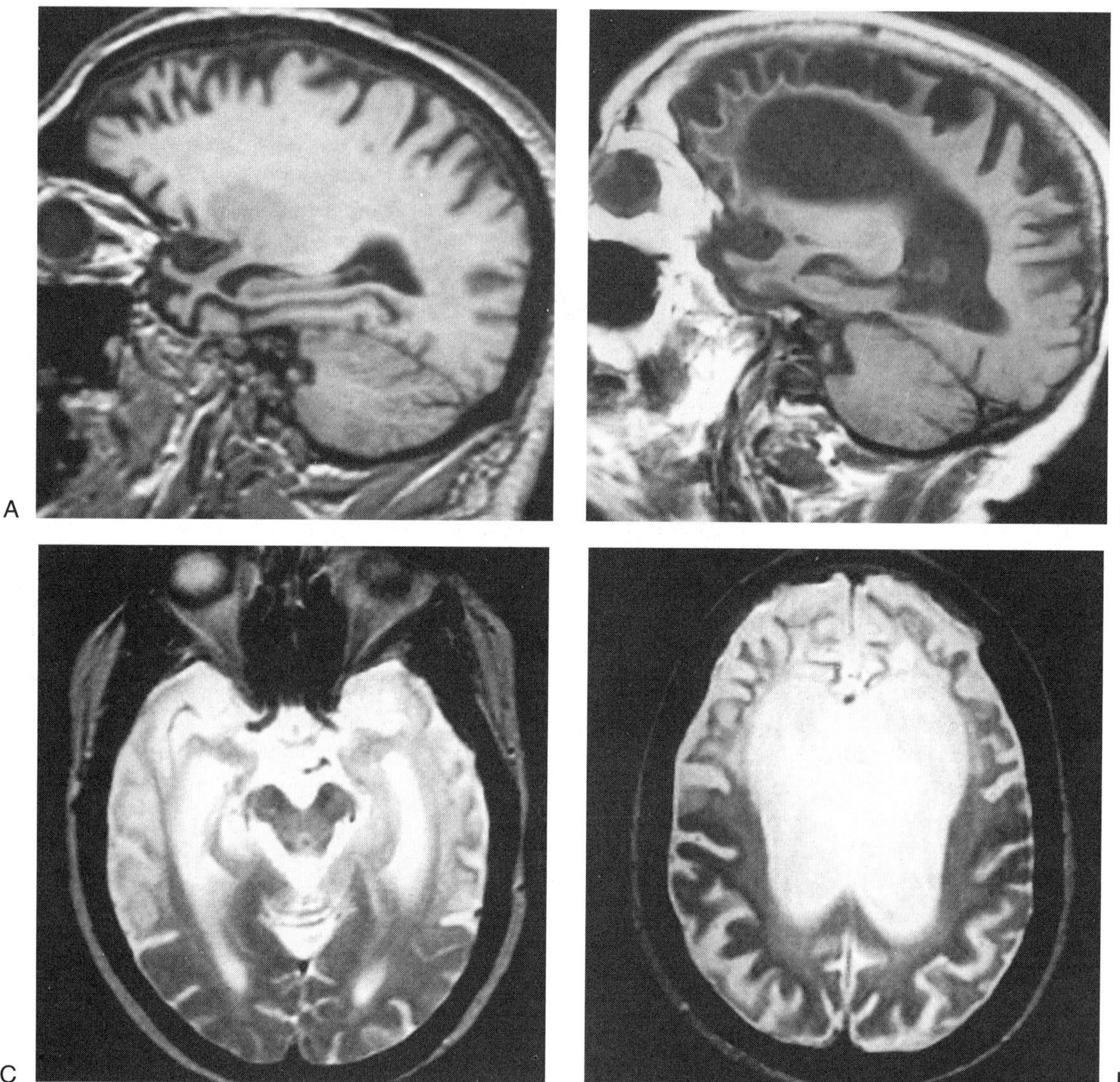

FIG. 3. FTD. In an initial case (**A**), the sagittal T1-weighted image on the right hemisphere shows mild to moderate frontal and more severe temporopolar atrophy. In a much more advanced case (**B** to **D**), marked frontal and temporal atrophy, with knife edge gyri in the anterior frontal and temporopolar regions (**B,** sagittal T1-weighted image on the right hemisphere), is present. This patient is a sister of a proven case of Pick's disease. Axial T2-weighted images (**C** and **D**) show an atrophic cortex in the anterior regions with marked hyperintensity also involving the subjacent white matter, fading posteriorly. The heads of the caudate nuclei are atrophic, with ballooning of the frontal horns (**D**). In the midbrain, there is atrophy of the medial part of the cerebral peduncles with consequent widening of the interpeduncular cistern (**C**).

A certain number of patients with MSA have simultaneous involvement of the infratentorial structures and of the basal ganglia, or isolated or strongly prevalent involvement of the extrapyramidal system (MSA-striatonigral degeneration type = MSA-SND) (Fig. 4).

In the SND type of MSA the pathological abnormalities are mostly located in the putamen, particularly in its posterior lateral part (19–23). The putamina become shrunk and discolored, with neuronal and myelin loss, gliosis, and deposition of iron, manganese, neuromelanin, and

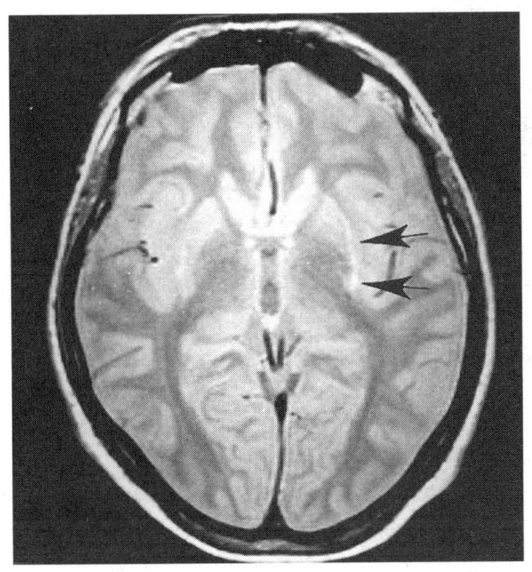

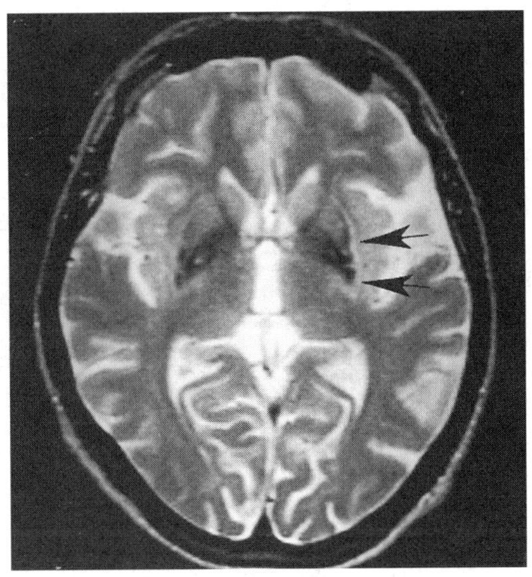

FIG. 4. MSA-SND. 1.5 T MRI. Axial proton density (**A**) and T2-weighted (**B**) images through the basal ganglia in a 55-year-old woman show T2 hypointensity consistent with iron deposition in the putamina; compare with the normal putaminal signal intensity of the PSP patient, of age 61, of Fig. 2 D. A thin rim of hyperintensity is visible in the most lateral part of the putamina, more evident on the left side (*arrows*).

hematin pigments. The putamina are, therefore, the structure that we have to observe for possible MRI abnormalities.

In 1986, Pastakia et al. (24) and Drayer et al. (25) simultaneously described loss of signal intensity in T2-weighted images at high field intensity MRI in the putamina, owing to magnetic susceptibility effects of ferric iron or other paramagnetic substances. The putamina become hypointense to the same or to a more marked degree than the pallida, where iron is normally present (Fig. 4 B). We observed that even lower field intensity MRI can demonstrate abnormalities in the putamina, which consist of high signal intensity related to increased water content (consistent with cell loss and gliosis) not masked at this field intensity (0.5 T or less) by the opposite effect of iron (8). We also observed that a thin rim of hyperintensity may sometimes remain visible also at 1.5 T MRI in the most lateral part of the putamen, not masked by the magnetic susceptibility effects of iron (Fig. 4); on the other hand, the iron deposition may occasionally be marked enough to be detected as a hypointensity even in 0.5 T MRI studies (8,9,17).

An important problem remains to be settled: How often are these findings present in clinically diagnosed SND? In other words, do they have a diagnostic value, and may support the clinical diagnosis, or are they found only in such advanced cases that their detection becomes unimportant?

In the review of 42 MSA cases that we published in 1993 (26), putaminal abnormalities were present in all the nine cases with clinical diagnosis of SND, in three of the 13 OPCA cases that all had infratentorial abnormalities, and were present in 17 of the 20 cases considered probable MSA, because parkinsonism poorly responding to L-dopa, cerebellar signs, and autonomic failure were present; 13 of these 20 patients also had infratentorial abnormalities characteristic of OPCA. In this group of 20 MSA patients, we had three patients with extrapyramidal signs with no detectable putaminal abnormalities at MRI.

In more recent MSA-SND cases we also occasionally found normal putamina at MRI, but signal abnormalities were present in most of the cases. However, we did not quantify these data and we had not yet specifically investigated sensitivity and specificity of these MRI findings. Schrag et al. in their recent review (18) found hyperintense putaminal rim on 1.5 T and putaminal hyperintensity on 0.5 T only in patients with MSA and in none of the control subjects or the patients with idiopathic Parkinson's disease (positive predictive value of 100%); however, these findings and putaminal hypointensity on 1.5 T were present only in a minority of their patients with MSA; in SND, basal ganglia abnormalities were present in 41% of the patients at 0.5 T, and 59% at 1.5 T. They conclude that sensitivity of the MRI findings in SND is limited and that absence of these changes does not exclude the diagnosis of MSA. We agree with this last point; the difference from our previous series may be partly explained by a different selection of the patients, since our cases might have been more severely affected, but further studies are needed to assess the sensitivity and specificity of the putaminal abnormalities.

ALZHEIMER'S DISEASE

Alzheimer's disease (AD) is the most common degenerative disorder of the brain and the most common cause of dementia; it hardly requires CT or MRI scans to support the diagnosis. Cerebral atrophy with more marked involvement of the temporal lobes is demonstrated by both imaging techniques. However, with its coronal sections, MRI is more demonstrative of the complete distribution of atrophy.

There is considerable overlapping between the atrophy of AD and that of the normal aging population, at least in the initial stages. However, longitudinal studies show that the progression of atrophy is faster in AD patients (27). Because of the prevalent temporal involvement, the suprasellar cisterns, the sylvian fissures, and the temporal horns become particularly enlarged (15,28) (Fig. 5). More subtle signs, well demonstrated only by coronal MRI, are dilatation of the choroidal fissure and atrophy of the hippocampus itself, which is less affected in normal aging (29,30). Measurements of the hippocampal or amigdalohippocampal volume have been proposed (15,31,32), but are not applicable in a clinical setting.

Signal abnormalities consisting of hyperintensity in proton density and T2-weighted images may be occasionally seen in the hippocampus and adjacent mesial temporal structures (33,34); they probably reflect the histopathology of AD, with neuronal loss, gliosis, senile plaques, etc., prominent in these regions. Other signal changes,

A 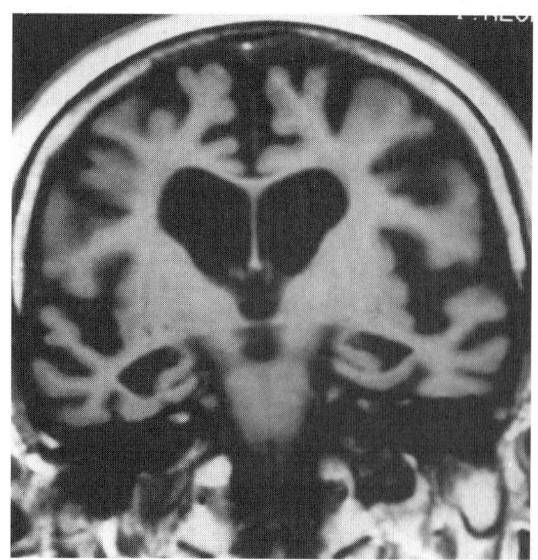

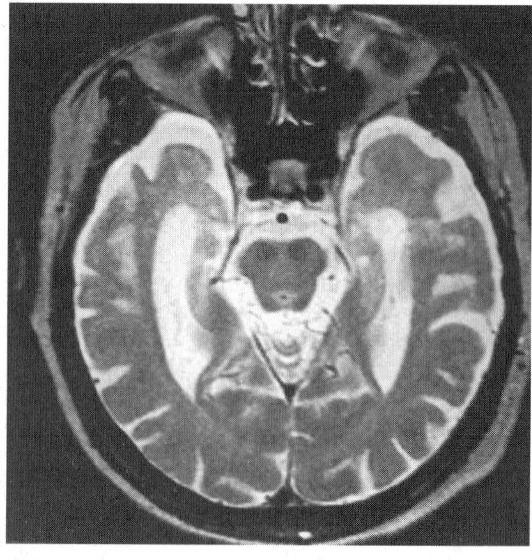 B

FIG. 5. AD. Coronal T1-weighted section (**A**) shows diffuse atrophy more marked in the temporal lobes, particularly of the hippocampi. Axial T2-weighted image (**B**) confirms severe atrophy of the temporal lobes with enlargement of the sylvian fissures, ambiens and perisellar cisterns, without definite signal abnormalities.

such as periventricular hyperintensities possibly representing incomplete white matter infarctions, seem to be more frequent in AD patients than in normal elderly subjects (33,35), but this difference is not found in other series (36).

In conclusion, distribution of atrophy in the temporal regions, and particularly atrophy of the hippocampus, are the best support to the diagnosis of AD; they are best demonstrated by coronal MRI. The search of a simple measurement that can be made on routine MRI, able to differentiate AD from normal aging, remains elusive (37,38).

CONCLUSIONS

MRI may give a strong support to the diagnosis of many neurodegenerative diseases, both in the group of motor disorders and dementias. The ability of MRI to show the entire brain in different planes is extremely useful, because it allows the recognition of the distribution of the signal abnormalities that very likely reflects the distribution of the pathological changes. The distribution of certain pathologies can vary, thus accounting for certain "atypical" presentations of various pathological disorders; however, the occurrence of "atypical" presentations implies that typical cases are fortunately the rule.

Obviously, many pathological changes, particularly in the degenerative diseases, may not have an MRI correlate, but it is hard to believe that signal abnormalities do not have a pathological correlate. Since the distribution of histopathological changes is hard to obtain from most pathological reports that often explore only a limited number of structures, the value of MRI is indubitable. Knowledge of the distribution of pathological changes, that often is so well demonstrated by MRI, is particularly important when we consider Neary's comments regarding frontotemporal degeneration, Pick's disease, and corticobasal degeneration (12): If the brain has a limited repertoire of responses to a variety of degenerative processes of different origin, the demonstration of the *distribution* of the involved areas obtained by MRI is indeed important and allows clinical correlations, no matter what the exact histopathological processes.

REFERENCES

1. Caselli RJ, Jack CR Jr, Petersen RC, Wahner HW, Yanagihara T. Asymmetric cortical degenerative syndromes: clinical and radiological correlations. *Neurology* 1992;42:1462–1468.
2. Giménez-Roldán S, Mateo D, Benito C, Grandas F, Pérez-Gilabert Y. Progressive supranuclear palsy and corticobasal ganglionic degeneration: differentiation by clinical features and neuroimaging techniques. *J Neural Transm* 1994;42:(suppl)79–90.
3. Grisoli M, Fetoni V, Savoiardo M, Girotti F, Bruzzone MG. MRI in corticobasal degeneration. *Eur J Neurol* 1995;2:547–552.
4. Savoiardo M, Grisoli M. Magnetic resonance imaging of movement disorders. In: Jankovic J, Tolosa E, eds. *Parkinson's disease and movement disorders.* Baltimore: Williams & Wilkins, 1998:967–990.
5. Litvan I, Agid Y, Goetz C, et al. Accuracy of the clinical diagnosis of corticobasal degeneration: a clinicopathologic study. *Neurology* 1997;48:119–125.
6. Litvan I, Agid Y, Jankovic J, et al. Accuracy of clinical criteria for the diagnosis of progressive supranuclear palsy (Steele-Richardson-Olszewski syndrome). *Neurology* 1996;46:922–930.
7. Schonfeld SM, Golbe LI, Sage JI, Safer JN, Duvoisin RC. Computed tomographic findings in progressive supranuclear palsy: correlation with clinical grade. *Movement Disorders* 1987;2:263–278.
8. Savoiardo M, Strada L, Girotti F, D'Incerti L, Sherna L, Soliveri P, et al. MR imaging in progressive supranuclear palsy and Shy-Drager syndrome. *J Comput Assist Tomogr* 1989;13:555–560.
9. Savoiardo M, Girotti F, Strada L, Ciceri E. Magnetic resonance imaging in progressive supranuclear palsy and other parkinsonian disorders. *J Neural Transm* 1994;42:(suppl)93–110.
10. Aiba I, Hashizume Y, Yoshida M, Okuda S, Murakami N, Ujihira N. Relationship between brainstem MRI and pathological findings in progressive supranuclear palsy—study in autopsy cases. *J Neurol Sci* 1997;152:210–217.
11. Brun A, Englund B, Gustafson L, et al. Clinical and neuropathological criteria for frontotemporal dementia. *J Neurol Neurosurg Psychiatry* 1994;57:416–418.
12. Neary D. Frontotemporal degeneration, Pick disease, and corticobasal degeneration. One entity or 3? 3. *Arch Neurol* 1997;54:1425–1427.
13. Kitagaki H, Mori E, Hirono N, et al. Alteration of white matter MR signal intensity in frontotemporal dementia. *Am J Neuroradiol* 1997;18:367–378.
14. Kitagaki H, Mori E, Yamaji S, et al. Frontotemporal dementia and Alzheimer disease: evaluation of cortical atrophy with automated hemispheric surface display generated with MR images. *Radiology* 1998;208:431–439.
15. Frisoni GB, Beltramello A, Geroldi C, Weiss C, Bianchetti A, Trabucchi M. Brain atrophy in frontotemporal dementia. *J Neurol Neurosurg Psychiatry* 1996;61:157–165.
16. Tomlinson BE, Corsellis JAN. Ageing and the dementias. In: Hume Adams J, Corsellis JAN, Duchen LW, eds. *Greenfield's neuropathology, 4th ed.* New York: Wiley, 1984:951–1025.
17. Savoiardo M, Strada L, Girotti F, et al. Olivopontocerebellar atrophy: MR diagnosis and relationship to multisystem atrophy. *Radiology* 1990;174:693–696.

18. Schrag A, Kingsley D, Phatouros C, et al. Clinical usefulness of magnetic resonance imaging in multiple system atrophy. *J Neurol Neurosurg Psychiatry* 1998;65:65–71.
19. Borit A, Rubinstein LJ, Urich H. The striatonigral degenerations: putaminal pigments and nosology. *Brain* 1975;98:101–112.
20. Oppenheimer DR. Diseases of the basal ganglia, cerebellum and motor neurons. In: Hume Adams J, Corsellis JAN, Duchen LW, eds. *Greenfield's neuropathology.* 4th ed. New York: Wiley, 1984:699–747.
21. Fearnley JM, Lees AJ. Striatonigral degeneration. A clinicopathological study. *Brain* 1990;113:1823–1842.
22. Dexter DT, Carayon A, Javoy-Agid F, et al. Alterations in the levels of iron, ferritin and other trace metals in Parkinson's disease and other neurodegenerative diseases affecting the basal ganglia. *Brain* 1991;114: 1953–1975.
23. Goto S, Matsumoto S, Ushio Y, Hirano A. Subregional loss of putaminal efferents to the basal ganglia output nuclei may cause parkinsonism in striatonigral degeneration. *Neurology* 1996;47:1032–1036.
24. Pastakia B, Polinsky R, Di Chiro G, Simmons JT, Brown R, Wener L. Multiple system atrophy (Shy-Drager syndrome): MR imaging. *Radiology* 1986;159:499–502.
25. Drayer BP, Olanow W, Burger P, Johnson GA, Herfkens R, Riederer S. Parkinson plus syndrome: diagnosis using high field MR imaging of brain iron. *Radiology* 1986; 159:493–498.
26. Testa D, Savoiardo M, Fetoni V, et al. Multiple system atrophy. Clinical and MR observations on 42 cases. *Ital J Neurol Sci* 1993;14:211–216.
27. de Leon MJ, George AE, Reisberg B, et al. Alzheimer's disease: longitudinal CT studies of ventricular change. *Am J Neuroradiol* 1989;10:371–376.
28. Le May M. CT changes in dementing diseases: a review. *Am J Neuroradiol* 1986;7:841–853.
29. de Leon MJ, Golomb J, George AE, Convit A, Tarshish CY, McRae T. The radiologic prediction of Alzheimer disease: the atrophic hippocampal formation. *Am J Neuroradiol* 1993;14:897–906.
30. Drayer BP. Imaging of the aging brain. Part II. Pathologic conditions. *Radiology* 1988;166:797–806.
31. Jack CR Jr, Petersen RC, O'Brien PC, Tangalos EG. MR-based hippocampal volumetry in the diagnosis of Alzheimer's disease. *Neurology* 1992;42:183–188.
32. Mori E, Yoneda Y, Yamashita H, Hirono N, Ikeda M, Yamadori A. Medial temporal structures relate to memory impairment in Alzheimer's disease: a MRI volumetric study. *J Neurol Neurosurg Psychiatry* 1997;63: 214–221.
33. Fazekas F, Chawluk JB, Alavi A, Hurtig HI, Zimmerman RA. MR signal abnormalities at 1.5 T in Alzheimer's dementia and normal aging. *Am J Neuroradiol* 1987; 8:421–426.
34. Lexa FJ, Trojanowski JQ, Braffman BH, Atlas SW. The aging brain and neurodegenerative diseases. In: Atlas SW, ed. *Magnetic resonance imaging of the brain and spine.* 2nd ed. Philadelphia: Lippincott-Raven, 1996: 803–870.
35. Bowen BC, Barker WW, Loewenstein DA, Sheldon J, Duara R. MR signal abnormalities in memory disorder and dementia. *Am J Neuroradiol* 1990;11:283–290.
36. Kobari M, Meyer JS, Ichijo M, Oravez WT. Leukoaraiosis: correlation of MR and CT findings with blood flow, atrophy, and cognition. *Am J Neuroradiol* 1990;11: 273–281.
37. Howieson J, Kaye JA, Holm L, Howieson D. Interuncal distance: marker of aging and Alzheimer disease. *Am J Neuroradiol* 1993;14:647–650.
38. Osborn AG. *Diagnostic neuroradiology.* St. Louis: Mosby, 1994.

Corticobasal Degeneration.
Advances in Neurology, Vol. 82,
edited by I. Litvan, C. G. Goetz, and A. E. Lang.
Lippincott Williams & Wilkins, Philadelphia © 2000.

19

Functional Imaging Studies in Corticobasal Degeneration

David J. Brooks

MRC Cyclotron Unit, Imperial College School of Medicine, London W12 0NN, United Kingdom

INTRODUCTION

The diagnosis of corticobasal degeneration (CBD) can pose considerable problems in life when clinical criteria alone are applied. Combinations of ideomotor apraxia, parkinsonism, dystonia, and myoclonus may be features of Pick's and Alzheimer's disease, prion disorders, diffuse Lewy body disease, striatonigral degeneration, and hemiatrophy-hemiparkinsonism syndrome, whereas supranuclear gaze problems, pseudobulbar dysfunction, parkinsonism, and gait instability are all features of PSP. Given this, it clearly would be helpful to have additional means of distinguishing CBD *in vivo* from other akinetic-rigid and apraxic syndromes in order to define a homogeneous patient population.

Structural brain imaging (MRI/CT) can be of diagnostic help in CBD if asymmetric frontoparietal atrophy is evident (1). In practice, however, only around 50% of suspected cases show such atrophy and it can be fairly subtle when present. Functional imaging (PET, SPECT, magnetic resonance spectroscopy [MRS]) provides a sensitive means of detecting and characterising regional changes in resting brain metabolism and receptor binding associated with the various parkinsonian syndromes. PET and MRI can also be used to study brain activation, as evidenced by local changes in blood flow, during performance of tasks or experience of sensory stimuli. This chapter will review the changes in regional cerebral blood flow, metabolism, and dopamine receptor binding reported in association with CBD.

RESTING METABOLIC STUDIES IN CBD

Sawle and coworkers (2) studied resting levels of regional cerebral oxygen metabolism ($rCMRO_2$) with $^{15}O_2$ PET for six patients aged 57 to 79 who were clinically diagnosed as having probable CBD. All had an asymmetrical non–L-dopa responsive akinetic-rigid syndrome with limb apraxia, whereas four had a supranuclear gaze palsy, three had limb myoclonus, and three exhibited alien limb phenomenon. One of these six cases subsequently had the diagnosis confirmed with a frontal brain biopsy. None of the six were demented at the time of PET but four had frontal lobe release signs and one showed expressive dysphasic and speech comprehension difficulties. Five out of the six had generalized cerebral atrophy on CT, whereas radiology was normal in the sixth. PET findings were compared with those of six age-matched controls.

Cortical oxygen metabolism ($rCMRO_2$) was globally reduced for the CBD group. In order to minimize the effect of global on focal $rCMRO_2$ variance these workers normalized all regional brain $rCMRO_2$ data to values measured for primary visual cortex, an area spared by CBD pathology, prior to statistical analysis. Relative reductions in oxygen metabolism were seen in superior prefrontal cortex (17%), both lateral (16%) and mesial premotor (19%) areas, and in sensorimotor (16%), inferior parietal (16%), and superior temporal (21%) cortex. In contrast to the reported metabolic changes in Pick's disease, the reductions in cortical metabolism were strikingly asymmetrical in these CBD cases and inferior frontal and temporal cortex were relatively spared (Fig. 1). The only significantly affected subcortical area was the thalamus where metabolism was reduced 15%, again in a strikingly asymmetrical pattern.

Eidelberg and coworkers (3) measured side-to-side asymmetry of regional cerebral glucose metabolism (rCMRGlc) in five cases of clinically probable CBD, mean age 68, one of whom had the diagnosis subsequently confirmed at necropsy. All five patients had progressively worsening unilateral limb rigidity or tremor resistant to levodopa associated with apraxia (4), cortical sensory impairment (4), and pyramidal signs (5). Three of the five manifested possible alien limb phenomena and one was dysphasic intermittently. No intellectual decline or supranuclear gaze difficulties were evident. Two (40%) patients had asymmetrical cortical atrophy, one had symmetrical cortical atrophy, and the other two had normal structural imaging. PET findings were compared with those obtained for 18 age-matched controls and nine patients with asymmetrical Parkinson's disease.

Brain glucose metabolism was globally reduced by 38% in CBD and lateral temporal, inferior parietal and frontal opercular regions were focally targeted. Left-right metabolic asymmetries were significantly increased in inferior parietal, medial temporal, and thalamic regions compared with both normal and PD cohorts. Individually, all of the five CBD patients showed a greater than 5% side-to-side asymmetry in parietal rCMRGlc, although, surprisingly, no significant asymmetry in striatal rCMRGlc was noted. In contrast, none of the nine PD patients showed a greater than 5% side-to-side rCMRGlc asymmetry in any brain region, although all these subjects had asymmetrical parkinsonism.

Blin and coworkers (4) reported ^{18}FDG PET findings for five patients, mean age 62 years, with clinically probable CBD. Again, all their patients had a progressive non–L-dopa responsive asymmetric akinetic-rigid syndrome associated with apraxia. Four patients had a dystonic limb and two exhibited alien phenomena. All showed evidence of postural instability but none had a supranuclear gaze paresis. Although none of these subjects were demented, three showed "frontal" behavior patterns. Four of these five subjects had normal MRI findings, whereas the fifth showed mild left hemisphere atrophy. PET findings were compared with those obtained for five age-matched controls.

As previously noted, mean resting levels of glucose metabolism were significantly reduced

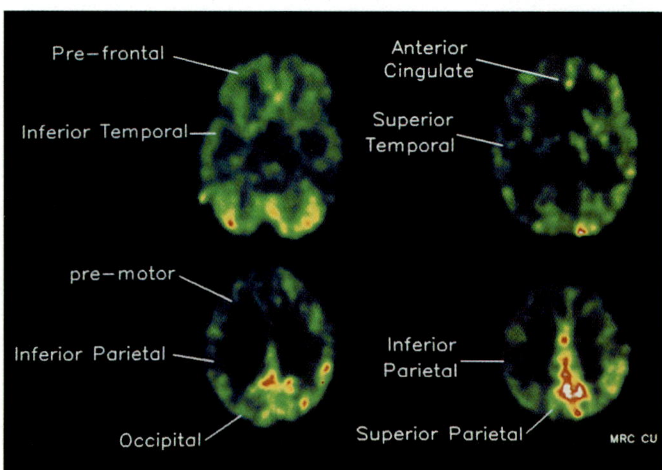

FIG. 1. PET images of $^{15}O_2$ uptake showing asymmetrically reduced oxygen metabolism in superior frontal, superior temporal, inferior parietal, and thalamic areas of a patient with probable CBD (image, courtesy of GV Sawle).

in frontal, temporal, sensorimotor, and parietal areas. Subcortically, caudate, lenticular, and thalamic metabolism were also impaired. There was a clear asymmetry in these metabolic reductions, the hemisphere contralateral to the clinically more affected side being more affected (Table 1).

Nagasawa and colleagues (5) have studied six cases of clinically probable CBD with ^{18}FDG PET. All six had progressive limb rigidity and apraxia and three exhibited alien limb phenomena. One was demented and another aphasic and none of the six responded to L-dopa therapy. MRI showed mild symmetrical cortical atrophy in five and right frontotemporal atrophy in the sixth. These workers reported asymmetrically reduced levels of rCMRGlc in parietal and sensorimotor cortex, thalamus, caudate nucleus, and putamen contralateral to the dominantly affected limbs. Occipital, inferior frontal, and temporal cortex were relatively spared, as previously noted.

The changes in regional cerebral blood flow (rCBF) associated with CBD have been studied with ^{99m}Tc-HMPAO SPECT. Markus and coworkers (6) compared SPECT findings for eight clinically probable CBD patients with those obtained for 12 age-matched PD patients and 12 normal controls. The eight CBD cases all had asymmetric, non–L-dopa responsive limb rigidity, whereas seven had apraxia, four exhibited alien limb phenomena, four had a cortical sensory deficit, and three had limb myoclonus. Six out of the eight cases showed cerebral atrophy on MRI but this was felt to be asymmetrical in only one of the eight patients.

Compared with controls, the rCBF images of the CBD patients all showed a striking asymmetry and there were significant reductions of rCBF in the more affected hemisphere targeting posterior frontal cortex (12%), the parietal lobe (10 to 13%), caudate (9%), putamen (10%), and thalamus (9%). ^{99m}Tc-HMPAO uptake was normal in temporal and occipital cortex. Individually, seven of the eight CBD cases showed significant reductions in contralateral parietal rCBF. A similar but less severe pattern of impairment was also evident in the other hemisphere of these patients.

TABLE 1. *Mean percentage reductions in rCMRGlc in five cases of CBD*

Brain region	Contralateral	Ipsilateral
Frontal cortex	25	19
Temporal cortex	33	22
Sensorimotor cortex	39	27
Lentiform nucleus	25	15
Thalamus	28	18

After Blin et al. (4).

Storey and coworkers (7) have reported ^{99m}Tc-HMPAO SPECT findings for seven of eight patients with probable CBD who presented with asymmetric upper limb rigidity and dystonia accompanied by ipsilateral ideomotor apraxia, cortical sensory disturbance, and sensory reflex myoclonus. SPECT revealed contralateral fronto-parietal perfusion defects out of proportion to the focal or generalized atrophy demonstrated on MRI scans. The authors concluded that SPECT scanning appeared to be a useful confirmatory investigation in patients presenting with probable CBD and capable of separating them from patients with other causes of asymmetric rigid syndromes, such as Parkinson's disease.

Okuda and coworkers (8) have reported ^{123}I-IMP SPECT findings for two cases of possible CBD. Both patients had increased limb rigidity with apraxia, which was felt to be limb-kinetic in one case and constructional in character in the other. SPECT showed reduced levels of resting rCBF in perirolandic areas and posterior parietal cortex.

Regional cerebral metabolism has been studied with proton magnetic resonance spectroscopy (PMRS) in nine patients with probable CBD (9). These cases all had a progressive asymmetrical parkinsonian syndrome that was unresponsive to dopaminergic medication with associated limb dystonia, myoclonus, apraxia, or cortical sensory loss. Eight of the nine cases had cortical atrophy, although this was not noted to be asymmetrical. No midbrain atrophy was evident. The *N-acetylaspartate*:creatine (NAA/Cr) ratio was reduced in the centrum semiovale of CBD cases but not in cortical regions or the basal ganglia. The NAA/choline ratio, however, was significantly reduced in both parietal cortex and the lentiform nucleus.

To summarize, PET and SPECT studies on patients with clinically probable CBD have all shown strikingly asymmetrical reductions in resting levels of brain metabolism and blood flow. The dysfunction is most severe in the brain hemisphere contralateral to the more affected limbs and particularly targets posterior frontal, inferior parietal, and superior temporal regions, and also thalamus and striatum. PMRS has also demonstrated reduced NAA/Cho ratios in the parietal cortex and lentiform nucleus in CBD.

DOPAMINERGIC STUDIES IN CBD

At autopsy, a uniform loss of nigral cells and reduction in caudate and putamen dopamine levels has been reported in CBD (1). Striatal uptake of the PET tracer ^{18}F-6-fluorodopa (^{18}F-dopa) reflects the capacity of the caudate and putamen to decarboxylate L-dopa and retain exogenous dopamine and so provides a functional measure of the integrity of nigro-striatal dopaminergic terminals.

Sawle and coworkers (2) measured striatal ^{18}F-dopa uptake for their six CBD patients and found that both caudate and putamen influx constants (Ki) were reduced in an asymmetric fashion, reductions being greatest in the structures contralateral to the clinically more affected limbs Figs. 2 and 3. Overall there was a similar mean 34% reduction in caudate and 38% reduction in putamen Ki associated with CBD. These workers also measured mesial frontal ^{18}F-dopa uptake; this was reduced by 37% in their patients suggesting that the function of both mesofrontal and nigrostriatal dopaminergic projections is affected in this condition.

Eidelberg and coworkers (3) studied one of their five CBD cases with ^{18}F-dopa PET. Striatal Ki values were reduced to 31% and 45% of the normal mean—individual caudate and putamen influx constants were not reported. Nagasawa et al. (5) studied four of their six CBD cases with ^{18}F-dopa PET. In agreement with Sawle and coworkers, these workers found an asymmetric reduction in striatal Ki. Caudate and putamen ^{18}F-dopa uptake were equivalently affected and reduced to around 25% of normal in the most affected hemisphere.

There have been two ^{123}I-IBZM SPECT case reports on striatal dopamine D_2 receptor binding in CBD. Frisoni et al. (10) scanned a 44-year-old male with an apraxic, akinetic-rigid left arm, sensory inattention and reflex myoclonus. The MRI showed right sided cortical atrophy and basal ganglia ^{123}I-IBZM uptake was asymmetric (14% lower in the right striatum relative to the left). Schwarz and colleagues (11) noted that a case of CBD amongst their nine cases out of 65 patients with *de novo* parkinsonism who failed to respond to dopaminergic medication had reduced striatal IBZM binding. Case details, however, were not formally presented.

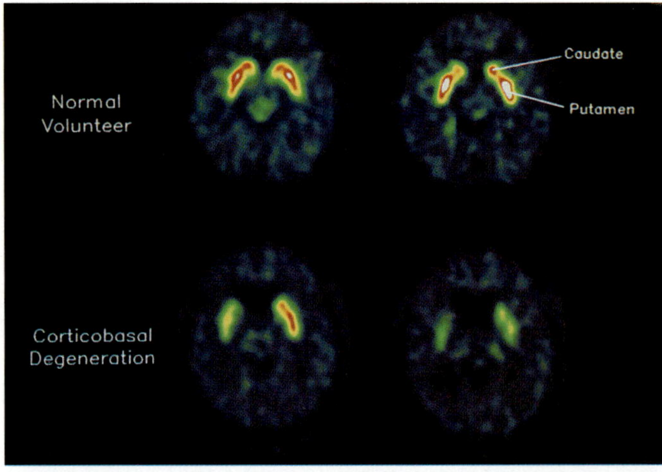

FIG. 2. PET images of striatal ^{18}F-dopa uptake in a normal subject. PD and CBD patients. It can be seen that although striatal dopaminergic function is asymmetrically reduced in both PD and CBD, caudate and putamen are equivalently affected in the latter (image, courtesy of GV Sawle).

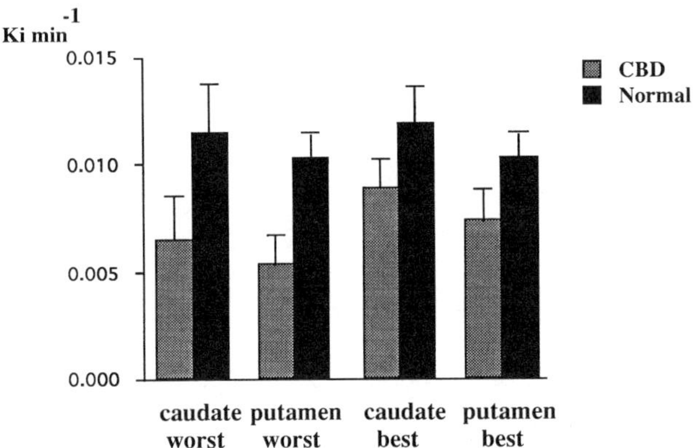

FIG. 3. A column graph showing mean levels of striatal ^{18}F-dopa uptake in CBD.

To summarize, striatal ^{18}F-dopa uptake can be reduced as low as 25% of normal in CBD and caudate and putamen are invariably similarly affected. Mean striatal dopamine D_2 receptor binding is also moderately reduced in CBD, which may help to explain the L-dopa resistant akinetic-rigid syndromes of these patients, although it is likely that degeneration of downstream pallidal and brainstem projections is also a contributor.

COMPARISON WITH PARKINSON'S DISEASE AND OTHER PARKINSONIAN SYNDROMES

Metabolic Studies

Several studies have directly compared the patterns of resting regional cerebral glucose metabolism or blood flow seen in CBD and PD. The pattern of metabolic derangement in CBD is characterized by asymmetric hypometabolism and hypoperfusion of inferior parietal, posterior frontal, superior temporal, thalamic, and striatal regions. This contrasts with PD where: (a) no asymmetry of cortical or striatal metabolism is generally evident despite the lateralization of the clinical involvement (3,6); and (b) levels of striatal metabolism are invariably preserved (12).

In their PMRS study, Tedeschi and coworkers (9) found that levels of lenticular NAA/Cr and NAA/Cho metabolite ratios did not reliably discriminate CBD and PD. Their CBD cases, however, showed reduced NAA levels in parietal cortex and centrum semiovale in contrast to the PD patients.

Nagahama and colleagues (13) directly compared the pattern of rCMRGlc in eight patients with clinically probable CBD and eight patients thought to have progressive supranuclear palsy (PSP). When compared with the PSP cases, the CBD cohort showed relatively reduced levels of inferior parietal, striatal, and thalamic glucose metabolism in their worst affected hemispheres. This was true even when the comparison was run against the five most asymmetric PSP cases.

Dopaminergic Studies

Although the nigra is uniformly involved in CBD, in PD the Lewy body degeneration targets the ventrolateral nigral dopaminergic projections to dorsal putamen (14) and, as a consequence, putamen dopamine levels fall to half those remaining in the head of caudate (15). Given this, one would expect relative levels of caudate: putamen ^{18}F-dopa uptake to discriminate CBD from PD. This is certainly the case for PSP and PD where ^{18}F-dopa PET can discriminate 90% of PSP cases from PD on the basis of their relatively lower caudate dopamine storage capacity (16).

To date, only one study has directly compared ^{18}F-dopa PET findings in CBD and PD. Eidelberg et al. (3) contrasted striatal ^{18}F-dopa uptake for a single case of CBD with that of 11 PD patients. These workers found that there was no significant difference in the level of striatal Ki or degree of side-to-side Ki asymmetry in their CBD case from the PD cohort. Unfortunately, however, these workers were not able to compare

TABLE 2. *PET findings in akinetic-rigid syndromes*

	PD	Diffuse LBD	SND	PSP	CBD	Picks
FDG	Normal	Low parietal/ temporal	Low striatal/ post frontal	Low striatal/ post frontal	Low thal/str inf par/post fr	Low striatal/ inf fr/inf temp
F-dopa	Putamen < caudate	Putamen < caudate	Putamen < caudate	Putamen = caudate	Putamen = caudate	Normal
Putamen D_2 binding	Raised (untreated) normal (treated)		Normal/low	Normal/low	Low	Normal

relative levels of caudate and putamen ^{18}F-dopa uptake in CBD and PD, which might have provided greater discrimination. Even though there are no directly comparative studies, it seems clear from the findings of Sawle et al. (2) and Nagasawa et al. (5) that caudate and putamen reductions are equivalent in CBD, whereas many groups have now demonstrated that putamen ^{18}F-dopa uptake is around half that of caudate in PD (17). Given this, the finding of an asymmetrical reduction in striatal Ki affecting putamen and caudate equally severely should be regarded as being strongly supportive of a presumptive diagnosis of CBD.

There is also the possibility that measurements of striatal D_2 binding may help distinguish CBD from PD though this has never been formally investigated. *De novo* PD patients have mildly raised putamen dopamine D_2 binding when assessed with ^{11}C-raclopride PET, which subsequently normalizes after chronic exposure to L-dopa therapy (18). In contrast, two cases of CBD have been reported to show reductions in striatal ^{123}I-IBZM uptake (10,11).

Further studies are required to establish whether measures of striatal dopamine receptor binding will prove to be a valuable means of discriminating CBD from PD.

Table 2 summarizes reported PET findings in CBD and compares these with other parkinsonian disorders.

FUTURE PERSPECTIVES

Although functional imaging has shown distinctive patterns of resting metabolic and dopaminergic dysfunction in CBD, there have been no formal discriminant analysis studies designed to determine how effectively CBD can be separated from other parkinsonian disorders. It is likely, however, that the majority of CBD patients can be reliably discriminated by a combination of: (a) asymmetrically reduced inferior parietal and thalamic blood flow/glucose metabolism and striatal ^{18}F-dopa uptake/dopamine transporter binding, and (b) equivalently reduced caudate and putamen dopamine terminal function. This will no doubt be formally confirmed in future series.

The majority of functional imaging ligand studies concerning parkinsonian syndromes have concentrated on the dopaminergic system. In the future it will be possible to explore other neuromodulatory systems, such as cholinergic, noradrenergic, opioid, and serotonergic function. It is already becoming clear that muscarinic and opioid receptor binding is differentially affected in PD and PSP (19,20) and this may also be true for CBD. Perhaps, more excitingly, it is now becoming possible to examine changes in neurotransmitter fluxes with PET and SPECT as evidenced by alterations in receptor availability to ligands after pharmacological and behavioral challenges. In the future it will be possible to directly assess *in vivo* the ability of dopaminergic and other pathways to release neurotransmitters in degenerative diseases and so directly quantify their functional impairment.

REFERENCES

1. Riley DE, Lang AE, Lewis A, et al. Cortical-basal ganglionic degeneration. *Neurology* 1990;40:1203–1212.
2. Sawle GV, Brooks DJ, Marsden CD, Frackowiak RSJ. Corticobasal degeneration: a unique pattern of regional cortical oxygen metabolism and striatal fluorodopa uptake demonstrated by positron emission tomography. *Brain* 1991; 114:541–556.
3. Eidelberg D, Dhawan V, Moeller JR, et al. The metabolic landscape of corticobasal ganglionic degeneration: regional asymmetries studied with positron emission

tomography. *J Neurol Neurosurg Psychiat* 1991;54: 856–862.
4. Blin J, Vidhailhet M-J, Pillon B, Dubois B, Feve J-R, Agid Y. Corticobasal degeneration: Decreased and asymmetrical glucose consumption as studied by PET. *Move Dis* 1992;7:348–354.
5. Nagasawa H, Tanji H, Nomura H, et al. PET study of cerebral glucose metabolism and fluorodopa uptake in patients with corticobasal degeneration. *J Neurol Sci* 1996;39:210–217.
6. Markus HS, Lees AJ, Lennox G, Marsden CD, Costa DC. Patterns of regional cerebral blood flow in corticobasal degeneration studied using HMPAO SPECT—comparison with Parkinson's disease and normal controls. *Move Dis* 1995;10:179–187.
7. Storey E, Lichtenstein M, Desmond P, Lloyd J. Clinical features and SPECT scanning in presumed corticobasal ganglionic degeneration. *J Clin Neurosci* 1995;2:321–328.
8. Okuda B, Tachibana H, Takeda M, Kawabata K, Sugita M, Fukuchi M. Focal cortical hypoperfusion in corticobasal degeneration demonstrated by three-dimensional surface display with ^{123}I-IMP: a possible cause of apraxia. *Neuroradiology* 1995;37:642–644.
9. Tedeschi G, Litvan I, Bonavita S, et al. Proton magnetic resonance spectroscopic imaging in progressive supranuclear palsy, Parkinson's disease and corticobasal degeneration. *Brain* 1997;120:1541–1552.
10. Frisoni GB, Pizzolato G, Zanetti O, Bianchetti A, Chierichetti F, Trabucchi M. Corticobasal degeneration—neuropsychological assessment and dopamine D-2 receptor SPECT analysis. *Eur Neurol* 1995;35:50–54.
11. Schwarz J, Tatsch K, Gasser T, et al. ^{123}I-IBZM binding compared with long-term clinical follow up in patients with de novo parkinsonism. *Move Dis* 1998;13:16–19.
12. Eidelberg D, Takikawa S, Moeller JR, et al. Striatal hypometabolism distinguishes striatonigral degeneration from Parkinson's disease. *Ann Neurol* 1993;33:518–527.
13. Nagahama Y, Fukuyama H, Turjanski N, et al. Cerebral glucose metabolism in corticobasal degeneration: Comparison with progressive supranuclear palsy and normal controls. *Move Dis* 1997;12:691–696.
14. Fearnley JM, Lees AJ. Ageing and Parkinson's disease: Substantia nigra regional selectivity. *Brain* 1991;114: 2283–2301.
15. Kish SJ, Shannak K, Hornykiewicz O. Uneven pattern of dopamine loss in the striatum of patients with idiopathic Parkinson's disease. *N Engl J Med* 1988;318:876–880.
16. Burn DJ, Sawle GV, Brooks DJ. The differential diagnosis of Parkinson's disease, multiple system atrophy, and Steele-Richardson-Olszewski syndrome: discriminant analysis of striatal 18F-dopa PET data. *J Neurol Neurosurg Psychiat* 1994;57:278–284.
17. Brooks DJ. Functional imaging in relation to parkinsonian syndromes. *J Neurol Sci* 1993;115:1–17.
18. Turjanski N, Lees AJ, Brooks DJ. PET studies on striatal dopaminergic receptor binding in drug naive and L-dopa treated Parkinson's disease patients with and without dyskinesia. *Neurology* 1997;49:717–723.
19. Asahina M, Suhara T, Shinotoh H, Inoue O, Suzuki K, Hattori T. Brain muscarinic recptors in progressive supranuclear palsy and Parkinson's disease: a positron emission tomographic study. *J Neurol Neurosurg Psychiat* 1998;65:155–163.
20. Burn DJ, Rinne JO, Quinn NP, Lees AJ, Marsden CD, Brooks DJ. Striatal opioid receptor binding in Parkinson's disease, striatonigral degeneration, and Steele-Richardson-Olszewski syndrome: an ^{11}C-diprenorphine PET study. *Brain* 1995;118:951–958.

Corticobasal Degeneration.
Advances in Neurology, Vol. 82,
edited by I. Litvan, C. G. Goetz, and A. E. Lang.
Lippincott Williams & Wilkins, Philadelphia © 2000.

20

Therapeutic Approaches

Katie Kompoliti* and Christopher G. Goetz†

**Department of Neurological Sciences, Rush University, Chicago, Illinois 60612; and †Department of Neurological Sciences, Rush-Presbyterian-St Luke's Medical Center, Chicago, Illinois 60612*

THERAPEUTIC APPROACHES

Introduction

Although great interest has been generated by the unusual constellation of clinical findings of corticobasal degeneration (CBD) and the pathological findings that CBD shares with other neurodegenerative diseases, the disease remains progressive and by in large untreatable. As with other neurodegenerative diseases, there is no therapeutic approach that can alter the natural history of CBD, and even symptomatic treatment is only modestly beneficial for certain clinical elements of the disorder. Until recently, treatment recommendations were based on the anecdotal experience of movement disorder clinic physicians and the few published case reports (1–3).

In 1995, an international congress was organized by the Movement Disorders Society to focus on CBD. As part of this effort, groups working with CBD patients joined efforts to consolidate their small series into a larger sample. As a result, we described a review of the pharmacological response of 147 patients diagnosed as CBD by movement disorders experts (4).

Patients and Methods

Movement disorders specialists from eight centers collected all clinically diagnosed cases of CBD with or without autopsy confirmation seen in their centers until 1995. There were no *a priori* entry criteria but all submitted cases had been diagnosed by movement disorders specialists as CBD. The complete medical records were reviewed with respect to clinical history, pharmacological intervention, and side effects. Clinical signs and response to medications were called present or absent based on a movement disorders specialist's opinion as documented in the chart. The participating physicians were given a structured checklist with clinical signs, medications, and side effects to complete. The centers participating were the following: Mayo Clinic, Rochester, MN, 38 cases; the National Hospital for Neurology and Neurosurgery, Queen Square, London, England, 30 cases; Columbia-Presbyterian Medical Center, New York, NY, 19 cases; Cleveland Clinic, Cleveland, OH, 18 cases; University of South Florida College of Medicine, Tampa, FL, 13 cases; Rush-Presbyterian-St. Luke's Medical Center, Chicago, IL, 10 cases; Albany Medical College, Albany, NY, 10 patients; Mount Sinai Medical Center, Cleveland, OH, nine cases.

The data were compiled by the primary investigator (4). Signs were categorized into the following domains: parkinsonian features, other movement disorders, and higher cortical dysfunction. Recording of medication response was based on the reporting investigator's rating and amelioration of at least one clinical area of disability was considered as clinical improvement. In all instances, drug response was defined as associated with objective improvement. Because reporting investigators did not collect the data in a standardized manner, we were comfortable assessing the presence but not the degree of drug improvement. Because of methodological limitations, information on medication initiation with respect to disease onset and precise duration of benefit were not documented. Data analysis was done using descriptive statistics. Subgroup analyses were performed using two-sided Fisher's exact test. Comparisons were done for tables with marginal total more or equal to 5. Bonferroni adjustment was used to correct for multiple comparisons.

Results

Medications

Ninety-two percent of the patients received some kind of dopaminergic medication (Tables 1 and 2). Eighty-seven percent received levodopa with a peripheral decarboxylase inhibitor, 25% a dopaminergic agonist, either bromocriptine or pergolide, 20% selegiline, and 16% amantadine. Other medications used were benzodiazepines (32%), anticholinergics (27%), baclofen (19%), antidepressants (11%), anticonvulsants (9%), propranolol (8%), and neuroleptics (4%). Botulinum toxin injections were given to 6% of the patients.

Clinical improvement occurred in 24% of patients receiving dopaminergic medications, no improvement occurred in 71%, and 5% experienced drug associated worsening of parkinsonian features, dystonia, myoclonus, or gait dysfunction. No patient experienced drug-related worsening of higher cortical dysfunction. Median levodopa dose used was 300 mg with a range from 100 to 2,000 mg. Levodopa/carbiolopa produced clinical improvement in 26% who received the drug. Bradykinesia and rigidity were the elements that improved the most. The worsening experienced by a small percentage of patients was owing to increased dystonia, myoclonus, or gait dysfunction.

Agonist dose was 0.82 mg of pergolide equivalent (1 mg of pergolide = 10 mg of bromocriptine, range: 0.15 to 3.0). Only 6% of the patients receiving an agonist experienced clinical improvement of their parkinsonism. Eleven percent reported medication-associated worsening of their symptoms, with parkinsonism being the element worsening in 8%. Selegiline was used in 30 patients and produced improvement in 10%. Parkinsonian features improved the most, but individuals showed improvement in other movement disorders. Similarly, amantadine had a beneficial effect in 13% of patients, with rigidity, tremor, and gait being the domains that improved the most.

Clinical improvement occurred in 40% of patients on benzodiazepines. Clonazepam was the agent used the most, but lorazepam, diazepam, and alprazolam were occasionally prescribed. Nineteen percent of these patients experienced improvement of their parkinsonism, specifically tremor and rigidity. Myoclonus improved in 23% and dystonia in 9%.

TABLE 1. *Exposure/response**

Medication given	Number exposed (%)	Number with clinical improvement (%)	Number with clinical worsening (%)
Dopaminergic agents	135 (92)	33 (24)	7 (5)
Levodopa/ Carbiolopa	128 (87)	33 (26)	7 (6)
Agonist	33 (25)	2 (6)	4 (11)
Selegiline	30 (20)	3 (10)	1 (3)
Amantadine	24 (16)	3 (13)	—
Benzodiazepines	47 (32)	19 (40)	5 (11)
Anticholinergics	38 (27)	8 (21)	3 (8)
Baclofen	28 (19)	2 (7)	1 (4)
Antidepressants	16 (11)	1 (6)	—
Anticonvulsants	13 (9)	3 (23)	—
Propranolol	11 (8)	2 (18)	—
Neuroleptics	6 (4)	4 (67)	—
Botulinum toxin	9 (6)	6 (67)	—

* Values are numbers (percentages). — = No improvement reported.

TABLE 2. *Specific areas of improvement**

Medication	Exposed	Clinical improvement	Parkinsonism	Dystonia	Myoclonus	Alien hand	Pyramidal
Levodopa/ Carbiolopa	128 (87)	33 (26)	25 (20)	1 (1)	—	1 (1)	—
Agonist	33 (25)	2 (6)	1 (3)	—	—	—	—
Selegiline	30 (20)	3 (10)	1 (3)	—	—	—	—
Amantadine	24 (16)	3 (13)	3 (13)	—	—	—	—
Benzodiazepines	47 (32)	19 (40)	9 (19)	4 (9)	11 (23)	—	—
Anticholinergics	38 (27)	8 (21)	4 (10)	3 (8)	—	—	—
Baclofen	28 (19)	2 (7)	2 (7)	2 (7)	—	—	2 (7)
Antidepressants	16 (11)	1 (6)	—	—	—	—	—
Anticonvulsants	13 (9)	3 (23)	3 (23)	—	—	—	—
Propranolol	11 (8)	2 (18)	2 (18)	—	—	—	—
Neuroleptics	6 (4)	4 (67)	—	—	1 (17)	—	—
Botulinum toxin	9 (6)	6 (67)	—	6 (67)	—	—	—

* Values are numbers (percentages). — = No improvement reported.

Anticholinergics, trihexiphenidyl and benztropine, produced clinical improvement in 21%. Parkinsonism, specifically rigidity and tremor, improved in 10%, and dystonia lessened in 8%. Baclofen improved rigidity, dystonia, or pyramidal symptoms in 7% of the patients.

Although no patient had seizures, 13 patients received anticonvulsant medications, including primidone, phenytoin, carbamazepine, divalproex sodium, and gabapentin. Three patients experienced improvement of tremor, two with primidone and one with carbamazepine. Eleven patients received propranolol with improvement of tremor in two of them.

Antidepressants, in the form of tricyclic antidepressants (TCAs), selective serotonin reuptake inhibitors (SSRIs), and buproprion, were given to 16 patients with improvement of depression in one of the patients who received fluoxetine.

Of the nine patients given botulinum toxin injections, six experienced improvement of their dystonia. Neuroleptics were given in six patients with improvement in four. Two patients experienced nonspecific improvement, one improvement of the myoclonus and one of the dysarthria.

Medical Side Effects

The most frequent and disabling central nervous system side effects of drug trials in these patients were somnolence in 24 patients, confusion in 16 patients, and hallucinations in five patients. Dyskinesias, either choreic or stereotypic, did not occur, even in patients who received high doses of dopaminergic drugs. Peripheral side effects included gastrointestinal complaints, 23 patients; dizziness, 12 patients; dry mouth, five patients. Levodopa's most frequent side effect was gastrointestinal complaints in 15% of the patients, followed by confusion (4%), somnolence (4%), dizziness (4%), and hallucinations (2%). Agonists resulted in confusion in 14%, gastrointestinal complaints in 11%, and dizziness in 11% of the patients. Benzodiazepines and anticonvulsants produced somnolence in 26% and 15% of the patients, respectively.

Subgroup Analysis

Three subgroup comparisons were made and no significant differences were detected for any of the following comparisons: autopsy proven cases (n = 7) versus other cases (n = 140), for medication responses; levodopa (n = 33) versus other cases (n = 95), for clinical signs and medication responses; clinically prototypic patients who had the triad of parkinsonism, other movement disorder, and higher cortical dysfunction (n = 115) versus other patients (n = 32), for medication responses.

Discussion

The majority of the patients in this population received a dopaminergic medication, in most instances levodopa/carbiodopa and approximately one-fourth experienced clinical improvement. Given the retrospective design of this study, there is no specific information available on the magnitude or duration of the response, although in most cases it was annotated in the clinic charts as modest and short-lived. The other dopaminergic agents (dopaminergic agonists, selegiline, amantadine) were used less frequently and produced less consistent improvement.

In this population of patients, there was a notable absence of dyskinesias despite high doses of antiparkinsonian medications in some patients. Dyskinesias are common in Parkinson's disease after only a few years of treatment. In CBD, drug-induced dyskinesias have not been reported in the literature, although Anthony Lang reported having seen one patient with levodopa-induced dyskinesias in his clinic (personal communication). Based on this large series of drug treated patients without dyskinesias, we suggest that the absence of dyskinesias may be useful as a differentiating factor between CBD and Parkinson's disease when levodopa/carbiodopa is used on a chronic basis on a high dose. Nevertheless, the absence of dyskinesias would not help differentiate CBD from other parkinsonian syndromes, such as (PSP), since dyskinesias are also very infrequent in those syndromes.

Anticonvulsants and propranolol were used frequently and were often helpful in ameliorating tremor. Tremors in CBD are mostly action and postural and rarely resting. Although each center's experience with these drugs was small, the combined series permits a conclusion that these drugs are worth trying in CBD patients with tremors. Likewise, botulinum toxin injections, although not tested in a large number of patients at any one center, were effective in alleviating dystonic spasms and the pain associated with them. Because the akinetic-rigid-dystonic limbs of CBD are usually functionally impaired at the time of botulinum injections, there were no dose related limitations with regard to weakness caused by the toxin. These combined data suggest that botulinum toxin may be used more widely in the future.

Finally, approaching specific areas of impairment, myoclonus, dystonia, or pyramidal signs, medications traditionally used for these phenomena are of clinical interest and had some limited success. The most remarkable was the response of myoclonus to clonazepam. Until an overall therapy for CBD is available, these data suggest that the clinician can help patients by dissecting the individual elements of disability and treating them with focused therapies. As such, treatments for myoclonus (clonazepam), dystonic signs (clonazepam, anticholinergics, baclofen, botulinum toxin injections), or pyramidal signs (baclofen) should be tried in cases where such signs predominate in the clinical picture.

This study represents the first attempt to present the clinical manifestations of a large number of patients with the diagnosis of CBD, and to summarize the combined experience of the therapeutic outcome of drug trials in this patient population. Advantages of the study are the large number of patients presented and the fact that they were assessed by doctors specializing in the diagnosis and treatment of parkinsonian disorders. Because there was no specific drug protocol, the data represent patterns of clinical practice in large university-based centers where these patients are generally referred. The study is limited because the data were collected retrospectively and there was no specific data collection methodology other than complete chart review. Since CBD continues to be an under- and misdiagnosed entity (5), this report may alert clinicians to the typical signs and gamut of findings in this condition and suggest rational therapies based on empiric observations from this large clinical series.

When managing patients with neurodegenerative diseases, there are two ways to approach the problem, symptomatic or neuroprotective management. In the case of CBD, the patient's disability appears to be the cumulative result of multiple cortical and basal ganglia deficits rather than a single anatomic or neurotransmitter defect. Therefore, a simple neurotransmitter replacement approach fails to address the multiple dimensions of the problem.

To date therapeutic attempts have focused on addressing specific areas of impairment, such as parkinsonism, tremor, myoclonus, dystonia, or depression. These therapies have met with modest success at best. In the future, research efforts should focus on identifying the causes of selective focal degeneration, the environmental insults that predispose to such a process, and the genetically determined factors, if any, that provide an increased susceptibility substrate upon which environmental factors act. Therapeutic attempts should then be directed toward reducing or eliminating those factors that predispose to disease, aiding the nervous system in regenerating or bypassing genetic defects.

In addition to pharmacological therapies, allied health professionals may provide significant assistance to their patients. Although the impact of these interventions has not been systematically studied, physical therapists can help with gait training, occupational therapists often devise strategies to accommodate for the patient's disability, speech therapy may be helpful in counteracting dysarthria or for dietary manipulation to deal with dysphagia, and social workers are sources of information about relevant community programs and skilled nursing facilities, if needed. Finally, the physician should guide the patient and the family in addressing issues such as the use of gastrostomy tubes and the use of "extraordinary measures" to treat acute, life-threatening illnesses in the face of a relentlessly progressive degenerative disease.

REFERENCES

1. Gibb WR, Luthert PJ, Marsden CD. Corticobasal degeneration. *Brain* 1989;112:1171–1192.
2. Greene PE, Fahn S, Lang AE, Watts RL, Eidelberg D, Powers JM. What is it? Case 1, 1990: progressive unilateral rigidity, bradykinesia, tremulousness, and apraxia, leading to fixed postural deformity of the involved limb. *Mov Disord* 1990;5:341–351.
3. Riley DE, Lang AE, Lewis A, et al. Corticalbasal ganglionic degeneration. *Neurology* 1990;40:1203–1212.
4. Kompoliti K, Goetz CG, Boeve BF, et al. Clinical presentation and pharmacological therapy in corticobasal degeneration. *Arch Neurol* 1998;55:957–961.
5. Litvan I, Agid Y, Goetz C, et al. Accuracy of the clinical diagnosis of corticobasal degeneration: a clinicopathologic study. *Neurology* 1997;48:119–125.

Corticobasal Degeneration.
Advances in Neurology, Vol. 82,
edited by I. Litvan, C. G. Goetz, and A. E. Lang.
Lippincott Williams & Wilkins, Philadelphia © 2000.

21

Diagnostic Controversies: Is CBD Part of the "Pick Complex"?

Andrew Kertesz* and David G. Munoz†

** Cognitive Neurology and Alzheimer Research Centre, St. Joseph Health Centre, London, Ontario N6A 4V2, Canada; and †Department of Pathology, London Health Sciences Centre, London, Ontario N6A 5A5, Canada*

INTRODUCTION

When Arnold Pick (1–5) described several cases of aphasia, apraxia, and personality disorders in various combinations associated with fronto-temporal atrophy, the histological picture was not specified. Therefore, Pick's disease (PiD) is an appropriate clinical term for fronto-temporal dementia. The convention of defining PiD only on the basis of Pick bodies on histological examination came later (6), resulting in the paradox of a clinical entity diagnosable only on autopsy. Although many pathologists accepted cases with frontotemporal atrophy, superficial spongiosis, neuronal loss, and gliosis without Pick bodies as a variant of PiD (7–10), many insist on the distinction (11, 12). Some clinicians repeatedly encountering the pathological verdict of "not Pick's disease" coined the new names dementia of frontal lobe type (FLD) (13), primary progressive aphasia (PPA) (14), and frontotemporal dementia (FTD) (15). Various facets of clinical PiD are described as distinct entities, in addition to variations on the pathological descriptions (Table 1) creating a profusion of terminology hampering the recognition of the condition as a unitary one. We suggested the term Pick complex to avoid the controversial clinical-pathological dichotomy of PiD, and the restriction of FTD to a cortical disease.

In the initial description of corticodentatonigral degeneration (16), the authors recognized the resemblance of the pathological features, especially the swollen neurons to PiD, but considered it a new entity clinically characterized by unilateral rigidity, cortical sensory loss, and apraxia. Later the disease was renamed corticobasal degeneration (CBD) by Gibb et al. (17), who pointed out the similarity of ballooned neurons and nigral basophilic inclusions to PiD. Other names such as corticobasal ganglionic degeneration (CBGD) (18) and cortical-basal ganglionic degeneration (19) were coined. Certain clinical features such as supranuclear gaze palsy, alien limb, and reflex myoclonus were further elaborated. The asymmetrical extrapyramidal apractic syndrome, unresponsive to L-dopa, was subsequently described mainly in movement disorder clinics. We, among others, recognized the pathological and clinical similarities between PPA, FTD, CBD, and PiD. We suggested the term Pick complex to avoid the confusing dichotomy in the use of PiD (20–22). Pick complex is meant to refer to both the pathological and clinical spectrum of these diseases. This concept has been validated by the discovery of chromosome 17 linked FTD (23,24) and associated tau mutations (25, 26) with a clinical and pathological spectrum similar to Pick complex.

TABLE 1. *Glossary of Pick complex**

Circumscribed cerebral atrophy	Dementia lacking distinctive histology (DLDH)
Pick's disease (PiD)	Semantic dementia
Lobar atrophy	Frontal lobe dementia with motor neuron disease
Progressive subcortical gliosis (PSG)	Primary progressive apraxia
Corticodentatonigral degeneration	Nonspecific familial dementia
Generalized Pick's disease	Atypical presenile dementia
Frontal lobe dementia (FLD)	Spongiform encephalopathy of long duration
Primary progressive aphasia (PPA)	Hereditary dysphasic dementia
Corticobasal degeneration (CBD)	Frontotemporal dementia (FTD)
Corticobasal ganglionic degeneration (CBGD)	Disinhibition—dementia—amyotrophy—Parkinsonism

* Terms presented in their historical order of first use.

The evidence is presented in favor of CBD being part of Pick complex under the following five categories:

1. Clinical PiD and FTD are often associated with extrapyramidal features.
2. Frontotemporal behavior disorder and progressive aphasia are commonly seen in corticobasal degeneration syndrome (CBDs).
3. The pathology of CBD and PiD significantly overlap.
4. The histological picture of CBD may be found with FTD and PPA with or without the extrapyramidal-apractic CBDs.
5. The clinical syndrome of CBDs may be found with typical Pick body or Pick variant pathology.

CLINICAL PICK'S DISEASE AND FRONTOTEMPORAL DEMENTIA ARE OFTEN ASSOCIATED WITH EXTRAPYRAMIDAL FEATURES

Extrapyramidal features in PiD have, in fact, been described on numerous occasions before CBD was isolated (8,27–30), but this has not been recognized in most of the CBD publications. Ferraro and Jervis (31) stated extrapyramidal symptoms were common in PiD, and subsequently others confirmed this (9,29). Sometimes unilateral rigidity and parkinsonism were the first symptoms to attract attention and this was known as the "Akelaitis variety" of PiD. The clinical overlap between PPA, CBD, and PiD is increasingly recognized (20). The occurrence of extrapyramidal features is also recognized in FTD (32). Although the extrapyramidal syndrome is considered a late feature in FTD (15), at times its prominence and early appearance are noted (33). PPA is also seen at times with definite extrapyramidal features (20,34,35). Extrapyramidal symptoms appear prominent in several of the pedigrees of familial frontotemporal dementia linked to chromosome 17. The original family where the linkage was found was called disinhibition dementia parkinsonism amyotrophy complex (36). Parkinsonism was added to chromosome 17-linked FTD in many subsequent publications (FTDP-17) (25).

We have observed the appearance of extrapyramidal features in 9/27 of our cases of PPA and 5/17 cases of FLD. In two of the cases of FLD, the extrapyramidal features appeared simultaneously with the cognitive or behavioral change. It was difficult to categorize these cases as primary CBD syndrome or FLD. In the other cases, the extrapyramidal syndrome was observed 1 to 7 years after the onset of the cognitive or personality changes. In four cases, the CBDs emerged as the tertiary or third set of symptoms, one of these rather late, 11 years after the onset of FLD (37).

FRONTOTEMPORAL BEHAVIOR DISORDER AND PROGRESSIVE APHASIA ARE COMMONLY SEEN IN THE CBD SYNDROME (CBDS)

The interest focused on the extrapyramidal syndrome may have led to the belief that behavioral changes are uncommon and dementia occurs only in a minority of cases of CBD (38). When the descriptions are specifically reviewed, however, dysexecutive syndrome, language disturbances, and personality changes suggestive of frontal and temporal lobe involvement seem to be frequent features during the course of the disease.

The first described case in the seminal article by Rebeiz et al. (16) began to show personality changes one year after her initial motor symptoms. She became "quiet and appeared depressed." Two years later, she became "fretful, querulous, and progressively withdrawn," although she had been a very social person. At that time she started to misuse a word at times. However, 1 year later, her language had worsened and "she spoke less and less, only occasionally answering questions in monosyllables." A pneumoencephalographic study showed frontal horn enlargement. Case 2 showed "normal memory and judgement" during the early stages of his disease, which at that time was characterized by stiffness and involuntary movements of his left limbs. However, he had become "mentally slower," "was undertaking fewer activities than previously," and seemed to have lost the ability to solve new or difficult problems. Neuropsychological testing 5 years after the onset showed intellectual decline "beyond that expected for his age." In the third case presented, the patient had noticed her memory was "less reliable" and her "thought processes were becoming slower." Two of the three cases by Gibb et al. (17) also had behavioral and cognitive deficit, such as poor thinking, verbal memory, fluency presentation, anomia, apathy, slurred speech, and poor performance on intellectual tasks.

Among the 15 cases (13 with a clinical diagnosis and two histologically proven) reported by Riley et al. (19), four were demented, 3/15 showed aphasia, and 9/15 had "frontal lobe reflexes." Detailed description of the clinical picture is given for only four cases. Their patient #2 had a "normal mental status examination" 4 years after his first symptoms. Two years later, he was emotionally incontinent and "his mental function began to deteriorate." Patient #10 showed personality change with aggression in the early stages of his disease. The largest clinical series of CBD cases from one site published to date (38) includes 36 patients, six of whom had neuropathological diagnosis. Thirty of these patients were followed for a mean period of 5.2 years and cognitive deficits were detected in nine of them. Two of these cases showed frontal lobe dysfunction in formal neuropsychological testing and a third patient presented "prominent personality and behavioral changes with impulsiveness and excessive eating and drinking." The authors admitted, "Sometimes formal testing was difficult because of dysarthria, apraxia, and loss of function of the dominant hand." A combined chart review of eight movement disorders centers yielded 147 cases of clinically diagnosed CBD (39). In this series, 25% was recorded to have dementia and 10% as aphasia, but apraxia occurred in 82% of cases. The authors admitted the predominance of parkinsonian signs may represent a selection bias among specialists of movement disorders. Furthermore, two case control studies have reported significantly low frontal scores on neuropsychological testing in patients with CBD as compared to controls (40,41).

We have seen 12 cases of extrapyramidal apractic disorders corresponding to the clinical syndrome of CBD (CBDs). All of the 12 patients presented with either an extrapyramidal disorder ($n = 6$) or apraxia followed closely by either an alien hand syndrome or extrapyramidal disorder or both ($n = 6$). Eleven of the 12 had one side or the other predominate in the extrapyramidal or alien hand symptomatology (R = 6, L = 5). Eleven out of the 12 developed a secondary cognitive syndrome, eight had progressive aphasia, and three a frontal lobe type apathy/disinhibition syndrome. One of the patients with progressive aphasia also developed FLD, and three of the FLD syndromes with CBDs also developed progressive aphasia subsequently. Forgetfulness and behavioral problems accompanied the extrapyramidal presentation in three of the cases. Forgetfulness on further questioning was often revealed to be inattentiveness, "forgetting to remember," and a general disinterest. Eight of the patients had language impairment either at the time when they were seen first or on the second follow-up a year later. Seven of the 12 patients developed significant personality changes compatible with the frontal lobe syndrome consisting of disinhibition, inattention, executive dysfunction, or atrophy. Detailed neuropsychological examination was carried out in four patients. Cognitive changes were mainly in the domain of language. MRI and CT scans were carried out in all showing asymmetrical or bilateral frontotemporal and parietal atrophy in various combinations. All three of the patients who had an autopsy showed typical CBD changes.

THE PATHOLOGY OF CBD, PID, AND FTD SIGNIFICANTLY OVERLAP

In this review of the pathological aspects, the term PiD will be reserved for dementia with Pick bodies. The neuropathological overlap between PiD and CBD, initially suggested by Rebeiz et al. (16), has been repeatedly demonstrated and goes far beyond the mere presence of focal atrophy and ballooned neurons (17,20,42–44). Most prominently, the cytoplasmic inclusions in CBD cortical neurons often adopt a rounded morphology, and thus are indistinguishable from Pick bodies on Bielchowsky stains, or for that matter most tau immunostains. Moreover, the inclusions preferentially involve small neurons in cortical layers II and III in both CBD and PiD, in contrast to the preferential involvement of large neurons in deep cortical layers seen in Alzheimer's disease. At the ultrastructural level, the inclusions in both CBD (45) and PiD (46) consist of 15 nm-wide straight tubules. It is not surprising that many cases of what now is recognized as CBD have been reported in the literature as atypical PiD. However, the argyrophilic rounded inclusions in CBD spare the dentate gyrus, which is always involved in PiD. The hippocampus proper almost always shows Pick bodies in PiD, but does not demonstrate inclusions in CBD. Furthermore, the Gallyas method stains the inclusions in CBD, but not those in PiD. Conversely, Pick bodies demonstrate chromogranin A immunoreactivity in PiD, but not in CBD. The absence of ubiquitin labeling of CBD inclusions, proposed by some as a diagnostic criterion, has been in our hands useless in separating PiD from CBD, since Pick bodies are equally nonreactive (47).

Involvement of subcortical nuclei is almost as common in PiD as in CBD, as several series have shown degeneration of the striatum, and particularly the substantia nigra in more than 70% of the cases of PiD (48–50). Additionally, the subthalamic nucleus and locus ceruleus are usually affected in both conditions. Furthermore, in both diseases the main cytoskeletal abnormality in subcortical nuclei is the presence of globose neurofibrillary tangles (47). These are the inclusions observed on H & E stains by Gibb et al. (17) in one of the original reports of the condition, where they were labeled corticobasal inclusions and construed as unique (17). Silver stains reveal their true nature. Subcortical pathology in PiD is not necessarily associated with extrapyramidal symptomatology (8,46).

Astrocytic argyrophilic inclusions that bind tau antibodies are a shared feature of CBD and PiD. The most common type, called thorny astrocyte because of its shape on Gallyas stains is common to both, but CBD demonstrates a unique type of astrocytic abnormality, which is pathognomonic of the condition. These so-called glial plaques appear on silver stains as clusters of argyrophilic threads not associated with amyloid. The astrocytic cell body from which they emerge is revealed by tau immunostains only (43).

The oligodendroglia is affected by the same type of pathology in both conditions. Silver stains reveal argyrophilic inclusions filling the cytoplasm and processes and tightly embracing the nucleus (thus, the name coiled bodies). Electron microscopy reveals 15 nm-wide straight tubules, similar to those seen in the neuronal inclusions (45,51). These lesions are much more common in CBD, where they result in the formation of the pervasive network of threads revealed by the Gallyas stain in the gray and white matter, which constitutes one of the hallmarks of the disease.

Other pathological changes of CBD are shared by all varieties of Pick complex. This include superficial linear spongiosis, neuronal loss preferentially involving the supragranular layers, cortical gliosis, and white matter gliosis, as well as the slightly more distinctive presence of ballooned neurons (47). Ballooned neurons are frequently seen in the brains of PPA and FLD patients when appropriate immunohistochemical techniques are applied (20,52–54). These patients often show subcortical atrophy too. Constantinidis et al. (9) described extrapyramidal involvement particularly in "group B" patients, and Mann et al. (55) in 8/12 of FLD patients. This has led Rinne et al. (38) to suggest that patients belonging to groups B and C2 of Tissot et al. (56) might well represent patients with CBD.

Dementia lacking distinctive histopathology, considered the pathological substrate of frontal lobe dementia, has no obvious inclusions, and thus the relationship to CBD would appear to be limited to the distribution of atrophy and the presence of ballooned neurons; however, tau immunostains sometimes demonstrate diffuse labeling of neurons (57). Consequently, the neuropathological overlap between PiD and CBD seems extendable to FTD and PPA.

Other entities within the Pick complex show additional points of congruence. What Munoz-Garcia and Ludwin (46) called the generalized form of Pick's disease is currently known as basophilic inclusion body disease; Munoz (47) shows a similar distribution of cortical and subcortical atrophy, the latter preferentially involving the substantia nigra, but sparing the cholinergic neurons of the nucleus basalis of Meynert.

Abnormalities of the microtubule associated protein tau are central to both CBD and PiD, to the point that they may be viewed as tauopathies (43,58). Although this is in favor of considering them related disorders, there are histochemical and biochemical differences argued as a reason for distinction (43,59,60). Tau is aberrantly phosphorylated in both PiD and CBD, but the isoform pattern is different: PiD shows a doublet at 64 and 55 kDa, and a weak band at 69 kDa, whereas the doublet of CBD is located at 64 and 69 kDa, with a minor band at 74 kDa (59,60). However, this area of tau biochemistry and the newly discovered tau mutations are in a developing stage, and the significance of these differences, exciting as they may be, remains to be determined. Some of these differences can be regarded as biologically more important than others.

The recent discovery of tau mutations in chromosome 17 linked frontotemporal dementia (FTDP-17) highlights the importance of this structural protein in the pathogenesis of these familial forms of Pick complex (25,26,61). Many of the FTDP-17 related dementias appeared to have CBD type of pathology, although their morphology overlaps with PiD and FTD (26,62). In fact, the differences between CBD and PiD, as discussed in the preceding, must be viewed in light of the marked variation in the histopathology among families bearing the same mutation on the tau gene. Thus, the differences found do not exclude considering these entities as being part of a spectrum of disorders with more similarities than differences.

THE HISTOLOGICAL PATTERN OF CBD IS OFTEN FOUND IN CASES OF FRONTOTEMPORAL DEMENTIA AND PROGRESSIVE APHASIA

There are several cases of pathologically diagnosed CBD presenting as FTD with or without associated extrapyramidal symptoms (38,53, 63–68). Although some authors dismiss the clinical diagnosis of PiD when CBD pathology is shown on autopsy (69), clinical FTD is the same as clinical PiD and the clinical diagnosis of PiD is appropriate in these instances. Frontal lobe dysfunction with behavioral disturbances, poor performance on frontal lobe tests or both is described in 53% of the 62 patients with CBD pathology for which case reports were available in the literature (16,17,19,38,63–77). Most of the cases of Feany and Dickson (78) describing new cytoskeletal and glial changes in CBD had behavioral and cognitive presentation. Cooper et al. (53) found CBD pathology in four cases of their FTD series. Similarly, CBD pathology can present with a clinical picture of PPA (20,52,79–81). Bergeron et al. (44) found nine cases with CBD from a brain bank of cases with dementia (25% of the non-Alzheimer cases). In addition to cortical neuronal loss and gliosis, a large number of ballooned neurons were present, similar to their cases of PiD. Two of these cases have been published as CBD with unusual clinical presentations, namely frontal lobe dementia and PPA (68). The other seven cases also had cognitive changes, including language, diagnosed as AD during life. A neuropathologically selected series of 11 CBD patients all had cognitive involvement and four of them had early behavioral or language presentation. Only eight had CBDs diagnosed clinically (82).

Another study selecting cases with neuropathological criteria of CBD found clinicians diagnosed CBD from the clinical vignettes at a rather low sensitivity when they were blinded to the pathology (83). It appears the neuropathological diagnosis of CBD does not correspond necessarily to the syndrome of extrapyramidal apractic disorder but it can present clinically with something else, most often as the behavior personality disorder of frontal lobe dementia or progressive aphasia that are both part of the Pick complex.

We have now seen six cases with a histological picture of CBD on autopsy. One of these cases with PPA was previously published as a Pick variant pathology because of the presence of Pick bodies, as described herein (Case 1 in [20]). This reflects the evolutionary nature of histopathological diagnosis; the gold standard of neuropathology changes even within a single case as new histochemical techniques are applied. Three of the six cases presented as a movement disorder or a CBD syndrome. Two of these cases developed FLD, one simultaneously with the movement disorder, and the other one 6 months later. One case had progressive aphasia, also within 6 months of the onset of the movement disorder. Three other cases presented clinically with primary cognitive deficit, two with PPA, and one with FLD. One of the cases with PPA developed extrapyramidal symptoms 4 years after the onset, and another one 2 years after onset. The third case had FLD and progressive aphasia for 5 years before developing CBDs. In summary, in this series of six pathologically diagnosed CBD cases, all of them had cognitive syndromes, about half of them presenting with CBDs and closely followed by PPA or FLD, and the other half presenting with FLD or PPA with a variable length of time before developing extrapyramidal syndrome.

THE CLINICAL SYNDROME OF CBDS MAY BE SEEN WITH PICK BODY PATHOLOGY AND OTHER VARIANTS OF THE PICK COMPLEX

Some reports describe patients with the clinical syndrome of CBD and the pathological findings of PiD with Pick bodies (30,42,84–87). A series of nine cases with a clinical syndrome of CBD followed to autopsy found a variety of different pathological substrates resulting in a similar clinical profile. CBDs can occur in the absence of basal ganglia and nigral degeneration with only asymmetric parietal and frontal cortical degeneration as the main pathological finding. CBDs was also found without tau abnormalities or argyrophilic inclusions (88). Litvan et al. (83) also described PiD pathology "misdiagnosed" as CBD by primary neurologists and movement disorder specialists from clinical vignettes. Therefore, the clinical diagnosis of CBD is not always predictive of distinct CBD pathology. It would be useful to distinguish the clinical CBDs from CBD pathology by using the small "s" for the syndrome as we have done throughout this chapter.

DISCUSSION

Clinical descriptions of CBD initially from movement disorder clinics have emphasized its motor manifestations, such as extrapyramidal features, myoclonus, apraxia, gaze palsies, and alien hand syndrome. However, in our experience, other behavioral and cognitive features, especially those related to frontal lobe symptomatology and progressive aphasia, are common, and a review of the literature supports this.

Eleven of the twelve patients who presented with CBD syndrome (CBDs) to our movement disorder and behavioral neurology clinic had significant cognitive disorder. Of these 12 CBDs presentations, apraxia was the presenting feature in four patients and later on all patients had significant and severe apraxia. Some consider apraxia, of course, as a cognitive impairment (motor cognition): therefore, one could argue that one of the core features of CBDs is impairment of motor cognition.

The difficulty determining which syndrome came first also leads to the variation in reporting the frequency of these entities. Often subtle cognitive changes are evident on history that are overshadowed by the extrapyramidal features, or they may not be reported because they were not elicited or observed at the time of the visit. Not many patients are followed for sufficient time to determine the development of the secondary syndromes. All three of these factors will contribute to the impression that cognitive deficits are less frequent than they are in reality in CBD.

Just what constitutes dementia in CBD patients is variable from report to report. Although Rebeiz et al. (16), in their original report of the entity, claimed in the introduction that "mental faculties were relatively spared until the end," they contradicted this in the comments: "Two patients early became aware of decrease in intellectual efficacy and this was confirmed on psychological testing." Few patients have detailed cognitive and behavioral evaluations as these are often beyond the scope of many clinics. Increased awareness, however, of the behavioral-cognitive syndrome of the frontotemporal type and progressive aphasia will help clinicians to recognize the variations, which nevertheless form a compelling cohesion.

Application of sophisticated histochemical, biochemical, and genetic technologies has allowed increasing fractionation of the Pick complex at the same time as recognition of the different clinical presentations has expanded the entity. This may well be a case in which the obvious clinical commonality may in the end be more biologically relevant than the distinctions observed in the laboratory. There is no easy answer forthcoming to this nosological debate. All points of view need to be considered in order to advance science. However, when making new discoveries and discarding old methodologies we have to be careful not to lose the sight of the forest from the trees.

Pick complex is a significant segment of degenerative dementia, estimated to be 15% to 20% of all dementias, competing with Lewy body disease (LBD) for the second place after Alzheimer's disease. Nevertheless, LBD is less clearly identifiable *in vivo* than FTD, since most cases will not have all the distinguishing features and have been diagnosed as AD. The relationship of CBD to PSP is covered elsewhere. Some people believe CBD and PSP are closely related. This overlap is important nosologically and biologically, but at this time it is premature to consider PSP as part of the Pick complex.

This review of studies supports our experience and our contention that FLD and PPA are related to CBD clinically and pathologically, and patients with CBDs have either a significant behavioral and language deficit at the beginning, or develop such symptoms later in the course of their illness. Therefore, not only is CBD related pathologically to PiD, but also shows a major clinical overlap sooner or later in the course of the illness.

REFERENCES

1. Pick A. Über die Beziehungen der senilen Hirnatrophie zur Aphasie. *Prag Med Wochenschr* 1892;17:165–167.
2. Pick A. Senile Hirnatrophie als Gundlage von Herderscheinunger. *Wien Klin Wschr, Mschr Psychiatr Neurol* 1901;14:403–404.
3. Pick A. Über primäre progressive Demenz bei Erwachsenen. *Prag Med Wschr* 1904;29:417–420.
4. Pick A. Zur Symptomatologie der linksseitigen Schläfenlappenatrophie. *Mschr Psychiatr (Berlin)* 1905;16: 378–388.
5. Pick A. Über einen weiteren Symptomenkomplex im Rahmen der Dementia senilis, bedingt durch umschriebene stärkere Hirnatrophie (gemischte Apraxie). Vortrag, gehalten im Wiener Vereine für Psychiatrie und Neurologie. *Mschr Psychiatr (Berlin)* 1906;19:97–108.
6. Onari K, Spatz H. Anatomische Beitrage zur Lehre von der Pickschen umschriebenen Grosshirnrindenatrophie (Pisckschе Krankheit). *Zeitschr Ges Neurol Psychiatr* 1926;101:470–511.
7. Malamud N, Boyd DA. Pick's disease with atrophy of the temporal lobes—a clinicopathologic study. *Arch Neurol Psychiatry* 1940;43:210–222.
8. Winkelman NW, Book MH. Asymptomatic extrapyramidal involvement in Pick's disease. *Arch Neurol Psychiatry* 1944;8:30–42.
9. Constantinidis J, Richard J, Tissot R. Pick's disease: histological and clinical correlations. *Eur Neurol* 1974;11: 208–217.
10. Kosaka K. On aphasia of Pick's disease—a review of our own 3 cases and 49 autopsy cases in Japan. (in Japanese) *Seishin Igaku* 1976;18:1181–1189, as quoted by Ohashi (1983).
11. Brun A. Frontal lobe degeneration of non-Alzheimer type. I. Neuropathology. *Arch Geront Geriatr* 1987;6: 193–208.
12. Dickson DW. Pick's disease: a modern approach. *Brain Pathol* 1998;8:339–354.
13. Gustafson L. Frontal lobe degeneration of non-Alzheimer type. II. Clinical picture and differential diagnosis. *Arch Geront Geriatr* 1987;6:209–223.
14. Mesulam MM. Primary progressive aphasia—differentiation from Alzheimer's disease. *Ann Neurol* 1987;22: 533–534.
15. Lund and Manchester Groups. Clinical and neuropathological criteria for frontotemporal dementia. *J Neurol Neurosurg Psychiatry* 1994;57:416–418.
16. Rebeiz JJ, Kolodny EH, Richardson EP. Corticodentatonigral degeneration with neuronal achromasia. *Arch Neurol* 1968;18:20–33.
17. Gibb WRG, Luthert PJ, Marsden CD. Corticobasal degeneration. *Brain* 1989;112:1171–1192.
18. Watts RL, Mirra SS, Young RR, Burger PC, Villier JA, Heyman A. Corticobasal ganglionic degeneration (CBGD) with neuronal achromasia: clinical-pathological study of two cases [abstract]. *Neurology* 1989;39 (suppl 1):140.
19. Riley DE, Lang AE, Lewis A, Resch L, Ashby P, Horneykiewicz O, Black SI. Cortical-basal ganglionic degeneration. *Neurology* 1990;40:1203–1212.
20. Kertesz A, Hudson L, Mackenzie IRA, Munoz DG. The pathology and nosology of primary progressive aphasia. *Neurology* 1994;44:2065–2072.
21. Kertesz A, Munoz, D. Clinical and pathological characteristics of primary progressive aphasia and frontal dementia. Non-Alzheimer Dementias Symposium Proceedings. *J Neural Transm.* Wien: Springer Verlag, 1996; (suppl) 47:133–141.
22. Kertesz A, Munoz DG. Pick's disease, frontotemporal dementia, and Pick complex: emerging concepts. *Arch Neurol* 1998a;55:302–304.

23. Wilhelmsen KC, Lynch T, Pavlou E, Higgins M, Nygaard TG. Localization of disinhibition-dementia-parkinsonism-amyotrophy complex (DDPAC) to 17q 21–22. *Am J Hum Genet* 1994;55:1159–1165.
24. Wilhelmsen KC. Frontotemporal dementia is on the MAPtau. *Ann Neurol* 1997;41:139–140.
25. Hutton M, Lendon CL, Rizzu P, et al. Association of missense and 5′-splice-site mutations in tau with the inherited dementia FTDP-17. *Nature* 1998;393:702–705.
26. Spillantini MG, Murrell JR, Goedert M, Farlow MR, Klug A. Ghetti B. Mutation in the tau gene in familial multiple system tauopathy with presenile dementia. *Neurbiology* 1998;95:7737–7741.
27. von Branmühl A. Ueber Stammganglienveränderungen bei Pickscher Krankheit. *Ztschr Gesamte Neurol Psychiatrie* 1930; 124:214.
28. Löwenberg K. Pick's disease—a clinicopathologic contribution. *Arch Neurol Psychiatr* 1935;36:68–789.
29. Akelaitis AJ. Atrophy of basal ganglia in Pick's disease. *Arch Neurol Psychiatry* 1944;51:27.
30. Brion S, Plas J, Jeaunea A. Pick's disease. *Rev Neurol* 1991;147:693–704.
31. Ferraro A, Jervis GA. Pick's disease. *Arch Neurol Psychiatry* 1936;36:739–767.
32. Neary D, Snowden J. Frontotemporal dementia: nosology, neuropsychology, and neuropathology. *Brain Cogn* 1996;31:176–187.
33. Morris JC, Cole M, Banker BQ, Wright D. Hereditary dysphasic dementia and the Pick-Alzheimer spectrum. *Ann Neurol* 1984;16:455–466.
34. Goulding PJ, Northen B, Snowden JS, MacDermott N, Neary D. Progressive aphasia with right-sided extrapyramidal signs: another manifestation of localised cerebral atrophy. *J. Neurol Neurosurg Psychiatry* 1989;52: 128–130.
35. Kertesz A, Martinez-Lage P. Cognitive changes in corticobasal degeneration. In: Kertesz A, Munoz D, eds. *Pick's disease and Pick complex.* New York: Wiley & Sons, 1998;121–128.
36. Lynch T, Sarno M, Marder KS, et al. Clinical characteristics of a family with chromosome 17-linked disinhibition-dementia-parkinsonism-amyotrophy complex. *Neurology* 1994;44:1878–1884.
37. Kertesz A, Munoz DG. Clinical and pathological overlap in Pick complex. In: Kertesz A, Munoz D, eds. *Pick's disease and Pick complex.* New York: Wiley & Sons, 1998b;281–286.
38. Rinne JO, Lee MS, Thompson PD, Marsden CD. Corticobasal degeneration—a clinical study of 36 cases. *Brain* 1994;117:1183–1196.
39. Kompoliti K, Goetz CG, Boeve BF, Maraganore DM, Ahlskog JE, Marsden CA, et al. Clinical presentation and pharmacological therapy in corticobasal degeneration. *Neurology* 1998;55:957–961.
40. Vidailhet M, Rivaud S, Goudier-Khouja N, et al. Eye movements in Parkinsonian syndromes. *Ann Neurol* 1994;35:420–426.
41. Pillon B, Blin J, Vidailhet M, Deweer B, Sirigu A, Dubois B, Agid Y. The neuropsychological pattern of corticobasal degeneration: comparison with progressive supranuclear palsy and Alzheimer's disease. *Neurology* 1995;45:1477–1483.
42. Jendroska K, Rossor MN, Mathias CJ, et al. Morphological overlap between corticobasal degeneration and Pick's disease: a clinicopathological report. *Mov Disord* 1995; 10:111–114.
43. Feany MB, Mattiace LA, Dickson DW. Neuropathologic overlap of progressive supranuclear palsy, Pick's disease and corticobasal degeneration. *J Neuropathol Exp Neurol* 1996;55:53–67.
44. Bergeron C, Davis A, Lang AE. Corticobasal ganglionic degeneration and progressive supranuclear palsy presenting with cognitive decline. *Brain Pathol* 1998;8: 355–365.
45. Wakabayashi K, Oyanagi K, Makifuchi T, et al. Corticobasal degeneration: etiopathological significance of the cytoskeletal alterations. *Acta Neuropathol* 1994; 87:545–553.
46. Munoz-Garcia D, Ludwin SK. Classic and generalized variants of Pick's disease: a clinicopathological, ultrastructural and immunocytochemical study. *Ann Neurol* 1984;16:467–480.
47. Munoz DG. The pathology of Pick complex. In: Kertesz A, Munoz D, eds. *Pick's disease and Pick complex.* New York: Wiley & Sons, 1998;211–241.
48. von Bagh K. Anatomic findings in 30 cases of systematic atrophy of cortex (Pick's disease) with special consideration of basal ganglia and long descending nerve tracts, preliminary report. *Arch Psychiatrie* 1941; 114:68.
49. Kosaka K, Ikeda K, Kobayashi K, Mehraein P. Striatopallidonigral degeneration in Pick's disease: a clinicopathological study of 41 cases. *J Neurol* 1991;238: 151–160.
50. Uchihara T, Tsychiya K, Kosaka K. Selective loss of nigral neurones in Pick's disease. *Acta Neuropathol* 1990;81:155–161.
51. Ikeda K, Akiyama H, Haga C, Kondo H, Arima K, Oda T. Argyrophilic thread-like structure in corticobasal degeneration and supranuclear palsy. *Neurosci Lett* 1994; 174:157–159.
52. Lippa CF, Smith TW, Fontneau N. Corticonigral degeneration with neuronal achromasia. A clinicopathological study of two cases. *J Neurol Sci* 1990;98: 301–310.
53. Cooper PN, Jackson M, Lennox G, Lowe J, Mann DMA. τ-Ubiquitin, and αβ-crystallin immunohistochemistry define the principal causes of degenerative frontotemporal dementia. *Arch Neurol* 1995;52:1011–1015.
54. Jackson M, Lennox G, Lowe J. Motor neurone disease-inclusion dementia. *Neurodegen* 1996;5:339–350.
55. Mann DMA, South PW, Snowden JS, Neary D. Dementia of frontal lobe type: neuropathology and immunohistochemistry. *J Neurol Neurosurg Psychiatry* 1993;56: 605–614.
56. Tissot R, Constantinidis J, Richard J. Pick's disease. In: Frederiks JAM, ed. Handbook of Clinical Neurology, Vol. 2 (46): *Neurobehavioural disorders.* Amsterdam: Elsevier, 1985;233–246.
57. Scheltens P, Ravid R, Kamphorst W. Pathologic findings in a case of primary progressive aphasia. *Neurology* 1994;44:279–282.
58. Lowe J, Spillantini MG. Non-Alzheimer degenerative dementias. *Brain Pathol* 1998;8:295–297.
59. Buée-Scherrer V, Hof P, Buée L, Leveugle B, Vermesh P, Perl D, Olanow C, Delacourte A. Hyperphosphorylated tau proteins differentiate corticobasal degeneration and Pick's disease. *J Neuropathol Exp Neurol* 1996;91: 351–359.

60. Delacourte A, Sergeant N, Wattez A, Robitaille Y. The biochemistry of the cytoskeleton in Pick complex. In: Kertesz A, Munoz D, eds. *Pick's disease and Pick complex.* New York: Wiley & Sons, 1998;243–258.
61. Poorkaj P, Bird TD, Wijsman E, et al. Tau is a candidate gene for chromosome 17 frontotemporal dementia. *Ann Neurol* 1998;43:815–825.
62. Sima AAF, Defendini R, Keohane C, et al. The neuropathology of chromosome 17-linked dementia. *Ann Neurol* 1996;39:734–743.
63. Clark AW, Manz HJ, White III CL, Lehmann J, Miller D, Coyle JT. Cortical degeneration with swollen chromatolytic neurons: its relationship to Pick's disease. *J Neuropathol Exp Neurol* 1986;45:268–284.
64. Paulus W, Selim M. Corticonigral degeneration with neuronal achromasia and basal neurofibrillary tangles. *Acta Neuropathol* 1990;81:89–94.
65. Lennox G, Jackson M, Lowe J. Corticobasal degeneration manifesting as frontal lobe dementia. Abstract. *Ann Neurol* 1994;36:273–274.
66. Rey GJ, Tower R, Levin BE, et al. Psychiatric symptoms, atypical dementia, ad left visual field inattention in corticobasal ganglionic degeneration. *Mov Disord* 1995;10: 106–110.
67. Frisoni GB, Pizzolato G, Zanetti O, Bianchetti A, Chierichetti F, Trabucchi M. Corticobasal degeneration: Neuropsychological assessment and dopamine D2 receptor SPECT analysis. *Eur Neurol* 1995;35:50–54.
68. Bergeron C, Pollanen MS, Weyer L, Black SE, Lang AE. Unusual clinical presentations of cortical-basal ganglionic degeneration. *Ann Neurol* 1996;40:893–900.
69. Oda T, Ikeda K, Akamatus W, et al. An autopsy case of corticobasal degeneration clinically misdiagnosed as Pick's disease. *Seishin Shinkeigaku Zasshi* 1995; 97:757–769.
70. Anonymous Case records of the Massachusetts General Hospital. Weekly clinicopathological exercises. Case 38-1985. *NEJM* 1985;313:739–748.
71. Greene PE, Fahn S, Lang AE, Watts RL, Eidelberg E, Powers JM. Progressive unilateral rigidity, bradykinesia, tremulousness, and apraxia leading to fixed postural deformity of the involved limb. *Mov Disord* 1990; 5:341–351.
72. Eidelberg D, Dhawan V, Moeller JR, et al. *NEJM* 1991;54:856–862.
73. Sawle GV, Brooks DJ, Marsden CD, Frackowiak RSJ. Corticobasal degeneration. A unique pattern of regional cortical oxygen hypometabolism and striatal fluorodopa uptake demonstrated by positron emission tomography. *Brain* 1990;114:541–556.
74. Lerner A, Friedland R, Riley D, et al. Dementia with pathological findings of corticobasal ganglionic degeneration (Abstract). *Ann Neurol* 1992;32:271.
75. Muhiddin KA, Hardie RJ, Pearce VR, Kirby BJ. Corticobasal degeneration: a report of three cases. *J Roy Soc Med* 1994;87:359–360.
76. Leiguarda R, Lees AJ, Merello M, Starkstein S, Marsden CD. The nature of apraxia in corticobasal degeneration. *J Neurol Neurosurg Psychiatry* 1994;57:455–459.
77. Horoupian D, Chu PL. Unusual case of corticobasal degeneration with tau/Gallyas-positive neuronal and glial tangles. *Acta Neuropathol* 1994;88:592–598.
78. Feany MB, Dickson DW. Widespread cytoskeletal pathology characterizes corticobasal degeneration. *Am J Pathol* 1995;146:1388–1396.
79. Lippa CF, Cohen R, Smith TW, Drachman DA. Primary progressive aphasia with focal neuronal achromasia. *Neurology* 1991;41:882–886.
80. Marti-Masso JF, Lopez de Muniain A, Poza JJ, Urtasun M, Carrera N. Degeneracion corticobasal ganglionica: a proposito de siete observaciones diagnosticada clinicamente. *Neurologia* 1994;9:115–120.
81. Dobato JL, Mateo D, de Andres C, Gimenez-Roldan S. Degeneracion ganglionica corticobasal presentandose como un sindrome de afasia progresiva primaria. *Neurologia* 1993;8:141.
82. Schneider JA, Watts RL, Gearing M, Brewer RP, Mirra SS. Corticobasal degeneration: neuropathologic and clinical heterogeneity. *Neurology* 1997;48:959–969.
83. Litvan I, Agid Y, Goetz C, et al. Accuracy of the clinical diagnosis of corticobasal degeneration: a clinicopathologic study. *Neurology* 1997;48:119–125.
84. Cambier JJ. Masson M, Dairou R, Henin D. Etude anatomoclinique d'une forme parietale de maladie de Pick. *Rev Neurol* 1981;137:33—38.
85. Lang AE, Bergeron C, Pollanen MS, Ashby P. Parietal Pick's disease mimicking cortical-basal ganglionic degeneration. *Neurology* 1994;44:1436—1440.
86. Fukui T, Sugita K, Kawamura M, Shiota J, Nakano I. Primary progressive apraxia in Pick's disease: a clinicopathologic study. *Neurology* 1996;47:467—473.
87. Boeve BF, Maraganore DM, Parisi JE, et al. Disorders mimicking the "classical" clinical syndrome of corticobasal ganglionic degeneration: report of nine cases [abstract]. *Mov Disord* 1996;11:351.
88. Kawasaki K, Iwanaga K, Wakabayashi K, Yamada M, Nagai H, Idezuka J. et al. Corticobasal degeneration with neither argyrophilic inclusions nor tau abnormalities: a new subgroup? Acta Neuropathol 1996; 91:140—144.

Corticobasal Degeneration.
Advances in Neurology, Vol. 82,
edited by I. Litvan, C. G. Goetz, and A. E. Lang.
Lippincott Williams & Wilkins, Philadelphia © 2000.

22

Diagnostic Controversies: Another View

Charles Duyckaerts and Jean-Jacques Hauw

Laboratoire de Neuropathologie, Raymond Escourolle, Hôpital de la Pitié-Salpêtrière,
75651 Paris, Cedex 13 France

INTRODUCTION

Several diseases or syndromes are characterized by a primary progressive cognitive deficit, with or without parkinsonian features, among which are Pick disease (1), progressive supranuclear palsy (PSP) (2), corticobasal degeneration (CBD) (3,4), semantic dementia (5,6), primary progressive aphasia (7), frontotemporal dementia and parkinsonism linked to chromosome 17 (FTDP-17) (8), and finally, (degenerative) frontotemporal dementia (9,10) or dementia lacking distinctive histologic feature (11). The grouping of those disorders under the common labeling of "Pick complex" has been recently advocated "to cover a family of related conditions, of which Pick body dementia is but one of the components" (12,13). We believe (14) with others (15) that this new eponymous labeling should be discouraged since it is theoretically and practically confusing (What is a complex?). In addition, it adds a new meaning to the Pick eponym, already ambiguous (Pick atrophy, Pick disease, Pick body, Pick cell). We are willing to discuss our conclusion in the hope that this debate will help to clarify the questions that have been recently raised by the identification (or renaming) of new clinical syndromes and pathological markers. Our argument will develop the following points: a disease is a syndrome that has a cause. In the absence of a cause, clinical syndromes are but a set of indications pointing to the topography of a lesion and to a loosely defined mechanism (such as vascular, expansive, and degenerative lesions). Pathological markers are usually closer to the cause: in the last decade, numerous examples have shown that they may be clues to the pathogenesis. The synthetic view expressed in the term "Pick complex" is thus a regression since it lumps *diseases* that should be differentiated, into a poorly defined *syndrome* that hampers further analysis.

THE CAUSE MAKES THE DISEASE

The concept of disease has evolved over time and is ever changing. For more than two centuries (Morgagni, "*De sedibus et causis morborum per anatomem indagatis*" 1761) clinicopathological data have been used as criteria to delineate new disorders. Some clinical or pathological signs are indeed associated more often than by chance: those sets of frequently grouped signs are traditionally called "syndromes" in accordance with the etymology. Diseases are different from syndromes. The cause, indeed, makes the disease. To take a straightforward example, a chronic respiratory disorder, a rapidly progressive meningitis, and adrenocortical insufficiency are syndromes that could hardly be grouped under a common name, were the clinical data taken in isolation. However they all may be due to the same cause: tuberculosis. In the example mentioned before, tuberculosis may cause a nonspecific exudate, a granuloma with or without caseum, or a fibrous scar: pathology itself is not sufficient to define a disease. The identification of the causative pathogen, *M. tuberculosis,* is the sole reason to group all the previously listed symptoms, signs, and lesions under one and the same disease. This example is purposefully simple and does not exclude the possibility of multifactorial diseases in which several causes act synergistically. It is unfortunate that the term "disease" remains commonly attached to disorders having multiple causes, as in Alzheimer "syndrome," which is, as it is now known, a stereotyped manner in which the brain reacts to various pathogenetic events such as different mutations involving the genes of the amyloid precursor protein, of presenilin 1 and 2 or maybe repeated head trauma (dementia pugilistica). It should finally be stressed that physiopathology, between cause and syndrome, remains often obscure, although the key of treatment. Largely thanks to the progress of genetics during the last decade, the causes of a significant number of inherited neurodegenerative diseases have been unraveled. Old syndromes have been split into various diseases as in the autosomal dominant ataxias, or regrouped in one single disorder, as in Friedreich ataxia where atypical cases have been explained by smaller repeat expansions (16). On the other hand, clues furnished by the molecular analysis have allowed clinicians to recognize more accurately subtle differences that helped to delineate newly isolated diseases. To take the same example, the examination of eye movements in cerebellar ataxias, makes it now possible to predict the genotype with great accuracy (17): new diseases make new syndromes. The synthetic point of view, that is, linking together several diseases in the same syndrome, would be a regression in this context.

CLINICAL SYNDROMES AND PATHOLOGY

In many neurological disorders, however, only "syndromes" are identified. The clinical syndromes yield two types of information: symptoms and signs suggest the *topography* of the lesion; the course, its *mechanism*. Hemiplegia, to take a trivial example, indicates a lesion of the motor pathway; it may be sudden (suggestive of a vascular process) or progressive (common in expansive processes). The macroscopic examination (including neuroradiological investigations) and the microscopical study help to determine the *nature* of the mass lesion: tumor (meningioma, astrocytoma, glioblastoma), abscess, edematous plaque of sclerosis, and others. The hierarchical levels of description (15) are similar for a cognitive syndrome. Symptoms and signs point to the topography: aphasia to the language areas, executive syndrome to the frontal, and apraxia to the parietal lobes. The slow progression of the clinical signs suggests a degenerative process, a hypothesis that is reinforced by the finding of atrophy on the CT scan. Finally, the microscopic examination provides information on the nature of the pathogenetic process. Isolating Pick complex to describe a primary progressive deficit is, in our view, like identifying "progressive hemiplegia," a syndrome, not a disease. By neglecting pathology, it tells us little concerning the cause. The microscope, however, helps to confirm that the process is a degeneration and allows to dissect the pathogenetic mechanisms at work, with a precision that has dramatically increased in the last decade.

THE ALPHABET OF THE PATHOLOGICAL EXAMINATION IN PROGRESSIVE COGNITIVE DEFICIT

The information provided by the histopathological examination is of unequal value and includes two types of information: the quantitative changes (too few neurons, dendrites, synapses; too many astrocytes) and the presence of markers.

The Quantitative Changes

They are usually hard to ascertain and imply either a large experience or quantitative methods. The neuronal loss adds little to the clinical conclusions since this loss causes a clinical deficit that the examination of the patient has, in most cases, already demonstrated. It is, moreover, nonspecific, being the endpoint of many neurodegenerative processes. When only the distribution of the neuronal loss could be used as a diagnostic tool, the classification of the cases was a difficult, and often subjective, matter leading to a botanic type of taxonomy. Neuronal loss is accompanied by an increase in the density of fibrillar astrocytes. It also causes a dendritic loss and, in the projection areas, a deafferentation. Dendritic loss and deafferentation (18) are the two plausible mechanisms of laminar spongiosis, also a poorly specific sign since it is encountered in many different conditions such as Alzheimer disease or AIDS dementia as well as in "dementia lacking distinctive histology" (19).

The Markers

Neuropathological markers are visible accumulations of normal or abnormal material in the cells (e.g., abnormally phosphorylated tau in the neurons) or in the neuropile (e.g., Aβ peptide in the amyloid core of the senile plaque). The diagnostic or pathogenetic value of the markers is variable.

Chromatolytic neurons have lost (=lytic) their color (=chroma). The so-called color is actually due to the Nissl bodies, stained blue with anilin dyes. At the same time, the neurons enlarge—they are also called "ballooned" or "swollen"—and accumulate heat-shock proteins such as alpha-B crystallin (20). The presence of ballooned neurons suggests impairment of the axonal flow (such as encountered after axonal section). They have been reported mainly in Pick disease (21) (hence, the unfortunate term "Pick cell" which adds to the confusion surrounding the eponym) and in CBD (4,22). However, they have been also seen in many other conditions (Creutzfeldt-Jakob disease, amyotrophic lateral sclerosis, pellagra) (23,24). Therefore, the informative value of this marker is low.

More robust markers have been reported in cases of primary progressive cognitive deficits. They will be abundantly discussed in this book and this is not the place to go into details, similar diagnostic diagrams having been proposed in the literature (10,20,25,26). A rapid sketch is presented here for the sake of the discussion.

A high density of *senile plaques and neurofibrillary tangles* have been seen in many cases of apparently focal cognitive deficit, most noticeably of posterior cortical atrophy (27) and of primary progressive aphasia (28). They justify the diagnosis of Alzheimer disease.

Pick bodies, tau-positive, spherical inclusions found in the cytoplasms of neurons, particularly in the dentate gyrus (29), are associated with an abnormal migration of tau protein on Western immunoblots of brain extracts. Two bands (at 55 and 64 kDa) (30) are indeed identified instead of the six that are present in normal brains. Pick bodies have been reported in various clinical settings, mainly frontal syndromes, but also progressive aphasia (or "semantic dementia") as in one of the original cases of Pick (31) and in more recently reported cases of primary progressive aphasia (32). We endorse here the opinion that Pick bodies are necessary to the diagnosis of Pick disease, since it has repeatedly been shown that it clearly identifies a homogeneous group of sporadic cases of frontotemporal degeneration (29, 33–37).

Intracytoplasmic inclusions labeled by anti-ubiquitin antibodies have been described in cases of amyotrophic lateral sclerosis (ALS) with or without dementia (38,39). They are associated with ubiquitin neurites in cases of dementia without ALS (40).

Tau-positive inclusions have been seen in neurons and, more specifically, in astrocytes in cases of progressive supranuclear palsy (41) and of CBD (42). The tau-positive glial inclusions might be different in these two disorders: the tuft of abnormal fiber suggesting the former, the astrocytic plaque being more common in the latter (43). The Western immunoblotting of brain extracts have shown two tau bands (at 64 and 69 kDa) in progressive supranuclear palsy (PSP) (44) as well as in CBD (45), different from those seen in Pick disease (30). The delineation of these disorders is still a matter of discussion, echoed in several chapters of this book.

Tau-positive neurofibrillary pathology has been seen in FTDP-17. Its frequency is not yet strictly established—tau immunohistochemistry remains to be checked in some families (46). Mutations in the tau gene have been identified in several families (47). The phenotypic variation of FTDP-17 has been discussed (8).

As with the clinical signs, the pathological markers are grouped into syndromes: Pick bodies, for instance, generally occur in association with swollen neurons and severe neuronal loss. When no markers are present, the histopathological examination is of little help in the diagnosis, except in excluding the previously mentioned changes. The term dementia lacking distinctive histology (19) seems then the most appropriate. It will no doubt be used less often in the future years, with the isolation of new entities.

The list of markers mentioned here is by no means exhaustive and does not represent the immutable alphabet of the diagnosis as soon as it is accepted that the cause, rather than the histopathology or the clinical picture, defines the disease. The value of the markers has changed and will again with time: for instance, the discovery of a mutation of the tau protein gene establishes the diagnosis of FTDP-17 (47). The diagnostic value of the neurofibrillary tangles in that pathology has, at the same time, become weak. Their possible scientific value, however, has increased since it appears useful to determine if they are a necessary step between the genetic defect and the clinical sign.

The genetic heterogeneity and the variety of histopathological and biochemical changes warrant, in our view, the opinion that we are dealing with a group of highly differentiated diseases rather than with a common pathogenetic mechanism expressed in slightly different ways. However, this conclusion obviously depends heavily on the pathogenetic significance that is attributed to the marker.

IS HISTOPATHOLOGY CLOSER TO CAUSES? THE SIGNIFICANCE OF THE MARKERS

The importance that we have attributed to the markers could indeed be questioned by the reader. Should clinical homogeneity be taken as strong evidence of a common pathogenetic mechanism? Or, on the contrary, is it better justified to consider that the markers tell us something about the cause of a disease or that they are closer to it than the clinical signs? The recent history of neurology and neuropathology support a definitely positive answer to the last question. The relations between pathology and fundamental research have been a two-way dialogue: sometimes, the careful study of the markers opened new vistas; sometimes, the biological findings, opened the eyes of the microscopist, who was then able to uncover changes that were looked at but remained unseen for decades. The examples are numerous: the isolation of the Aβ peptide from the amyloid angiopathy (48) has allowed the discovery of mutations present in familial Alzheimer disease (49). Amyloid plaques, scrapie-associated fibrils (SAF), and rods have paved the way to the identification of the prion protein, its gene, and its mutations (50). The isolation of a gene mutated in a family of Parkinson disease has led to the discovery that the Lewy body contained α-synuclein (51) and to the surprising finding that the oligodendroglial inclusions of multiple system atrophy also contain them (52). The report of a polyglutamine expansion in Huntington disease and autosomal dominant spinocerebellar atrophies has permitted the identification of ubiquitinated nuclear inclusions containing the abnormal protein (53) previously overlooked (54,55). The mutated gene in FTDP-17 has been shown to code for tau (47), a protein that accumulates in the cytoplasm of neurons and glia in that pathology. These examples suggest that in many cases the histopathological markers are not innocent bystanders but indicators of the pathogenesis.

A final point can be made in discussing the importance of the markers. In some cases, the clinical and the pathological data are, apparently, dissociated. To take an example in other areas of medicine, miliary and chronic pulmonary tuberculoses have little in common from a clinical standpoint, although the pathology indicates a common origin, proved by bacteriology. Both clinical pictures obviously would be classified today as tuberculosis. The importance of the "marker" (caseum) supplanted the clinical feeling in that case. In a similar way, the presence of a common mechanism may eventually be disclosed in disorders that appear clinically different, but exhibit some common pathology. The question is raised for Parkinson disease and dementia with Lewy bodies as well as for PSP and CBD. In other words and to conclude, we believe that the pathology more easily unravels the pathogenetic mechanisms than the clinical data because it is located closer to the causes.

"PICK COMPLEX"

We understand the efforts made by the "lumpers" to synthetize the facts and to avoid the botanical style of splitting the pathological entities, a practice that was once common in neuropathology. However, as previously stated, we do not recommend the term "Pick complex".

The Term "Complex" Is Not Clearly Defined

"Complex" is ambiguous. Are we dealing with a disease, a group of diseases, or a syndrome? Does the term imply a common pathogenetic mechanism? The genetic heterogeneity of the diseases that are listed under that heading is against this hypothesis. Is it used to designate a common histopathological picture? This is clearly not the case. Pick bodies, neurofibrillary pathology, and ubiquitin cytoplasmic inclusions are distinctive pathological signatures. Is it, then, a purely clinical term, actually a synonym of syndrome, that should be taken as the chapter headline, preceding a more detailed analysis? If a term is to be chosen that avoids, at the bedside, a discussion of the pathology responsible for the symptoms, then it would be better if this term were purely clinical (as "hemiplegia") avoiding reference to any known disease (as to Pick disease). The term primary focal cognitive deficit, which we propose here, fulfills these conditions and avoids the confusion in the level of analysis, the major source of nosological problems (14,15). Alternatives have been proposed (15). We believe that the synthesis that the term Pick complex suggests represents regression rather than progress, since it apparently relies heavily on clinical ground. Neuropsychology (56), histopathology (57), and genomic analysis (47) clearly split the complex into several disorders. What is the use of having one term for several diseases: A researcher receiving a sample from a "Pick complex case" could be dealing as well with a chromosome 17-linked dementia as with a sporadic case with Pick bodies. Would a sample from a case with "progressive hemiplegia" be useful?

The Term "Pick Complex" Adds a New Meaning to the Already Overloaded Pick Eponym

The discovery of cerebral localization at the end of the last century (58) led to a considerable clinical curiosity—people were looking for the experiments of nature that would add new localization to the known functions of the cerebral cortex. Arnold Pick worked in this context; he described circumscribed atrophies of the left temporal lobe causing aphasia (31) and of the parietal lobe causing apraxia (59). The cause of the atrophies were barely considered ("dementia senilis" in the case of apraxia; senile atrophy is mentioned in one of the cases of aphasias). Those cases were not cases of "Pick diseases" as we understand it now, for several reasons. Pick did not describe a *disease;* he was studying circumscribed *atrophies* to elucidate cerebral localization. All of his studies were purely macroscopic without microscopic examination. The frontal syndrome, that is usually associated with Pick disease, was not mentioned in his cases. Pick disease is a later creation. In a case of "senile circumscribed atrophy," Alzheimer described a peculiar argyrophilic inclusion in the neuron, the "Kugel" (60), now known as "Pick bodies." Ganz, a Dutch neurologist, described cases of circumscribed atrophy of the frontal lobe under the name "Pick's atrophy of the frontal lobes" (61). The term Pick disease is owing to Onari and Spatz (1). Historically, the eponym has thus been attached to at least three different clinicopathological situations.

1. It has been used to designate any circumscribed atrophy; this was the original point of view of Pick himself (31,59,62,63) and of Alzheimer (60).
2. It has come to mean frontal lobe degeneration (64), with Pick bodies (type A), without Pick bodies but with ballooned cells (type B), without Pick bodies or ballooned cells (type C) (65).
3. Pick bodies are now often thought necessary to the diagnosis of Pick disease—a constraint that we endorse here with others (29, 33–37,57).

This point emphasizes that original articles may serve as the basis for the classical eponymous designations, but are not final arbiters of diseases profiles, which are subject to evolution and refinement (66). Is it useful to add some new meanings to the eponym by adjoining now a "complex" to the "atrophy" and to the disease? How will the eponym Pick finally be understood: a circumscribed atrophy (original meaning), a frontal syndrome with various pathologies (64,65), a chapter including several conditions as in Pick complex, a cell, an inclusion or a disease characterized by the presence of these inclusions? We would encourage its use only with the last meaning—in the sense of "Pick body dementia," a term used by A. Kertesz (12).

Only a few decades ago, three types of degenerative dementia were recognized—senile dementia, Alzheimer, and Pick diseases. The present-day classification is more complex and there is no doubt that the disorders that we believe homogeneous will be split again. The trunk will give more branches and the branches themselves more ramifications. The causes of the deficits will probably supersede the general, and thus poorly specific, terms. One may wonder, then, if it is useful to discuss terminology at length, when the scientific rules are so clear; as long as the clinical, pathological, and histological features of all reported cases are carefully documented, they can be reclassified into 1, 2, 3 or whatever number of entities eventually emerge (67).

REFERENCES

1. Onari K, Spatz H. Anatomische Beiträge zur Lehre von der Pickschen umschriebenen Grosshirnrinde-Atrophie ("Picksche Krankheit"). *Z Neurol* 1926;101:470–511.
2. Steele JC, Richardson JC, Olszewski J. Progressive supranuclear palsy: a heterogeneous degeneration involving the brain stem, basal ganglia and cerebellum with vertical gaze and pseudobulbar palsy, nuclear dystonia and dementia. *Arch Neurol* 1964;10:333–359.
3. Rebeiz JJ, Kolodny EH, Richardson EP. Corticodentatonigral degeneration with neuronal achromasia. *Arch Neurol* 1968;18:20–33.
4. Gibb WRG, Luthert PJ, Marsden CD. Corticobasal degeneration. *Brain* 1989;112:1171–1192.
5. Warrington EK. The selective impairment of semantic memory. *Q J Exp Psychol* 1975;27:635–657.
6. Snowden JS, Goulding PJ, Neary D. Semantic dementia: a form of circumscribed cerebral atrophy. *Behav Neurol* 1989;2:167–182.
7. Mesulam MM. Slowly progressive aphasia without generalized dementia. *Ann Neurol* 1982;11:592–598.
8. Foster NL, Wilhelmsen K, Sima AA, Jones MZ, D'Amato CJ, Gilman S. Frontotemporal dementia and parkinsonism linked to chromosome 17: a consensus conference. *Ann Neurol* 1997;41:706–715.
9. The Lund and Manchester groups. Clinical and neuropathological criteria for frontotemporal dementia. *J Neurol Neurosurg Psychiatr* 1994;57:416–418.
10. Jackson M, Lowe J. The new neuropathology of degenerative frontotemporal dementias. *Acta Neuropathol* 1996;91:127–134.
11. Knopman DS, Mastri AR, Frei WH, Sung JH, Rustan T. Dementia lacking distinctive histologic feature: a common non-Alzheimer degenerative dementia. *Neurology* 1990;40:251–256.
12. Kertesz A. Frontotemporal dementia, Pick disease, and corticobasal degeneration. One entity or 3? 1. *Arch Neurol* 1997;54:1427–1429.
13. Kertesz A, Munoz D. Pick's disease, frontotemporal dementia, and Pick complex: emerging concepts. *Arch Neurol* 1998;55:302–304.
14. Duyckaerts C, Dürr A, Uchihara T, Boller F, Hauw J-J. Pick complex: too simple? *Eur J Neurol* 1996;3:283–286.
15. Neary D. Frontotemporal degeneration, Pick disease, and corticobasal degeneration. One entity or 3? 3. *Arch Neurol* 1997;54:1425–1427.
16. Dürr A, Cossee M, Agid Y, et al. Clinical and genetic abnormalities in patients with Friedreich's ataxia. *N Engl J Med* 1996;335:1169–1175.
17. Rivaud-Pechoux S, Durr A, Gaymard B, et al. Eye movement abnormalities correlate with genotype in autosomal dominant cerebellar ataxia type I. *Ann Neurol* 1998; 43:297–302.
18. Duyckaerts C, Colle MA, Seilhean D, Hauw J-J. Laminar spongiosis of the dentate gyrus: a sign of disconnection, present in cases of Alzheimer disease. *Acta Neuropathol* 1998;95:413–420.
19. Knopman DS. Overview of dementia lacking distinctive histology: pathological designation of a progressive dementia. *Dementia* 1993;4:132–136.
20. Cooper PN, Jackson M, Lennox G, Lowe J, Mann DMA. Tau, ubiquitin, alpha-B crystallin immunohistochemistry define the principal causes of degenerative frontotemporal dementia. *Arch Neurol* 1995;52:1011–1115.
21. Lüers T, Spatz H. Picksche Krankheit. (Progressive umschriebene Grosshirnatrophie). In: Lubarsch O, Henke F, Rössle R, eds. *Hanbuch der speziellen pathologischen Anatomie und Histologie.* Berlin: Springer-Verlag, 1957.
22. Rebeiz JJ, Kolodny EH, Richardson EP. Corticodentatonigral degeneration with neuronal achromasia: a progressive disorder of late adult life. *Transact Am Neurol Assoc* 1967;92:23–26.
23. Hauw J-J, De Baecque C, Hausser-Hauw C, Serdaru M. Chromatolysis in alcoholic encephalopathies. Pellagra-like changes in 22 cases. *Brain* 1988; 111:843–857.
24. Kato S, Hirano A, Umahara T, Kato M, Herz F, Ohama E. Comparative immunohistochemical study on the expression of alphaB crystallin and stress-response protein 27 in ballooned neurons in various disorders. *Neuropathol Appl Neurobiol* 1992;18:335–340.
25. Hauw J-J, Duyckaerts C, Seilhean D, Camilleri S, Sazdovitch V, Rancurel G. The neuropathologic diagnostic criteria of frontal lobe dementia revisited. A study of ten consecutive cases. *J Neural Transm (Suppl)* 1996;47: 47–59.
26. Lowe J. Establishing a pathological diagnosis in degenerative dementias. *Brain Pathol* 1998;8:403–406.

27. Hof PR, Vogt BA, Bouras C, Morrison JH. Atypical form of Alzheimer's disease with prominent posterior cortical atrophy: a review of lesion distribution and circuit disconnection in cortical visual pathways. *Vision Res* 1997;37:3609–3625.
28. Greene JD, Patterson K, Xuereb J, Hodges JR. Alzheimer disease and nonfluent progressive aphasia. *Arch Neurol* 1996;53:1072–1078.
29. Hof PR, Bouras C, Perl D, Morrison JH. Quantitative neuropathologic analysis of Pick's disease cases: cortical distribution of Pick bodies and coexistence with Alzheimer's disease. *Acta Neuropathol (Berlin)* 1994; 87:115–124.
30. Delacourte A, Robitaille Y, Sergeant N, et al. Specific pathological Tau protein variants characterize Pick's disease. *J Neuropathol Exp Neurol* 1996;55:159–168.
31. Pick A. Ueber die Beziehungen der senilen Himatrophie zur Aphasie. *Prager Med Wschr* 1892; 17:15–17.
32. Graff-Radford NR, Damasio AR, Hyman BT, et al. Progressive aphasia in a patient with Pick's disease: a neuropsychological, radiologic and anatomic study. *Neurology* 1990;40:620–626.
33. Dickson DW. Pick's disease: a modern approach. *Brain Pathol* 1998;8:339–354.
34. Hauw J-J, Daniel SE, Dickson D, et al. Preliminary NINDS neuropathologic criteria for Steele-Richardson-Olszewski syndrome (Progressive Supranuclear Palsy). *Neurology* 1994;44:2015–2019.
35. Litvan I, Hauw JJ, Bartko JJ, et al. Validity and reliability of the preliminary NINDS neuropathologic criteria for progressive supranuclear palsy and related disorders. *J Neuropathol Exp Neurol* 1996;55:97–105.
36. Litvan I, DeLeo JM, Hauw J-J, et al. What can artificial neural networks teach us about neurodegenerative disorders with extrapyramidal features? *Brain* 1996.
37. Litvan I, Agid Y, Sastry N, et al. What are the obstacles for an accurate clinical diagnosis of Pick's disease? A clinicopathologic study. *Neurology* 1997;49: 62–69.
38. Okamoto K, Shunsaku H, Yamazaki T, Sun X, Nakazato Y. New ubiquitin-positive intraneuronal inclusions in the extra-motor cortice in patients with amyotrophic lateral sclerosis. *Neurosci Lett* 1991; 129:233–236.
39. Wightman G, Anderson VE, Martin J, et al. Hippocampal and neocortical ubiquitin-immunoreactive inclusions in amyotrophic lateral sclerosis with dementia. *Neurosci Lett* 1992;139:269–274.
40. Tolnay M, Probst A. Frontal lobe degeneration: novel ubiquitin-immunoreactive neurites within frontotemporal cortex. *Neuropathol Appl Neurobiol* 1995;21:492–497.
41. Hauw J-J, Verny M, Delaère P, Cervera P, He Y, Duyckaerts C. Constant neurofibrillary changes in the neocortex in progressive supranuclear palsy. Basic differences with aging and aging. *Neurosci Lett* 1990; 119: 182–186.
42. Feany MB, Dickson DW. Widespread cytoskeletal pathology characterizes cortico-basal degeneration. *Am J Pathol* 1995;90:37–43.
43. Komori T, Arai N, Oda M, et al. Astrocytic plaques and tufts of abnormal fibers do not coexist in corticobasal degeneration and progressive supranuclear palsy. *Acta Neuropathol* 1998;96:401–408.
44. Flament S, Delacourte A, Verny M, Hauw J-J, Javoy-Agid F. Abnormal tau protéins in progressive supranuclear palsy. Similarities and differences with the neurofibrillary degeneration of the Alzheimer type. *Acta Neuropathol* 1991;81:591–596.
45. Buée-Scherrer V, Hof PR, Buée L, Leveugle B, et al. Hyperphosphorylated tau proteins differentiate corticobasal degeneration and Pick's disease. *Acta Neuropathol (Berlin)* 1996;91:351–359.
46. Spillantini MG, Bird TD, Ghetti B. Frontotemporal dementia and parkinsonism linked to chromosome 17: a new group of tauopathies. *Brain Pathol.* 1998;8:387–402.
47. Hutton M, Lendon CL, Rizzu P, et al. Association of missense and 5′-splice-site mutations in tau with the inherited dementia FTDP-17. *Nature* 1998;393:702–705.
48. Glenner GG, Wong CW. Alzheimer's disease: Initial report of the purification and characterization of a novel cerebrovascular amyloid protein. *Biochem Biophys Res Commun* 1984;120:885–890.
49. Chartier-Harlin MC, Crawford F, Houlden H, et al. Early-onset Alzheimer's disease caused by mutations at codon 717 of the ß-amyloid precursor protein gene. *Nature* 1991;353:844–846.
50. Prusiner SB. Molecular biology and pathogenesis of prion diseases. *Trends Biochem Sci* 1996;21:482–487.
51. Spillantini MG, Schmidt ML, Lee VMY, Trojanowski JQ, Jakes R, Goedert M. Alpha-synuclein in Lewy bodies. *Nature* 1997;388:839–840.
52. Spillantini MG, Crowther RA, Jakes R, Cairns NJ, Lantos PL, Goedert M. Filamentous alpha-synuclein inclusions link multiple system atrophy with Parkinson's disease and dementia with Lewy bodies. *Neurosci Letts* 1998;251:205–208.
53. Davies SW, Beardsall K, Turmaine M, DiFiglia M, Aronin N, Bates GP. Are neuronal intranuclear inclusions the common neuropathology of triplet-repeat disorders with polyglutamine-repeat expansions? *Lancet* 1998;351:131–133.
54. Holmberg M, Duyckaerts C, Durr A, et al. Spinocerebellar ataxia type 7 (SCA7): a neurodegenerative disorder with neuronal intranuclear inclusions. *Hum Mol Genet* 1998;7:913–918.
55. Duyckaerts C, Dürr A, Cancel G, Brice A. Nuclear inclusions in SCA1. *Acta Neuropathol (Berl)* 1998, in press.
56. Pillon B, Dubois B, Agid Y. Cognitive deficits in non-Alzheimer's degenerative diseases. *J Neural Transm* 1996;47 (supp) 61–71.
57. Lantos PL. Overview of neuropathology. In: Rossor MN, ed. *Unusual dementias.* London: Baillière Tindall, 1992.
58. Broca P. Remarques sur le siège de la faculté du langage suivis d'une observation d'aphémie (perte de la parole). *Bull Mém Soc Anat (Paris)* 1861;36:330–357.
59. Pick A. Uber einen weiteren Symptomencomplex im Rahmen der Dementia senilis, bedingt durch umschriebene stärkene Hirnatrophie (gemischte Apraxie). *Mschr Psychiat Neurol* 1906;19:97–108.
60. Alzheimer A. Uber eigenartige Krankheitsfälle des späteren Alters. *Zentralblatt Gesam Neurol Psychiat* 1911;4:356–385.
61. Ganz A. Betrachtungen über Art und Ausbreitung des krankhaften Prozesses in einem Fall von Pickscher krankheit des Stirnhirns. *Zentralblatt Gesam Neurol Psychiat* 1923;80:10–28.
62. Pick A. *Beiträge zur Pathologie und pathologischen Anatomie des Zentralnervensystems.* Berlin: S. Karger, 1898.
63. Pick A. Senile Hirnatrophie als Grundlage von Herderscheinungen. *Wiener klinische Wschr* 1901;14:16–17.

64. Escourolle R. *La maladie de Pick. Etude critique d'ensemble et synthèse anatomo-clinique.* Paris: R. Foulon, 1958.
65. Constantinidis J, Richard J, Tissot R. Pick's disease. Histological and clinical correlation. *Eur Neurol* 1974;11: 208–217.
66. Henry JM. Neurons and Nobel prizes: a centennial history of neuropathology. *Neurosurgery* 1998,42: 143–156.
67. Hachinski V. Frontotemporal degeneration, Pick disease, and corticobasal degeneration. Three entities or 1? *Arch Neurol* 1997;54:1429.

Corticobasal Degeneration.
Advances in Neurology, Vol. 82,
edited by I. Litvan, C. G. Goetz, and A. E. Lang.
Lippincott Williams & Wilkins, Philadelphia © 2000.

23
Conclusions

Yves Agid

Fédération de Neurologie and INSERM U 289, Hôpital de la Salpêtrière, 75013 Paris, France

During a neurology course on corticobasal degeneration (CBD), a noisy student in the back of the room is disturbing the class. The professor is annoyed, and asks the student: "What is CBD"? "Humm . . . I knew what it was, but I don't remember." "*I regret that you have forgotten, because you must have been the only person to have ever known!*" says the professor. After reading this first and seminal book on CBD, however, we have learned a lot about this recently described and strange clinical entity. Let us look more closely at some of the principal observations reported in these excellent chapters.

First, can one imagine a more imprecise name for a disease? How many disorders in our discipline involve lesions of both the cortex and the basal ganglia? Very many, indeed. Too many! Therefore, the only word that is really useful is "degeneration," which indicates that there is a progressive and selective loss of neurons during the course of the disease. If Jean-Martin Charcot was really the first to point out this form of parkinsonism at the end of the last century (see Chapter 1), that is, 75 years before Rebeiz et al. described the three cases that became the archetype of the syndrome, it might perhaps be more reasonable to name this affliction Charcot-Rebeiz disease, at least until its mechanism and causes are discovered. I doubt that this can happen, but the eponym would be less ambiguous than CBD.

CBD is a rare disorder (see Chapter 5), in the order of 1% to 5% of patients with parkinsonism, although its true prevalence is unknown. Mean age of onset is 60 to 65 years; the youngest case reported is 45. No risk factors, genetic or other, have been detected. In one family, two brothers were diagnosed as having CBD, but there was no pathological confirmation of the diagnosis.

In the past, we believed that the diagnosis of CBD was evident when the following features were observed in a given patient: an akineto-rigid syndrome unresponsive to L-DOPA associated with dystonic postures, apraxia, and a marked asymmetry of symptoms. Indeed, the criteria by which a diagnosis of CBD is made consist of a progressive aggravation of the disease, a unilateral onset and asymmetric course of symptoms, and clinical manifestations reflecting dysfunction in both cerebral cortex (higher functions) and basal ganglia (movement disorders) (see Chapter 17). In the different chapters of this book, however, we have learned that the clinical picture of this disorder is more complex than previously thought (see Chapters 3 and 4), in part owing to the existence of several atypical cases.

Parkinsonism (plastic rigidity and bradykinesia) in CBD is indeed extremely common, but it is sometimes difficult to distinguish from paratonia (Gegenhalten rigidity modified by passive movements of the limbs) often seen in old subjects and in patients with various neurodegenerative disorders (see Chapter 6). It never significantly responds to L-DOPA and is usually associated with an asymmetric limb dystonia. Dystonia, particularly in one arm, is strongly suggestive of CBD (see Chapter 7) when it is associated with myoclonus (essentially action and reflex myoclonus), as seen during the course of the disease in half of the patients with CBD (see Chapter 8).

At a time when the concept of apraxia is changing as a result of a better understanding of the physiology of the sensori-motor cortex and basal ganglia, it nevertheless remains one of the most characteristic features of CBD (see Chapter 10). Apraxia needs to be assessed in the least affected limb as it is not always possible to demonstrate it in the severely rigid and immobile limb. Patients usually have a dysfunction of praxis production causing ideomotor (impaired timing, sequencing, and spatial organization of gestures, usually bilaterally) and limb-kinesic (impaired manipulation of fingers and hands, usually unilaterally) apraxia. A disrupted action conception (ideational apraxia) is rarely observed, except in advanced stages of the disease. In any case, the observation of apraxia, in a given patient, sometimes difficult to identify, especially in severely disabled patients with rigidity and dystonia, is not pathognomonic of CBD as limb apraxia has been described in other neurodegenerative disorders such as progressive supranuclear palsy (PSP).

The presence of other symptoms suggesting the involvement of the cerebral cortex may evoke the diagnosis of CBD. Aphasia (see Chapter 11) is not rare (its prevalence is close to 50% in autopsy series), and is usually of the nonfluent type, indicating that CBD pathology should be systematically envisaged as a possible neuropathological substrate for primary progressive aphasia. Aphasia is difficult to identify in advanced cases because of the presence of dysarthria (slurred dysarthric speech with extrapyramidal and pseudobulbar aspects (see Chapter 14) and, less frequently of buccofacial apraxia. Cortical sensory deficits (astereognosia, abnormal joint position, loss of sensitivity to light touch) should point towards CBD, once structural lesions of the parietal cortex are ruled out. The alien limb (see Chapter 12), defined as the "feeling that a limb is wandering uncontrollably together with observable autonomous motor activity of the affected limb" is usually subdivided into "callosal" (with intermanual conflict) and "frontal" (with a frontal syndrome) variants. This symptom is difficult to identify precisely because of the presence of additional sensory, dystonic and apraxic defects that develop as brain lesions spread during the course of the disease.

In association with motor and praxis disorders, patients with CBD exhibit moderate cognitive deterioration (see Chapter 9) with subcortico-frontal features (executive dysfunction and memory impairment with defective retrieval). This association of cognitive disorders of subcortical origin with instrumental dysfunction (praxis disorders more than linguistic and visuospatial dysfunction) is suggestive of CBD, where cognitive decline often does not reach the level of defined dementia.

Eye movements are often abnormal in CBD patients (see Chapter 15). Supranuclear palsy, that usually evokes a misdiagnosis of progressive supranuclear palsy, is found at late stage in about 50% of CBD patients. Electrooculography, when possible, can contribute to the differential diagnosis of CBD by showing characteristic increased latencies of reflexive visually guided saccades (more often ipsilateral to the apraxia).

Computed tomography (CT) and magnetic resonance imaging (MRI) can strongly support the diagnosis of CBD if atrophy of the cerebral cortex is asymmetrical with a focal distribution in the posterior frontal and parietal regions contralateral to the clinically most affected side (see Chapter 18). Abnormalities in the basal ganglia, including hypointensities in the lenticular nuclei (T2-weighted images) or mild atrophy of the midbrain, are less specific. Recent experience indicates, however, that asymmetrical atrophy of the cortex is sometimes not found in CBD cases with clinically bilateral presentation and that basal ganglia abnormalities are not specific for the disease. Whether functional imaging (fluorodeoxyglucose, F-DOPA, dopamine receptor binding) helps the clinician to diagnose CBD is still a matter of debate, as the patterns of dysfunction observed in CBD do not completely distinguish CBD from other neurodegenerative disorders (see Chapter 19).

The fact that there is no specific treatment for this disabling disorder does not mean that the patients cannot be helped (see Chapter 20). Professional assistance (physical, occupational, speech therapy), symptomatic pharmacological treatment (antidepressants, since depression is a common feature (see Chapter 13), social services and nursing facilities can all contribute to the welfare of the patients.

In sum, the association of an akineto-rigid syndrome with dystonia, apraxia, and an asymmetrical presentation of symptoms still constitutes the cardinal triad of CBD. The red flags against the diagnosis of CBD are: presentation before age 45; a sustained response to L-DOPA treatment; the presence of symptoms orienting the diagnosis toward other neurodegenerative disorders, including severe frontal lobe-like symptomatology with falls during the first year of the disease and the precocious development of vertical supranuclear palsy (PSP), autonomic dysfunction (multiple system atrophy), delusions and hallucinations (Lewy body disease), characteristic resting tremor (Parkinson's disease). There are no laboratory markers for the diagnosis of CBD, but three laboratory tests can be useful in difficult cases: a detailed neuropsychological examination, electrooculography, and nuclear magnetic resonance imaging (see the preceding).

Finally, CBD is difficult to diagnose as the characteristic clinical picture of CBD may have, in addition to the classical pathology of CBD, a variety of pathological causes, such as PSP, Pick's disease, Alzheimer's disease, basal ganglia infarctions, leucodystrophy, and perhaps others that remain to be discovered (see Chapters 16 and 17). Therefore, we can consider CBD not a unique entity but a clinically defined syndrome that reflects the histopathology of various disorders.

Like the signs and symptoms, the pathological markers of CBD can also be grouped into characteristic features including neuronal loss, spongiosis, and ballooned neurons (see Chapter 2): neuronal loss is focal, found in the frontal and parietal parasaggital cortex, and to a lesser degree in the basal ganglia and brainstem; spongiosis, associated with astrocytic gliosis, at the gray-white matter junction, is found in superficial atrophic cortical regions; ballooned neurons, classically considered to be the histological hallmark of CBD, are identical to "Pick cells" and are also seen in smaller numbers in a variety of disorders. The most distinctive pathological sign of CBD has been recently described, however, namely the presence of tau related lesions not only within neurons (perikaria and cell processes), but also in astrocytes (typical "astrocytic plaques") and oligodendroglia ("coiled bodies"). This newly described histological pattern of CBD allows the differentiation of CBD from other neurodegenerative disorders, although the latter have several morphological features in common. In Alzheimer's disease, the localization of the neuronal loss is mostly concentrated in the temporal region, with a distinctive pathology including the presence of amyloid plaques; in Pick's disease, the degenerative process is characteristically found in the limbic lobes, including the presence of Pick bodies (with a different tau isoform pattern); the limited cortical pathology, the absence of white matter lesions and the localization of tau-immunoreactive lesions in cell bodies seen in PSP is different from CBD; frontotemporal dementia and Parkinsonism linked to chromosome 17, which is pathologically close to CBD, is distinguished by the presence of a family history and the discovery of mutations in the tau gene. There is no need to say that the overlap in clinical and histopathological features in these disorders constitute a diagnostic challenge (see Chapter 17).

There is one source of controversy, however. Kertesz and Munoz (see Chapter 21) are struck by the pathological and clinical similarities between primary progressive aphasia, fronto-temporal dementia, Pick's disease, and CBD. Keeping in mind that at the end of the last century, Pick only described cases of aphasia, apraxia and personality disorders in various combinations, associated with fronto-temporal atrophy, but no specific histological picture, the authors estimate that Pick's disease is an appropriate term for fronto-temporal dementia. They present evidence to support the hypothesis that CBD is part of the so-called "Pick complex." On the other hand, Duyckaerts et al. (see Chapter 22) think that the term Pick complex adds few features to the Pick eponym. Does Pick refer to an inclusion? to a cell? to a circumscribed atrophy? to a frontal syndrome? The authors conclude that this concept, therefore, leads to a regression, "since it lumps together diseases that should be differentiated into a poorly defined syndrome." They usefully remind us that a disease is a syndrome that has a cause. The concept of clinical syndrome, which is simply "a set of indicators that evoke a topography of putative lesions and poorly defined mechanisms such as degeneration," nevertheless, helps to take care of patients. In the absence of the cause, most degenerative disorders, including CBD, still remain a clinical syndrome associated with classically defined histopathological stigmata. These morphological markers, grouped into histopathological syndromes, are indeed closer to the cause(s) of the disease. Unfortunately, at this time, we still do not know the cause(s) of CBD.

With our present knowledge, there are no clear routes for approaching the pathogenesis of CBD. Epidemiological studies are difficult to perform owing to the rarity of the disorder and to the absence of a suitable marker. We hope that an effort will be made by patients and families to set up active patient associations that would facilitate this type of research in the future. Today, we know of no existing strong research network that could investigate the cellular and molecular mechanisms of CBD. The histopathological approach is powerful, but, as we have seen, it may not be entirely specific. As for other common neurodegenerative disorders, genetics is very likely the best way to approach the causes of this disorder, which points out the urgency to identify familial cases if they exist. Let us hope that a vast collaborative international research program on the pathophysiology of CBD will soon be initiated.

In conclusion, CBD is a disorder that is distressing for patients and their families, with no specific spectacular treatment but that can be palliated by physicians and professional assistance; a disorder that is not so easy to identify with certainty among atypical parkinsonian syndromes, even if there is a good clinical examination; a disorder that still remains the challenge for neuropathologists given the overlap in the histological and molecular features; a rather mysterious disorder for neuroscientists who have, at present, only a few ideas on how to proceed to find the cause(s). I am sure, however, that our professor of neurology and his less than assiduous student will learn what CBD is in the very near future.

Subject Index

Note: Page numbers followed by f indicate figures; those followed by t indicate tables